OX                                      TIONS

Fitness for Work

U(

# FITNESS FOR WORK
## The Medical Aspects
SECOND EDITION

Edited by
R.A.F. Cox
with
F.C. Edwards and R.I. McCallum

### R.A.F. Cox
*Consultant Occupational Physician*
*Previously: Chief Medical Officer, CEGB and National Power*

### F.C. Edwards
*Formerly Senior Employment Medical Adviser,*
*Medical Division, Health and Safety Executive*

### R.I. McCallum
*Honorary Consultant in Occupational Medicine,*
*Institute of Occupational Medicine, Edinburgh*

A Publication of the
Faculty of Occupational
Medicine of the Royal College
of Physicians

Oxford    New York    Melbourne
OXFORD UNIVERSITY PRESS
1995

Oxford University Press, Walton Street, Oxford OX2 6DP

Oxford    New York
Athens    Auckland    Bangkok  Bombay
Calcutta Cape Town Dar es Salaam Delhi
Florence Hong Kong Istanbul Karachi
Kuala Lumpur Madras Madrid Melbourne
Mexico City Nairobi Paris Singapore
Taipei Tokyo Toronto

and associated companies in

Berlin    Ibadan

Oxford is a trade mark of Oxford University Press

Published in the United States
by Oxford University Press Inc., New York

First edition published 1987
by Oxford University Press

A catalogue record for this book is available from the British Library

Library of Congress Cataloging in Publication Data
(Data available on request)

ISBN 0  19  262344  3 (Hbk)
ISBN 0  19  262345  1 (Pbk)

Typeset by
EXPO Holdings, Malaysia.
Printed in Great Britain by
Biddles Ltd., Guildford & Kings Lynn

# Foreword

*Jean François Caillard*

President, The International Commission on Occupational Health

June 1994

Originally formed for the exclusive purpose of preventing workers' health from being impaired by their working conditions, occupational health today faces new problems, particularly in the most developed countries. On the one hand, for most of them, the survival of greater numbers of people into old age has great consequences for the health of the labour force, as workers remain in employment with the deficiencies and disabilities which accompany ageing. On the other hand, because of growing international economic competition, which demands more effort from everyone plus the massive introduction of new technologies in the workplace, the number of employees has significantly decreased, a trend which is not expected to be reversed in the near future.

All this means that deficient health poses a great threat of exclusion from the workplace whether for managers or manual workers. For we occupational health physicians, who have both to protect the individual's health and guarantee his medical reliability for his employer, it is necessary to utilize all the latest advances and the best therapy to maintain and prolong effective working life. That is one of the aims of this book, first published in 1988 and now revised, which brings together the latest scientific knowledge on the relations between health and work.

The book has been written collaboratively between occupational physicians who have unique knowledge of people and their working environments, and the medical consultants practising in the various clinical specialties. They have been ever mindful of medical ethics, which exists to protect the patient in the midst of society's changing values.

One of the essential qualities of this book is to provide information for practitioners in every medical specialty with sufficient diagnostic and prognostic guidance to assess any patient's capacity to work. This has been achieved without detailed physiological or clinical descriptions except where this is necessary to reach a proper conclusion regarding the patient's medical capability or whatever modifications of working conditions are necessary.

At the same time, it exemplifies the role of medicine in the difficult problems of occupational integration; medical treatment not only aims at relieving pain or prolonging life but also to a better blooming of people both in their professional and social lives.

It is a pleasure for a French occupational health specialist, who has been working in a country which legally requires him to furnish a certificate of work ability after every medical assessment, to congratulate his British colleagues, who are not under this constraint, except in rare cases, to have conceived and then produced such a useful book. I hope it will be read all over the world by a great number of people, and translated into many languages because the questions it addresses are universal and therefore its need is even more important in countries with little or no developed occupational health services. Indeed, it is an essential tool for those who need the knowledge and technology of occupational health. As with other specialized knowledge and technologies, the countries which own them have the duty to share them, a duty to which The International Commission on Occupational Health has committed itself.

# Preface to the second edition

The first edition of this book was published as a Report of the Royal College of Physicians in 1988. It clearly fulfilled a very real need and we have been greatly encouraged by the favourable comments and reviews which it received. With changes both in clinical medicine and in employment practice the contents of the Report required updating. In so doing, the book has become a reference textbook and is no longer a report of a large steering group. The general format has been retained with each chapter written by an occupational physician and a practising clinician in the respective specialty, but some of the chapters in the first edition have been divided for functional convenience. For example, a separate chapter on trauma has replaced part of the previous chapter on orthopaedics, while disorders of the spine now have a chapter to themselves. In addition, there are new appendices on fitness for work overseas, European Community legislation, ill-health retirement and ethics. All the addresses referred to in each chapter will be found in the appendix of useful addresses (Appendix 9).

The editors feel that the subject of ethics in occupational medicine is not only of great importance but is also often misunderstood by employers and even by occupational physicians. The Faculty of Occupational Medicine's *Ethics for Occupational Physicians*, has recently been published and we believed that this should be included in its entirety apart from some minor editing to save space (see Appendix 6). Copies of the booklet are available from the Faculty of Occupational Medicine.

A further concession to the need to keep the size of the book within the publisher's limits was to prune the number of references. The references which the editors have included, therefore, are selected for their interest and relevance and we have abandoned any attempt to make the list at the end of each chapter comprehensive. We apologize to any authors who may be offended by this decision and to any readers who may feel that the style of the book has been diminished but the limitation of references has enabled us to expand the breadth of the book.

Although it will be of particular value to doctors, nurses, managers, and personnel staff in the United Kingdom, we feel that most of the topics are covered in such a general way that it will also be a great help wherever in the world there is a need to make informed decisions about the medical aspects of fitness for work. It is particularly with this wider readership in mind that we are delighted that Professor Jean-François Caillard, Professor of Occupational Medicine, Director of Occupational Medicine in the University of Rouen, Chairman of the French Federation of Occupational Medicine, and the current President of the International Commission on Occupational Health (ICOH), has written the Foreword to this edition. We also feel that the book will have an even greater relevance and application in the United Kingdom in the light of the new DSS proposals on the medical assessment for Incapacity Benefit.

In fact, this book will be invaluable to anyone practising occupational medicine.

Although occupational medicine is one of the most rapidly expanding medical disciplines, and more doctors enter training for the specialty every year, the advice of occupational physicians is still not available widely enough, in the United Kingdom, to workers in industry and commerce, and to the self-employed. We hope that this book will, therefore, be of particular value to those people, whether general practitioners, nurses, personnel managers, trade unionists, or others such as the staff of the employment and careers services who need guidance on the medical aspects of employment and may not be able to obtain it from a specialist occupational physician.

R.A.F. Cox
F.C. Edwards
R.I. McCallum

*February 1995*

*Note*: The authors have used the male personal pronoun in the text where both genders are intended.

# Preface to the first edition

The stimulus for this report came originally from the Health and Safety Executive's Medical Division, who approached the Royal College of Physicians of London and its Faculty of Occupational Medicine. A steering group, under the Chairmanship of the late Dr Peter Taylor, was set up by the College and the Faculty to plan and produce the report, with the requirements of hospital specialists, general practitioners, and occupational physicians particularly in mind.

Apart from specific activities for which detailed guidelines exist, such as heavy goods vehicle drivers, airline pilots, and professional divers, the vast majority of jobs have no clear criteria of fitness and precise guidelines cannot be laid down. Thus the need for informed advice on medical aspects of fitness for work covering a wide range of medical conditions is evident. Some chronic diseases, while not excluding work altogether, can clearly limit the scope of employment, but the restrictions that may be imposed on such patients are often unnecessary and without any rational basis. While it must be accepted that there may be diverse views on employability in many medical conditions, such problems should always be the subject of informed discussion between the employer, occupational medical adviser, the patient's own doctor, and the patient. This report provides a basis for such discussions.

Occupational medicine is often thought of as being concerned only with the effects of work on health, i.e. the prevention of occupational disease and of the effects of exposure to various environmental hazards, but equally it is about the effects of health on work, the fitness for work, and the rehabilitation of the individual. Occupational medicine is essentially a clinical speciality and throughout this book authors emphasize the need for close collaboration between occupational physicians and their clinical colleagues. Each chapter has been written jointly by a clinician practising in the specialty and an occupational physician, and it is hoped that one outcome will be that clinicians and occupational physicians will be brought closer together, enabling them to see each other's point of view.

Most firms, particularly small ones, still have no occupational health service or medical advice of their own. Medical guidance on fitness for work usually comes from the patient's family or hospital doctor. Unfortunately, inappropriate advice may be given, either because not enough is known by doctors about the jobs their patients do, or because employers are unaware of the way in which advances in medical treatment have improved prognosis.

The up-to-date specialist opinion and background information given here on a number of medical conditions should improve both the relevance and consistency of advice. It should also reduce discrimination, often on irrelevant health grounds, against those who are at work or seeking work. As with any clinical judgement, the medical advice that is given on a patient remains the responsibility of the doctor concerned, and the general guidance contained in this book must always be interpreted in the light, not only of the effect of the illness or disability on the individual patient, but also of the special requirements of the job.

We hope that the report will be of use not only to doctors in occupational medicine, but also to those in general practice or hospital medicine, and of interest to occupational health nurses, managers, and personnel staff. It will provide an essential core of information and advice on the effects of health on work for doctors in training for the examination for Associateship of the Faculty of Occupational Medicine (AFOM).

It was decided to retain some overlapping sections in different chapters, for example those on haemophilia, cervical spondylosis, and ankylosing spondylitis, because these reflected the different approaches and expertise of the authors. In spite of the speed with which the picture of Acquired Immune Deficiency Syndrome (AIDS) is changing as further knowledge of the disease develops, the steering group felt strongly that it should be included in the book because of its importance in relation to public concern about employability and safety at work.

F.C.E.
April 1988                                                                    R.I.McC.

# Acknowledgements

So many people have helped with the production of this book that there is a danger, in compiling a list of acknowledgements, that someone will be omitted. If there is anyone who feels affronted, however slightly, because their name is not mentioned please accept our apologies and assurance that no offence was intended.

We would particularly like to thank the authors of the first edition, some of whom did not contribute to the second edition, because their contributions provided the foundations for the new authors' chapters. We would also like to thank all the contributors, not only for the contents of their chapters, but for responding so willingly and helpfully to our cajoling and criticisms.

The members of the Editorial Panel were Professor Ian McCallum, Dr Felicity Edwards, Dr David Slattery, Mr Bernard Lloyd, and Miss Julie Hoare, and their wise advice and comments throughout the production of the book were invaluable.

We have received unstinted assistance and financial support from the Royal College of Physicians who were represented on the Editorial Panel by Bernard Lloyd and, latterly, Diana Beaven to whom we owe special thanks. The staff of the Faculty Office were also of inestimable help and were gratifyingly tolerant of our periodic intrusions, and we are delighted to acknowledge their assistance.

The Employment Service Disability Services Branch provided us with information and assistance and Geoffrey Browne was most helpful in checking the ever changing titles of officers and departments in the Department of Health.

The Department of Social Security and the Health and Safety Executive have very generously assisted with the funding of production costs for this enterprise and we are greatly indebted to them. Esso Petroleum has kindly agreed to sponsor the launch of this edition on February 9, 1995, as they did with the first edition and, for that, we are very grateful.

Finally, and deliberately last, because her contribution has been so outstanding, we wish to thank Anna McNeil. She has worked with dedication beyond the call of duty, with commensurate efficiency, and with unfailing courtesy and good humour. Without Anna this edition would never have reached the publishers and every contributor would have been denied the pleasure of working with such an accomplished administrative assistant. With the completion of the book her home and family can return to a peaceful existence!

# Contents

# Contributors

*J.F.L. Aldridge*
Chairman, Ethics Committee,
Faculty of Occupational Medicine

*P.J. Baxter*
University of Cambridge and Addenbrookes Hospital,
Cambridge

*L. Beeley*
Retired—previously Consultant Clinical Pharmacologist,
Queen Elizabeth Hospital, Birmingham

*G. Bennett*
Lately Chief Medical Officer,
Civil Aviation Authority

*E.M. Botheroyd*
Senior Employment Medical Adviser,
Health and Safety Executive, Aberdeen

*I. Brown*
European Medical Director, DowElanco Europe, Oxfordshire.
Hon. Senior Lecturer, Institute of Occupational Health,
University of Birmingham

*J.T. Carter*
Health and Safety Executive,
Director Medical Services/Field Operations

*G.V.P. Chamberlain*
Professor of Obstetrics and Gynaecology,
St George's Hospital Medical School, London

*G.M. Cochrane*
Previously Consultant Physician in Rehabilitation
Medicine, Oxford

*A. Cockroft*
Consultant/Senior Lecturer in Occupational Medicine,
Royal Free NHS Trust and School of Medicine.

*R.R.A. Coles*
MRC Institute of Hearing Research,
Nottingham

*R.A.F. Cox*
Consultant Occupational Physician.
Previously: Chief Medical Officer CEGB and National Power

*N.F. Davies*
Chief Medical Officer,
Nuclear Electric plc

*D. Dean*
Chief Medical Officer,
Chamber of Shipping

*P.A.M. Diamond*
Formerly Director of Medical Services,
London Transport

*F.C. Edwards*
Formerly Senior Employment Medical Adviser,
Medical Division, Health and Safety Executive

*P.M. Emerson*
Consultant Haematologist,
John Radcliffe Hospital, Oxford

*C.J. English*
Senior Medical Officer,
Civil Service Occupational Health Service

*A. Fingret*
Consultant Physician, Occupational Medicine,
Royal Marsden Hospital, London

*N.M. Foley*
Department of Respiratory Medicine,
Royal United Hospital, Bath

*F.B. Gibberd*
Physician and Neurologist,
Chelsea and Westminster Hospital, London

*R. Gokal*
Consultant Nephrologist,
Hon. Lecturer University of Manchester

*P.G. Harries*
Formerly Chief Medical Officer,
Rank Hovis McDougall

*J.M. Harrington*
Professor of Occupational Health,
University of Birmingham

*D.J. Hendrick*
Consultant Physician Newcastle General Hospital;
Honorary Senior Lecturer
University of Newcastle Upon Tyne.

*G.S. Howard*
Barrister at Law

*W.J. Hunter,*
Director of Health and Safety Commission of the European Community.

*L.H. Kapadia*
Occupational Health Physician,
Marks & Spencer plc

*J.L. Kearns*
Formerly Head of Health and Safety,
J. Lyons Group of Companies

*M.S. Lipsedge*
Consultant Psychiatrist,
Guy's Hospital, London

*E.B. Macdonald*
Senior Lecturer in Occupational Health,
University of Glasgow

*D.P. Manning*
Retired Senior Medical Officer, Ford Motor Company,
Halewood, Liverpool

*L.J. Marks*
Consultant in Rehabilitation, Stanmore DSC,
Royal National Orthopaedic Hospital Trust

*J.A. Mathews*
Consultant Rheumatologist,
St Thomas' Hospital, London

*The Lord McColl*
Professor of Surgery
Guy's Hospital, London

*N.K.I. McIver*
Director
North Sea Medical Centre,
Gorleston, Great Yarmouth, Norfolk

*A. McNeil*
Committee Secretary

*C.G.F. Munton*
Consultant Ophthalmic Surgeon,
Kent County Ophthalmic & Aural Hospital, Maidstone.
Chairman, 1989–94 Visual Standards Sub-Committee,
Royal College of Ophthalmologists, London

*M.C. Petch*
Consultant Cardiologist,
Papworth Hospital

*K.J. Pilling*
Head of Occupational Health
Rover Group, Longbridge

*D. Prothero*
Consultant Psychiatrist and Medical Director,
Grovelands Priory Hospital, London

*D.A. Pyke*
Formerly Physician-in-Charge, Diabetic Department,
King's College Hospital, London

*I.G. Rennie*
Chief Medical Officer,
Kodak Ltd

*R.J.G. Rycroft*
Consultant Dermatologist, St John's Institute of
Dermatology, St Thomas's Hospital, London; and Senior
Employment Medical Adviser (Dermatology), Health and
Safety Executive, London.

*D.A. Scarisbrick*
Principal Medical Office,
British Coal Corporation, Mansfield

*S.D. Shorvon*
Reader in Neurology, Institute of Neurology, London
University; Consultant Neurologist, National Hospital for
Neurology and Neurosurgery; Medical Director, National
Society for Epilepsy

*A. Sinclair*
Consultant Occupational Physician,
Previously: Chief Medical Officer, British Steel plc

*G. Smith*
Chief Medical Officer,
British Railways Board

*D.C. Snashall*
Clinical Director, Occupational Health Services,
Guy's and St Thomas' Trust, Senior Lecturer UMDS

*J.F. Taylor*
Chief Medical Adviser,
Department of Transport, UK

*H.G. Vaile*
Chief Medical Officer,
BBC Occupational Health

*C.A. Veys*
Formerly Chief Medical Officer
Michelin Tyre plc,
Stoke on Trent.

*R.J. Wyke*
Consultant Gastroenterologist,
The Ipswich Hospital NHS Trust

# 1

# Introduction

*R.A.F. Cox and F. C. Edwards*

## Introduction

This book on medical aspects of fitness for work gathers together specialist advice on the medical aspects of employment and the majority of medical conditions likely to be encountered in the working population. Although personnel managers and others will find it of great help it is primarily written for doctors so that family practitioners, hospital consultants, and occupational physicians, as well as other doctors and occupational health nurses can best advise managers and others who may need to know how a patient's illness might affect his work. Although decisions on return to work or on placement must depend on many factors, it is hoped that this book, which combines the best clinical and occupational health practice, will be used by doctors and others as a source of reference and will remind them about the occupational implications of illness.

It must be emphasized that, apart from relieving suffering and prolonging life, the objective of most medical treatment, whether it is chemotherapy or a renal transplant is to return the patient to work. Much of the benefit of modern medical technology and the skills of physicians and surgeons will have been wasted if patients, who have been successfully treated, are denied work by employers, or doctors acting on their behalf, through ignorance or prejudice. A main aim of this book is to remove the excuse for denying work to those who have overcome injury and disease and deserve to work.

The book is arranged in chapters according to specialty, each chapter written jointly by a clinician and an occupational physician. For each specialty the chapter outlines the conditions covered; notes relevant statistics; discusses clinical aspects, including treatment that may affect work capacity; notes rehabilitation requirements or special needs at the workplace; discusses problems that may arise at work and any necessary work restrictions; notes any current advisory or statutory medical standards and makes recommendations on the employment aspects of the conditions covered. A chapter on the possible effects of medication on work performance is also included (Chapter 3). Appendices on driving, civil aviation, merchant shipping, offshore work and diving, fitness for work overseas, ethics, European legislation, ill-health retirement, and useful addresses conclude the book.

The first two chapters cover general aspects applicable to any condition. This chapter deals mainly with the principles underlying medical assessments of fitness for work, contacts between medical practitioners and the workplace, and confidentiality of medical information. Chapter 2 covers legal, administrative, and other aspects and outlines the services currently available to assist with employment in the U.K.

## Contacts between the patient's medical advisers and the workplace

The importance of contact between the patient's own medical advisers and the workplace cannot be overemphasized. We suggest that consultants, as well as family practitioners, ask the patient if there is an occupational health service at the workplace and, if so, obtain written consent to contact the occupational physician, or the occupational health nurse in the absence of a physician.

Where there is no occupational health service, early contact between the patient's doctor and management (usually the personnel manager) may also be valuable. It helps the employer to know when the patient is likely to be back at work, or whether some work adjustment will be needed, while family practitioners and consultants will be helped by having a better understanding of their patient's job.

Employers with about 100 people or more will probably have a member of the management team designated to look after the placing of individuals within the organization, who is often addressed as the 'Job Placement Officer'. Organizations with more than 300 employees will have a personnel manager detailed to supervise job placement, and possibly their own occupational health nursing staff. The occupational health nurse will usually have a considerable amount of responsibility, an extensive knowledge of the workings of the organization, and is a useful person to contact. Employers with 1000 or more employees should have either full-time or part-time medical advisers to whom recommendations should be directed.

### Confidentiality

Usually any recommendations and advice on placement or return to work are based on the functional effects of the medical condition, the diagnosis itself normally being unnecessary. A simple statement that the patient is medically 'fit' or 'unfit' for a particular job often suffices, but occasionally further information may need to be disclosed particularly if limitations on work are being imposed. The certificated reason for any sickness absence is usually known by personnel departments, who maintain their own confidential records.

**The patient's consent to the disclosure of confidential health information to other doctors, occupational health nurses, employers, or to other persons such as staff of the careers or employment services, for example, must be obtained, preferably in writing**. The purpose of this should be made clear to the patient; it may be to help him with suitable work, and/or to maintain his own, and others' health and safety. If the patient is found to be medically unfit for certain employment, a full explanation should be given to him of why the disclosure of unfitness is necessary. Further advice may be found in the Faculty of Occupational Medicine's *Guidance on ethics for occupational physicians* 1993[1] (see also Appendix 6).

## Impairment, disability, and handicap

It is usually found that disabled workers are often highly motivated, with excellent work and attendance records. When medical fitness for work is assessed, what matters is often not the medical condition itself, but the associated loss of function, and any resulting disability or handicap. It should be borne in mind that a disability seen in the consulting room may be irrelevant to the performance of a particular job. **The patient's condition should be interpreted in functional terms and in the context of the job requirements**. Handicap may result directly from an impairment (for instance, severe facial disfigurement) or more usually from the resulting disability.

To be consistent in the use of these terms, the simplified scheme of the World Health Organization's *International classification of impairments, disabilities, and handicaps*[2,3] should be used as follows. A disease, disorder or injury produces an *impairment* (change in normal structure or function). A *disability* is a resulting reduction or loss of an ability to perform an activity, for example climbing stairs, or manipulating a keyboard. A *handicap* is a social disadvantage, resulting from an impairment or disability, which limits or prevents the fulfilment of a normal role. For example:

1. A relatively minor impairment, the loss of a finger, would be both a major disability and an occupational handicap to a pianist, although not to a labourer.

2. A relatively common impairment, defective colour vision, limits the ability to discriminate between certain hues. This may occasionally be a handicap at work, although there are, in fact, very few occupations for which defective colour vision is a significant handicap.

## Prevalence of disability in populations of working age

Figures on the prevalence of disability and/or handicap in different populations vary according to the definitions and methods used and the groups sampled.[4] Much of the uncertainty about the numbers of disabled people in the workforce, or seeking work, arises from these variations in definition and ascertainment and (in some surveys) from the reluctance of people to register as disabled.

Differences between surveys may also be due to the inclusion of non-physical handicaps, and to different methods of reporting and sampling. Common to all is the rise in prevalence of disability with increasing age and, to a lesser extent, with manual as opposed to non-manual, social class, and/or occupational groups.

The most recent national population survey in Great Britain was undertaken between 1985 and 1987 by the Social Survey Division of the Office of Population Censuses and Surveys (OPCS). Six reports were published. The first described the prevalence of disability among adults,[5] the fourth dealt with services for, transport, and the employment of disabled adults,[6] and the fifth report described their financial circumstances. The other reports were concerned with disabled children and their families.

From the survey's findings it was estimated that there were about 6.5 million people of all ages in Great Britain with physical, sensory and/or mental disabilities, of whom 6.2 million (11.3 per cent of the whole population) were aged 16 years or more, and almost 2 million (3.5 per cent of the whole population) were aged between 16 and 59 years. The survey classified the severity of disability into 10 categories, category 1 being the least severe, and category 10 being the most severe. The survey found that 20 per cent of disabled adults aged between 16 and 59 years were classified in the higher five categories, i.e., they were considered to be severely or very severely disabled. Put another way, the findings suggest that there were about 17 severely or very severely disabled people per 1000 people aged 16 to 59 years and another 45 with minor or less severe disabilities. (For a description of the scales of severity and of the methods used in the OPCS surveys see the first report,[5] and for a summary of the prevalence figures see Warren.[7])

The OPCS report on employment[6] indicated that, of disabled adults under pension age living at home, about one-third were working, one-third were permanently unable to work, and one in ten were looking for work, while the remainder were not seeking work. Severity of disability was strongly related to employment status.

Specific work forces have also been studied and Table 1.1 summarizes the findings of two British[8–10] and two Scandinavian[11,12] studies. Taylor and Fairrie [8] found that the prevalence of disability was about 10 per cent of men working in the refinery they studied (Table 1.1). A markedly increased prevalence of disability/handicap with age, particularly over 50 years, was found. Substantial proportions of the workforce were found to be sufficiently incapacitated to need 'rehabilitation measures', such as work accommodation, and/or would have been restricted in their ability to perform if their jobs had been more demanding. The most common causes of disablement in all four studies were circulatory, respiratory, and musculoskeletal disorders. These were the main causes of ill-health retirement over a two-year period in British Steel,[13] while the main causes of ill-health retirement in coal miners (between 1981 and 1983) were musculoskeletal, psychological, cardiovascular, and respiratory conditions, in that order (Dr Roy Archibald, personal communication). The two earlier British studies[8–10] highlighted the inadequacies of the Register of Disabled Persons and the Quota Scheme (see Chapter 2, pp. 35, 36).

**Table 1.1** Prevalence of disability affecting working capacity in two British and two Scandinavian workforces

| Reference | Working population | | Chronic disability affecting employment | | |
| --- | --- | --- | --- | --- | --- |
| | Sample size | Workforce | No. | Percentage | Comment |
| Taylor and Fairrie (1968)[8,9] | 1995 (M) (Britain) | Oil refinery | 206 | 10.3 | |
| Taylor *et al.* (1970)[10] | 11 399 (M) | 7 companies | 1233 | 10.8 | |
| Jarvikoski and Tuunainen (1978)[12] | c.2300 (M & F) (responders) | Helsinki City employees (Finland) | Not given | 10–17 | Estimate of subjective need for rehabilitation |
| Heijbel (1978)[11] | 3846 (M & F) | Volvo Skovde Works (Sweden) | 527 | 13.7 | Physical reasons only: 'conditionally employable' |

## Fitness for work

**The primary purpose of a medical assessment of fitness for work is to make sure that an individual is fit to perform the task involved effectively and without risk to his own or to others' health and safety.** The main areas where medical conditions may impinge on work are as follows:

1. The patient's condition may limit, reduce or prevent him from performing the job effectively (e.g., musculoskeletal conditions that limit mobility, or manipulative ability).

2. The patient's condition might be made worse by the job (e.g., excessive physical exertion in some cardiorespiratory conditions; exposure to certain allergens in asthma).

3. The patient's condition is likely to make it unsafe for him to do the job (e.g., liability to sudden unconsciousness in a hazardous situation; risk of damage to the remaining eye or ear in a patient with monocular vision or monaural hearing in certain work environments).

4. The patient's condition is likely to make it unsafe both for him and others, whether fellow workers and/or the community (e.g., road or railway driving in someone who is liable to sudden unconsciousness or to behave abnormally).

5. The patient's condition might make it unsafe for the community (e.g., for consumers of the product, if a food-handler transmits infection).

There is usually a clear distinction between the first-party risks of (2) and (3) and the third-party risks of (5). In (4), first- and third-party risks may both be present.

Thus, when assessing a patient's fitness to work, his doctor must consider the following factors.

1. The level of skill, physical, and mental capacity, sensory acuity, etc., needed for effective performance of the work.

2. Any possible adverse effects of the work itself or of the work environment on the patient's health.

3. The possible 'health and safety' implications of the patient's medical condition when undertaking the work in question, for himself, fellow workers, and/or the community.

For some jobs it should also be remembered that there may be an 'emergency' component in addition to the 'routine' job structure, and higher standards of fitness may thus be needed on occasion for the former.

**Medical standards**

Medical standards may be advisory or statutory. Standards are often laid down where work entails entering a new environment which may present some hazard to the individual, such as the increased or decreased atmospheric pressures encountered in compressed-air work, diving, and flying, or work in the high temperatures of nuclear reactors. Standards are also laid down for work where there is a potential risk of a medical condition causing an accident, as in transport; or transmitting infection, as in food-handling. For onerous or arduous work, such as the Mines Rescue Service or the Fire Service, very high standards of physical fitness are needed. Specific medical standards will need to be met in such types of work: where relevant, such advisory and/or statutory standards are noted in each specialty chapter.

**Pension schemes**

Many doctors and personnel managers in industry still believe that their company pension fund requires high standards of medical fitness for new entrants. Direct enquiry to the pension fund administrators themselves usually demonstrates that this is not the case. Fortunately, most pension funds follow the general principle recommended by the Occupational Pensions Board: 'Fit for employment—fit for the pension scheme'.[14] It was the Board's view that 'The concern of an employer, when assessing a prospective employee, should be with ability to perform the job efficiently. There is no reason why pension scheme considerations should influence the employer's decision whether to employ him.' In general, a disease or disability should not *per se* be a reason for exclusion from pension schemes, nor used as an excuse to refuse employment, unless it adversely affects job performance or health and safety. For an approach to the calculation of disability pensions and current thinking on life underwriting the reader is referred to Brackenridge and Elder.[15] Where company schemes still operate against the disabled, attempts should be made to amend them. However with recent changes in legislation pensions can now be personal, flexible and mobile, and anyone with a medical disability may be well advised to negotiate a personal policy which he can retain permanently irrespective of his employer.

**When an assessment of medical fitness is needed**

An assessment of medical fitness may be needed for those who are

(1)  unemployed or employed, but being considered for a particular job (i.e., at recruitment or transfer or pre-employment assessment);

(2)    already in employment; and

(3)    unemployed and seeking work or training, but without a specific job in mind.

For (1) and (2), the assessment will be related to a particular job, or to a defined range of alternative work in a given workplace. The assessment is needed to help both employer and employee, and should be clearly related to the job in question. However, after a pre-placement or pre-employment medical examination, employers are entitled to know if there may be consequences from a medical condition which may curtail or restrict a potential employee's working life in the future. But, for (3), where there may be no specific job in view, the assessment must inevitably be more open-ended: health assessments may be required, for instance, by the employment or careers services in their attempt to find suitable work for unemployed disabled people. It is thus all the more important to avoid unnecessary medical restrictions or labels (e.g., 'epileptic'), as these tend to follow the individual in his search for work and may limit his future choice unduly.

## Recruitment and disclosure

Employers often use health questionnaires as part of their recruitment process. Such questionnaires should be marked 'medically confidential' and should be read and interpreted only by an occupational physician or nurse. A questionnaire which has to be returned to a non-medical person because an employer does not have an occupational health service, for example, is not protected by medical confidentiality and should not be so described. Some individuals may be reluctant to disclose a medical condition to a future employer (sometimes with their own doctor's support) for fear that this may lose them the job. Although understandable, it must be pointed out that should work capability be impaired or an accident arise due to the concealed condition, dismissal on medical grounds may follow. An industrial tribunal would be likely to support the dismissal if the employee had failed to disclose the relevant condition (see p. 28). It is not in the patient's interest to conceal any medical condition which could adversely affect his work.

It is noted above that for some jobs statutory medical standards exist (e.g., driving) and that for others employing organizations lay down their own advisory medical standards (e.g., food-handling or work in the offshore oil and gas industry). For the majority of jobs, however, no agreed advisory medical standards exist, and for many jobs there need be no special health requirements. Job application forms should be accompanied by an indication of any health standards or physical qualifications that are required and of any medical conditions that would be a bar to certain types of job, but no questions about health or disabilities should be included on job application forms themselves. If health information is necessary, applicants should be asked to complete a separate health declaration form or questionnaire which should be inspected and interpreted only by health professionals, and only after the candidate has been selected, subject to satisfactory health.[16]

**Employees**

The stages at which a health appraisal might be necessary for someone in employment are as follows:

1. *Job change*, although still working for the same employer, possibly for transfer or promotion. The employee should be told of any special health requirements or qualifications for the new post and the health appraisal should relate to these. Job change may include more seniority or responsibility, for instance, or include overseas posting with considerable increase in travel. All these factors might have to be taken into account.

2. *Periodic review* of individual health may be undertaken in some circumstances and will relate to specific requirements (for instance, regular assessment of visual acuity in some jobs).

3. *Return to work after illness or injury* usually merits a health assessment and is discussed further below.

4. Employees returning to work after *prolonged absence* often have special needs that should be taken into account where possible.

5. The question of *retirement on grounds of ill health* may need to be considered. (See also Appendix 8.)

**Young people**

Medical advice on occupation or training given to a young person who has not yet started his career often has a different slant from that given to an adult developing the same medical condition late in an established career. The later stages of a particular vocation may involve jobs incompatible with the young person's medical condition, or its foreseeable development. Also, the adult's experience may compensate for the possible disadvantages of a disease or disability that develops late. It is particularly important that young people entering employment are given appropriate and consistent medical advice when it is needed. For instance, although a school-leaver with epilepsy might be eligible for an ordinary driving licence at the time of recruitment, it would be most inadvisable for him to take up a position where vocational driving might be an essential part of his progress in that particular career.

**Severely disabled people**

Where a medical condition has so reduced the individual's employment abilities or potential that he is incapable either of continuing in his existing work or of working in any open competitive employment, then sheltered work of some kind may be the only alternative to premature medical retirement, on the one hand, or to continued unemployment on the other. Further details of sheltered employment are given in Chapter 2 (see p. 38).

## Assessment of medical fitness for work

### General framework for the assessment

The clinician's assessment should always be in terms of functional capacity and the actual diagnosis need not be reported. Even so, an opinion on the medical fitness of an individual is being conveyed to others and the patient's written consent is needed for the information to be passed on, in confidence.

To estimate the individual's level of function, general assessments of all systems should be made, with special attention both to those which are disordered and to those which may be relevant to the work. As well as physical systems, sensory and perceptual abilities should be noted, as well as psychological reactions, such as responsiveness, alertness, and other features of the general mental state. The effects of different treatment regimes on work suitability should also be considered; the possible effects of some medication on alertness, or the optimal position of an arthrodesis, are only two of the many examples. Each of the specialty chapters which follow, outlines the main points to be considered in the respective conditions, but a summary of the main features relevant to an assessment of fitness for work for use as a general framework, is listed here.

### FRAMEWORK FOR ASSESSING FITNESS FOR WORK

An evaluation of general physical and mental health forms the background to more specific assessments. Guiding principles throughout will be the *patient's residual abilities in terms of likely requirements at the workplace*. Many of these aspects are listed below. Not all will be relevant to any one individual, while some are relevant to more than one type of condition, or to more than one system or specialty.

Assessment should always include the results of relevant tests.

1. *General*: stamina; ability to cope with full working day, or shiftwork; liability to fatigue, etc.

2. *Mobility*: ability to get to work, and exit safely; to walk, climb, bend, stoop, crouch, etc.

3. *Locomotor*: general/specific joint function and range; reach of arms; gait; back/spinal function, etc.

4. *Posture*: ability to stand or sit for certain times; any postural restraints; work in confined spaces, etc.

5. *Muscular*: specific palsies or weakness; tremor; ability to lift, push or pull, with weight/time abilities if known; strength tests, etc.

6.  *Manual skill*: any defects in dexterity, ability to grip, or grasp, etc.

7.  *Co-ordination*: including hand/eye co-ordination if relevant.

8.  *Balance*: ability to work at heights; vertigo.

9.  *Cardiorespiratory limitations*, including exercise tolerance, and how this was tested; respiratory function and reserve; sub-maximal exercise tests, aerobic work capacity, if relevant.

10. *Liability to unconsciousness*, including nature of episodes, timing, any precipitating factors, etc.

11. *Sensory aspects*: may be relevant for the actual work, or in order to get about a hazardous environment safely.

    (a) *Vision*: ability for fine/close work, distant vision, visual standards corrected or uncorrected, any aids in use or needed. Visual fields. Colour vision defects may occasionally be relevant. Is the eyesight good enough to cope with a difficult working environment with possible hazards?
    (b) *Hearing*: each ear; can warning signals or instructions be heard?

    For both vision and hearing it is very important that if only one eye or one ear is functioning, this should be noted so that the remaining organ can be adequately protected against possible damage.

12. *Communication/speech*: two-way communication; hearing or speech defects; reason for limitation.

13. *Cerebral function* will be very relevant after head injury, cerebrovascular accident, some neurological conditions, and in those with some intellectual deficit: the presence of any confusion; disorientation; impairment of memory, intellect, verbal, or numerical aptitudes, etc.

14. *Mental state*: psychiatric assessments may mention anxiety, relevant phobias, mood, withdrawal, relationships with other people, etc.

15. *Motivation*: may well be the most important. With it, other defects may be surmounted; without it, difficulties may not be overcome. It can be particularly difficult to assess by a doctor who has not previously known the patient.

16. *Treatment of the condition*: special effects of treatment may be relevant, e.g., drowsiness, inattention, as side-effects of some medication; implications of different types of treatment in one condition (e.g., insulin as opposed to oral treatment for diabetes).

17. *Further treatment*: if further treatment is planned, e.g., further orthopaedic or surgical procedures, these may need to be mentioned.

18. *Prognosis*: if the clinical prognosis is likely to affect work placement, e.g., likely improvements in muscle strength, or decline in exercise tolerance, these should be indicated.

19. *Special needs*: these may be dietary; need for a clean area for self-treatment, e.g., injection; or relate to time, e.g., frequent rest pauses, no paced or shift work, etc.

20. *Aids or appliances* in use or needed. Implanted artificial aids may be relevant in the working environment (pacemakers and artificial joints). Aids to mobility may have implications for work (e.g., wheelchair). Prostheses/orthoses should be mentioned. Artificial aids or appliances that could help at the workplace should be indicated.

21. *Special third-party risks* that could be transmitted to other workers or to the community, e.g., via the product such as infection in food-handlers, etc.

**Requirements of the task**

These may relate not only to the present job but also to the future career. Some of the following aspects may be relevant:

1. *Work demands*: physical (e.g., mobility needs; strength for certain activities; lifting/carrying; climbing/balancing; stooping/bending; postural constraints; reach requirements; dexterity/manipulative ability, etc., see the next section for further details); *intellectual/perceptual demands*; types of skill involved in tasks.

2. *Work environment*: physical aspects; risk factors (e.g., fumes/dust) chemical or biological hazards; working at heights.

3. *Organizational/social aspects*, e.g., working in small groups or alone; intermittent or regular pressure of work; need for tact in public relations, etc.

4. *Temporal aspects*, e.g., need for an early start; type of shiftwork; day or night work; arrangements for rest pauses or breaks, etc.

5. *Ergonomic aspects*: workplace (e.g., need to climb stairs; distance from toilet facilities, access for wheelchairs, etc.); workstation (e.g. height of workbench, adequate lighting, type of equipment or controls used, etc.). Adaptations of equipment that could help at the workplace should be indicated.

6. *Travel*, e.g., need to work in areas remote from health care or where there are risks not found in the United Kingdom. (See also Appendix 5.)

**Requirements of the job**

The ability to perform physical work, and even intellectual occupations involve some physical work, depends ultimately on the ability of muscle cells to transform chemically bound energy from food into mechanical energy. This, in turn, depends upon the intake, storage, and mobilization of nutrients (fuel), and the uptake of oxygen and its delivery by the cardiovascular system to the muscles where the fuel is oxidized to release energy. This chain of activities and processes is influenced at every juncture by other factors both endogenous and external or environmental.

Factors which may influence work performance directly, or indirectly, include:

1. Training and adaptation.

2. The general state of health of the individual.

3. Sex, e.g., the maximal strength of women's leg muscles is only 65–75 per cent of that of men.

4. Body size.

5. Age. The maximal muscle strength of a 65-year-old man is, on average, only 75–80 per cent of that when he was 20 and at his peak.

6. Nutritional state—particularly important when working in cold environments.

7. Individual differences.

8. Attitude.

9. Motivation.

10. Sleep deprivation. This causes a marked deterioration in mental performance and releases emotional effects.

11. Stress.

12. Type of work (physical or mental).

13. The work itself.

14. Work load.

15. Fatigue.

16. Work schedules.

17. The environment:
Heat
Cold
Humidity
Air velocity
Altitude
Hyperbaric pressure
Noise
Vibration
Air pollution

These factors are summarized in Fig. 1.1 which is taken from Rodahl's *The physiology of work* which is recommended for further reading.[17]

Too often, medical statements simply state 'fit for light work only'. The dogmatic separation of work into 'light', 'medium', and 'heavy' often results in an individual being unduly limited in his choice of work. A refinement of this broad grading is adopted by the US Department of Labor in its *Dictionary of Occupational Titles*.[18] Jobs are graded according to physical demands, environmental conditions, certain levels of skill and knowledge, and specific vocational preparation (training time) required.

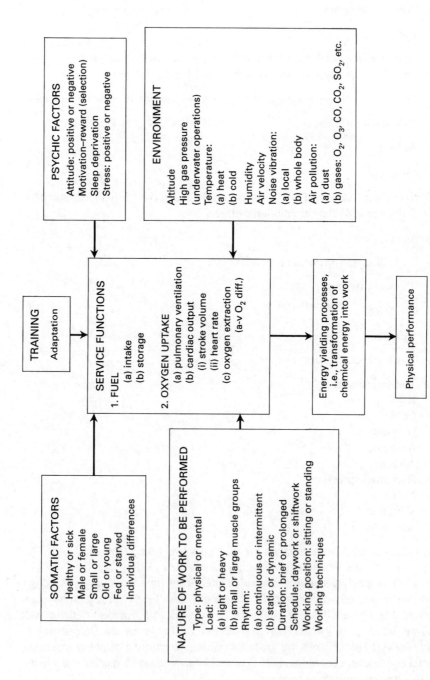

**Fig. 1.1** Requirements for the job (from Rodahl 1989).

If the energy or metabolic requirements of a particular task are known, the individual's work capacity may be estimated and, if expressed in the same units, a comparison between the energy demands of the work and the physiological work capacity of the individual may be made. This has been used in assessing work capacity of patients with heart disease.[19] (See also Chapter 14, p. 274.) Energy requirements of various tasks have been estimated and are often expressed in metabolic equivalents, or 'Mets'. (The 'Met' is an arbitrary unit recommended by the American Heart Association: 1 'Met' is the approximate energy expended while sitting at rest, and is defined as the rate of energy expenditure requiring an oxygen consumption of 3.5 ml/kg body weight/min).

The metabolic demands of many working activities have been published and the equivalents for the five grades of physical demands in terms of muscular strength adopted by the US Department of Labor[18] are included in the list below. Work physiology assessments in occupational medicine provide a quantitative way of matching the patient to his work[20] and are frequently used in Scandinavia and the United States.

## Physical demands

The physical demands listed below serve as a means of expressing both the physical requirements of the job and the physical capacities (specific physical traits) which a worker must have to meet those required by many jobs, e.g., perceiving by the sense of vision. The name of the specific capacity possessed by most people, e.g., having the power of sight is also defined. The worker must possess physical capacities at least in an amount equal to the physical demands made by the job.

PHYSICAL DEMANDS (FROM US DEPARTMENT OF LABOR 1981[18])

### 1. Strength

This factor is expressed in terms of sedentary, light, medium, heavy, and very heavy. It is measured by involvement of the worker with one or more of the following activities:

(a) Worker position(s):
   (i) standing: remaining on one's feet in an upright position at a workstation without moving about;
   (ii) walking: moving about on foot;
   (iii) sitting: remaining in the normal seated position.

(b) Worker movement of objects (including extremities used):
   (i) lifting: raising or lowering an object from one level to another (includes upward pulling):
   (ii) carrying: transporting an object, usually holding it in the hands or arms or on the shoulder;

(iii) pushing: exerting force upon an object so that the object moves away from the force (includes slapping, striking, kicking, and treadle actions);

(iv) pulling: exerting force upon an object so that the object moves toward the force (includes jerking).

The five degrees of Physical Demands Factor No. 1 (strength), (estimated equivalents in Mets, see p. 15) are as follows:

S  *Sedentary work (under 2 Mets)*: Lifting 10 lbs. (4.55 kgs) maximum and occasionally lifting and/or carrying such articles as dockets, ledgers, and small tools. Although a sedentary job is defined as one which involves sitting, a certain amount of walking and standing is often necessary in carrying out job duties. Jobs are sedentary if walking and standing are required only occasionally and other sedentary criteria are met.

L  *Light work (2–3 Mets)*: Lifting 20 lbs. (9.1 kg) maximum with frequent lifting and/or carrying of objects weighing up to 10 lbs. Even though the weight lifted may be only a negligible amount, a job is in this category when it requires walking or standing to a significant degree, or when it involves sitting most of the time with a degree of pushing and pulling of arm and/or leg controls.

M  *Medium work (4–5 Mets)*: Lifting 50 lbs. (22.75 kg) maximum with frequent lifting and/or carrying of objects weighing up to 25 lbs. (11.38 kg).

H  *Heavy work (6–8 Mets)*: Lifting 100 lbs. (45.5 kg) maximum with frequent lifting and/or carrying of objects weighing up to 50 lbs. (22.75 kg).

V  Very heavy work (over 8 Mets): Lifting objects in excess of 100 lbs. (45.5 kg) with frequent lifting and/or carrying of objects weighing 50 lbs. (22.75 kg) or more.

**2. Climbing and/or balancing**

(a) Climbing: ascending or descending ladders, stairs, scaffolding, ramps, poles, ropes, and the like, using the feet and legs and/or hands and arms.

(b) Balancing: maintaining body equilibrium to prevent falling when walking, standing, crouching, or running on narrow, slippery, or erratically moving surfaces; or maintaining body equilibrium when performing gymnastic feats.

**3. Stooping, kneeling, crouching, and/or crawling**

(a) Stooping: bending the body downward and forward by bending the spine at the waist.

(b) Kneeling: bending the legs at the knees to come to rest on the knee or knees.

(c) Crouching: bending the body downward and forward by bending the legs and the spine.

(d) Crawling: moving about on the hands and knees or hands and feet.

**4. Reaching, handling, fingering, and/or feeling**

(a) Reaching: extending the hands and arms in any direction.

(b) Handling: seizing, holding, grasping, turning, or otherwise working with the hand or hands (fingering not involved).

(c) Fingering: picking, pinching, or otherwise working with the fingers primarily (rather than with the whole hand or arm as in handling).

(d) Feeling: perceiving such attributes of objects and materials as size, shape, temperature, or texture, by means of receptors in the skin, particularly those of the fingertips.

## 5. Talking and/or hearing

(a) Talking: expressing or exchanging ideas by means of the spoken word.

(b) Hearing: perceiving the nature of sounds by the ear.

## 6. Seeing

Obtaining impressions through the eyes of the shape, size, distance, motion, color or other characteristics of objects. The major visual functions are: (a) acuity, far and near, (b) depth perception, (c) field of vision, (d) accommodation, and (e) color vision. The functions are defined as follows:

(a) Acuity, far—clarity of vision at 20 feet [6 m] or more; acuity, near—clarity of vision at 20 inches [50 cm] or less.

(b) Depth perception—three-dimensional vision. The ability to judge distance and space relationships so as to see objects where and as they actually are.

(c) Field of vision—the area that can be seen up and down or to the right or left while the eyes are fixed on a given point.

(d) Accommodation—adjustment of the lens of the eye to bring an object into sharp focus. This item is especially important when doing near-point work at varying distances from the eye.

(e) Color vision—the ability to identify and distinguish colors.

## Objective tests

The result of any objective tests of function relevant to the working situation should be noted. For instance, the physical work capacity of an individual may be estimated ergometrically using standard exercise tests, step tests, or different task simulations. Cardiorespiratory function may be relevant. Muscular strength and lifting ability can be assessed objectively by using either dynamic or static strength tests.

## Presentation of the assessment

If a written report is needed it should be legible, clearly laid out, and should be signed and dated. The report should mention any functional limitations and outline activities that may, or may not, be undertaken. Any health or safety implications should be noted and the assessment should aim at a positive statement about the patient's abilities. Any adaptations or ergonomic alterations to the work that would be helpful should be indicated (work accommodation is discussed on p. 20). Recommendations on restriction or limitation of employment particularly for health and/or safety reasons, should be unambiguous and precise, and should only be made if definitely indicated.

Many standard functional profiles of individual abilities have been used in North America and Scandinavia, and in the U.K. mainly in the armed services. These profiles, which resemble each other, are known by acronyms of the initial letters of the parts of the body assessed, e.g., PULHEEMS, GULHEMP, PULSES. In the case of the GULHEMP profile each division is graded from 1 to 7. Other profiles have combined the evaluation of physical abilities with indications of the frequency with which certain activities may be undertaken.[21] Although such profiles are relatively objective and systematic, and allow for consistent recordings on the same individual over a period of time, they take time to complete and much of the information may not be needed. Many doctors in industry who have tried to introduce a PULHEEMS type of system have found that it does not always help when dealing with the practical, and often complex, problems affecting individual employees.

Other simpler classifications are often used in clinical settings, e.g., the New York Heart Association's Impairment of Cardiac Functions. Graded in terms of symptoms, such classifications are of less use in assessing occupational fitness than in recording clinical progress or deterioration. Other scales (e.g., the Barthel Index) used to grade degree of damage or recovery after stroke, for instance, are used to assess outcome after different rehabilitation procedures, and often form part of occupational therapy assessments.

### Matching the individual with the job

A functional assessment of the individual's capacities will be of most use when as much is known about the job as about the individual assessed. Ideally, the requirements of the task should be categorized, so that a match can be made with the individual's capacity. There are wide variations in the practice of occupational medicine in different countries and both in France and in Germany job-matching of this kind is used formally in some work settings, but formal job analysis and matching is rarely done at the workplace in Britain. However, an Activity Matching Ability System (AMAS), which was developed in Britain, is being used by Remploy in a sheltered work setting (see Chapter 2, p. 38). In British industry, however, this ideal is often met in practice when personnel staff and managers, company doctors, and supervisors discuss the placement needs of their disabled employees and, as both worker abilities and task requirements are well known to them, a theoretical match is often superfluous. Outside the workplace itself, more formal assessments may be made in medical rehabilitation or occupational therapy departments; and in the Employment Service's Ability Development Centres where occupational skills can be tested using standard equipment, as well as by work rehearsal in different settings. (See Chapter 2, p. 37)

**It is essential that the occupational physician or nurse who is assessing medical suitability for employment has an intimate understanding of the job in question**.

### Recommendations following assessment

*If the patient is employed*, it should be possible to make a medical judgement on whether he is:

(1)  capable of performing the work without any ill effects;

(2)  capable of performing the work but with reduced efficiency and/or effectiveness;

(3)  capable of performing the work although this may adversely affect his medical condition;

(4)  capable of performing the work but not without unacceptable risks to the health and safety of himself, other workers, or the community; and

(5)  physically or mentally incapable of performing the work in question.

For the employed patient, where the judgement is (2)–(5), the options include work accommodation; alternative work on a temporary or permanent basis; sheltered work; or, in the last resort, retirement on medical grounds.

*If the patient is unemployed but is being given a pre-employment assessment* for recruitment to a particular job, the same range of options (1)–(5) also applies. *However, if the unemployed patient is not being considered for a specific job*, then the recommendation following the assessment cannot relate to specific job requirements and it is particularly important that no unnecessary medical restrictions are imposed.

### The return to work

Even if the patient is assessed as medically fit for a return to his previous job without modification, medical advice may still be needed on the time of return to work. A clear indication by the consultant or family practitioner to the patient, or to the employer or occupational physician, on when work may be resumed, should be given wherever possible. Work should be resumed as soon as the individual is physically and mentally fit enough, having regard to his own and others' health and safety. Return to work at the right time can assist recovery, while undue delay can aggravate the sense of uselessness and isolation that so often accompanies incapacity due to major illness or injury.

The contact between the patient's doctor and his employer or occupational physician, which was stressed earlier in the chapter, will ensure that preparations for the patient's return to work can be put in hand. Recommendations on when work may be resumed and on the patient's functional and work capacities should be clear and specific.

## Work accommodation

The patient's condition may be such that his previous work needs to be modified, either temporarily or permanently. Two aspects of the job are usually involved, place and time. Simple features such as bench height, type of chair or stool, or lighting, may need adjustment, or more sophisticated aids or adaptations may be required. The workplace environment may need adapting, for example by building a ramp or widening a doorway to improve access for wheelchairs. Financial assistance may be available from the Employment Service. Further details are included in Chapter 2, p. 38.

Information on equipment should be available from several voluntary organizations, such as RADAR (Royal Association for Disability and Rehabilitation), the DLF (Disabled Living Foundation), and the DIT (Disability Information Trust). (See the list of addresses in Appendix 9.) The Disability Information Trust has recently published a comprehensive volume on employment and the workplace.[22]

Certain time features of the work may need adjustment, for instance more flexible working hours, more frequent rest pauses, alterations to shift work or arrangements to avoid rush-hour travel. A short period of unpaced work may be necessary before resuming paced work. In some instances, the way in which the patient relates to fellow workers may need attention.

## Alternative work

In many occupations, work accommodation or job restructuring is not possible and some type of suitable alternative work, possibly only temporary, is recommended which may need to be discussed with both management and unions. This is usually judged individually by the occupational physician who can keep the employee under regular review. Where there are no occupational health services, the Employment Service's Disability Employment Advisers (DEAs) can visit the workplace to advise on work accommodation or alternative work; the Employment Medical Advisory Service (EMAS) can provide medical advice. Further details of these services can be found in Chapter 2, p. 40.

## Premature medical retirement

This may have to be considered as a last resort, if suitable alternative or sheltered work cannot be provided or if the employee will not accept it. After illness or injury the gradual recovery of fitness can be regarded as crossing the 'threshold of employability' determined by the task requirements. This 'threshold' may be lowered by work accommodations or by alternative work. Persistent or increasing disability may mean that the 'threshold' of fitness for a particular job is unlikely to be attained, or only after further treatment (Dr K.H. Nickol, personal communication). It may then be necessary for the doctor to recommend retirement on medical grounds, particularly if further treatment is impossible, ineffective, or is declined. Other reasons for medical retirement include increasingly severe mobility problems, as well as the non-availability of suitable alternative work. **A management decision on premature retirement on grounds of ill health should never be made without a supporting medical opinion that has taken the requirements of the job fully into account**. (See Appendix 8.) Other aspects of premature medical retirement in relation to the law are discussed in Chapter 2, p. 34.

### Incapacity Benefit

At the time of going to press the DSS have issued a consultation document on the Government's proposals to introduce a new Incapacity Benefit which will replace Sickness and Invalidity Benefit from April 1995. The new system will operate as follows:

1. During the first six months of incapacity for work the claimant's general practitioner (GP) will provide a certificate of incapacity if the person is unable to perform his or her normal occupation.

2. After six months a new medical test of incapacity will be applied which will be based purely on the effects of the medical condition and will not take account of such things as education and work experience. The objective nature of the test will mean that it will be readily understood by both patients and those who have to apply it. When the test is applied it will consider the person's ability to perform any work and not just his or her own job. There will be clear thresholds above which the capacity to work will be considered to be substantially reduced.

3. Under the new system, the patients will be asked to complete a questionnaire detailing the limits of their abilities over a range of functional categories. The G P will be asked to give information on the diagnosis(es) and on the disabling effects of any conditions present. However, no opinion will be sought on whether or not the patient is capable of work. There will, however, be a number of people who will not have to go through this process such as those whose capacity for work is not really in doubt, e. g., the terminally ill and those with severe mental illness. It is expected that most of the completed questionnaires will be referred to Benefits Agency Medical Advisers who will decide whether the evidence indicates that incapacity for work is not in doubt or, alternatively, that a medical examination should be carried out. In any examination, the criteria developed in the new medical test will be applied.

4. Patients' GPs will no longer be asked to supply repeated sickness statements once the 'all work test' has been applied.

Related to this but not part of the discussion document is a change in policy regarding the payment of Statutory Sick Pay (SSP) which is now, in the case of larger employers, (i.e. those with National Insurance contribution liability in excess of £20, 000) not recoverable by the employer from the first day of incapacity as it was in the past.

## Maintenance of fitness

From the viewpoint of the occupational physician, fitness for work does not end with medical assessment; an employee must remain fit which means attention to those factors which will prevent deterioration of health. This may include policies or advice on smoking, exercise, diet, and alcohol consumption. The subjects of health promotion, health screening, and general prevention of ill health are not considered in this volume although these concerns are important aspects of the activities of doctors in the workplace. The prevention of vascular disease, cardiac, cerebral, and peripheral is particularly important because these diseases take a very high toll of the working population and because simple initiatives are very effective.

The recent (July 1992) Department of Health document '*The Health of the Nation*' mentions some of the factors which can be addressed by occupational physicians although, unfortunately, the booklet contains insufficient emphasis on the importance of the work environment in the prevention of ill health.

Doctors have a duty to discourage smoking at work and smoking should be banned absolutely, on health grounds, in places where non-smoking employees would be subject to the tobacco fumes of others. Smoking causes more than a quarter of all deaths in men and women of working age and it is the cause of more than half the total deaths of those who indulge in the habit. Most of the deaths are from vascular diseases.

In the prevention of vascular disease diet is also important. Cholesterol and high intakes of animal fat increase the risk of developing these diseases. The occupational physician should, therefore, concern himself, not only with the education of employees on these matters but also with ensuring that proper, healthy food is available in eating places at work and, perhaps especially, in executives' dining rooms.

They should also encourage employers to provide facilities for employees to take exercise. This does not necessarily mean the provision of exercise gymnasia but it does mean ensuring that changing and showering facilities are available for those employees who wish to pursue their own exercise programmes, whether these are cycling to and from work or running in the lunch break.

The long-term prevention of ill health, by whatever means is as important to the prudent employer as ensuring that a new employee is fit for work.

Although the topics in this book have been approached mainly from a European point of view, a very useful treatise from an American perspective can be found in Himmelstein and Pransky.[23]

## Conclusion

Medical fitness is relevant when illness or injury reduce performance, or affect health and safety at the workplace; it may also be specifically relevant to certain onerous or hazardous tasks for which medical standards exist. Medical fitness should always be judged in relation to the work, and not the pension scheme. It has little relevance in a wide range of employment: very many medical conditions, and virtually all minor health problems have minimal implications for work and should not prevent employment. Medical fitness for employment is not an end in itself—it must be maintained.

### Acknowledgement

We are most grateful to Professor Michael Warren for his helpful advice on the prevalence of disability and the recent statistics and to the DSS Benefits Agency for their help with the new Incapacity Benefit proposals.

### Selected references and further reading

1. Faculty of Occupational Medicine of the Royal College of Physicians (1993), *Guidance on ethics for occupational physicians*, (4th edn). Royal College of Physicians, London.
2. WHO (World Health Organization) (1980). *International classification of impairments, disabilities and handicaps*. WHO, Geneva.
3. Wood, P.H.N. (1980). The language of disablement: a glossary relating to disease and its consequences. Int. Rehab. Med, **2**, 86–92.
4. Taylor, D.G. (1977). *Physical impairment: social handicap*. Office of Health Economics, London.
5. Martin, J., Meltzer, H., and Elliot, D. (1988) *The prevalence of disability among adults*. OPCS surveys of disability in Great Britain. Report No.1. HMSO, London.
6. Martin, J., White, A., and Meltzer, H. (1989). *Disabled adults: services, transport and employment*. OPCS surveys of disability in Great Britain. Report No. 4. HMSO, London.
7. Warren, M.D. (1989). The prevalence of disability. *J. Roy. Coll. Phys.*, **23**, 171–5.
8. Taylor, P.J. and Fairrie, A.J. (1968). Chronic disabilities and capacity for work. A study of 3299 men aged 16–24 in a general practice and an oil refinery. *Brit. J. Prev. Soc. Med.*, **22**, 86–93.
9. Taylor, P.J. and Fairrie, A.J. (1968). Chronic disability in men of middle age. A study of 165 men in a general practice and a refinery. *Brit. J. Prev. Soc. Med.* **22**, 183–92.

10.  Taylor, P.J. *et al.* (1970). A combined survey of chronic disability in industrial employees. *Trans. Soc. Occup. Med.*, **20**, 98–102.
11.  Heijbel, C.A. (1978). Occurrence of personal handicaps in an industrial population, survey and appraisal: Physical demands and the disabled. *Scand. J. Rehab. Med.*, **10**, (suppl. 6), 182–92.
12.  Jarvikoski, A. and Tuunainen, K. (1978). The need for early rehabilitation among Finnish municipal employees. *Scand. J. Rehab. Med.* **10**, 115–20.
13.  Fanning, D. (1981). Ill health retirement as an indicator of morbidity. *J. Soc. Occup. Med.*, **31**, 103–11.
14.  Occupational Pensions Board (1977). *Occupational pension scheme cover for disabled people.* Cmnd. 6849. HMSO London.
15.  Brackenridge, R.D.C. and Elder, W.J. (1992) *Medical selection of life risks*, (3rd edition). Macmillan Stockton Press, London and New York.
16.  Floyd, M. and Espir, M.L.E. (1986). Assessment of medical fitness for employment: the case for a code of practice. *Lancet*, **ii**, 207–9.
17.  Rodahl, K. (1989). *The physiology of work.* Taylor & Francis, London.
18.  US Department of Labor (1981). *Selected characteristics of occupations defined in the Dictionary of Occupational Titles.* US Government Printing Office, Washington, DC.
19.  Long, C. (ed.) (1980). *Prevention and rehabilitation in ischemic heart disease.* Williams & Wilkins, Baltimore.
20.  Erb, B.D. (1981). Applying work physiology to occupational medicine. *Occup. Hth. Safe.*, **50**, 20–4.
21.  Hanman, B. (1958). The evaluation of physical ability. *New Engl. J. Med.*, **258**, 986–93.
22.  Barrett, J. and Herriotts, P. (1994). *Employment and the workplace.* Disability Information Trust.
23.  Himmelstein, J.S. and Pransky, G.S. (ed.) *State of the art reviews. Occupational Medicine. Worker fitness and risk evaluations*, Vol. 3, No. 2, April–June 1988. Hanley and Belfus Inc., Philadelphia.

# 2

# Legal aspects and services for the disabled

## J.T. Carter and G.S. Howard

## Introduction

This chapter outlines the various facets of the law which may affect the employment of people with disabilities. The influence of common law judgments and of the Health and Safety at Work, etc., Act 1974 are reviewed. The effects of industrial tribunal decisions on practice is discussed. Details of the statutory and voluntary services available for assessment and rehabilitation for employment are given and the relationship of these to the Disabled Persons (Employment) Acts described.

## The common law

The English Legal System is based on common law. The legal system in Scotland is based on Roman Law but all the employment protection legislation mentioned in this chapter applies in Scotland. Common law developed from the decisions of the judges whose rulings over the centuries have created precedents for other courts to follow and these decisions were based on the 'custom and practice of the Realm'. Common law can be contrasted with statute law (passed by Parliament) and Equity (the body of rules administered by the Court of Chancery).

The system of binding precedent means that any decisions of the House of Lords (the highest Court in the United Kingdom) will bind all the lower courts unless the lower courts are able to distinguish the facts of the current case and argue that the old decision cannot apply due to the difference in the facts of the two cases.

### Common law duties of employers

At common law the employer has an obligation to take *reasonable care* of all his employees. This is judged in the light of the 'state of the art' knowledge of the employer—either that which he knows or ought to know (this is known as 'constructive knowledge').

The duty is summarized as:

(a)  the employer must take positive steps to ensure the safety of his employees in the light of the knowledge which he has or ought to have;

(b)   the employer is entitled to follow current recognized practice unless in the light of common sense or new knowledge this is clearly unsound;

(c)   where there is developing knowledge, the employer must keep reasonably abreast with it and not be too slow in applying it;

(d)   if he has greater than average knowledge of the risk, he must take greater than average precautions;

(e)   he must weigh up the risk (in terms of the likelihood of the injury and the possible consequences) against the effectiveness of the precautions to be taken to meet the risk and the cost and inconvenience.

### Higher duty of care for the vulnerable

The employer owes a higher duty of care to any particularly vulnerable employee with a known, pre-existing medical condition. This is defined as the 'egg shell skull' principle and a classic example of this can be seen in the case of *Paris* v. *Stepney Borough Council*.[1] Here, the Council employed a labourer with only one eye. They failed to ensure that he was wearing eye goggles and as a result he suffered an injury to his other eye at work and was blinded. The Courts held that his employers owed him a much higher duty of care as he was an individual with extra susceptibility to serious injury. (See also Chapter 8 regarding employees suffering from epilepsy.)

### Advice for employers

Employers may need to use competent advisers (normally qualified occupational health professionals) to assess the fitness for work, any disabilities which might affect the work or the health and safety of the individual or others, and whether any special arrangements, precautions or restrictions are needed. The Management of Health and Safety at Work Regulations (1992) include a duty to use competent advisers where appropriate.[2]

   The standard of care expected of a professional man e.g., an occupational health practitioner, general practitioner (GP), etc., was stated recently in the Court of Appeal[3] in this way:

A professional man should command the corpus of knowledge which forms part of the professional equipment of the ordinary member of his profession. ... He should be alert to the hazards and risks inherent in any professional task he undertakes to the extent that other ordinarily competent members of his profession would be alert. He must bring to any professional task he undertakes no less expertise, skill and care than other ordinarily competent members of his profession would bring, but need bring no more. The standard is that of the reasonable average. The law does not require of a professional man that he be a paragon combining the qualities of a polymath and prophet.

## The Health and Safety at Work, etc., Act 1974[4]

The employer's general responsibilities are more clearly defined in this Act, the culmination of over a century of legislation. The Health and Safety at Work Act is superimposed on earlier Acts and the duties imposed by some of these (e.g., the Mines and Quarries Act, 1954; the Factories Act 1961; and the Offices, Shops and Railway Premises Act 1963) must still be met, although most of their enforcement provisions have been replaced in the new legislation.

The Health and Safety Commission (HSC) was set up by the Act and is responsible for policy, while the Health and Safety Executive (HSE) together with local authority environmental health officers are responsible for enforcing the Act's requirements.

The Act covers everyone at work, including the self-employed, but excludes domestic servants in private households.

### Employers' duties

The Act imposes general duties on both employers and employees. Under Section 2, the employer has to ensure 'so far as is reasonably practicable' the health, safety, and welfare at work of all his employees, and must avoid putting at risk the health and safety of others through his work activities. The Act does not refer specifically to disabled employees, but applies equally to all employees, whatever their state of health.

The employer thus has a statutory duty under the Act to an employee disadvantaged by illness or injury, assuming that the employer knows, or ought reasonably to have known, of the disability. The employer should assess any problems likely to arise from the disability and make proper arrangements to avoid risks or hazards, e.g., by taking certain precautions or allocating particular work. He therefore needs informed advice on an employee's health in jobs where some medical conditions might impose health and safety risks.

### Employees' duties

Under Section 7 of the Act, the employee, while at work, must take 'reasonable care' for the health and safety of himself and of other persons who may be affected by his acts or omissions at work. This duty could be taken to include disclosing a medical condition which he knew might have health and safety risks in the work in question although, apart from those jobs where statutory medical standards apply (see Chapter 1 and Appendices 1–4), there is no implied obligation under the contract to disclose matters of health to an employer or to a prospective employer. If, however, an employee failed to disclose that he had epilepsy, for instance, when working in a job where this could pose a hazard, he might be in breach of his statutory duty under Section 7 of the Health and Safety at Work Act. Although no prosecutions of this nature have apparently occurred under the Act, lying, as opposed to failing to volunteer information about material health problems, has been accepted as being a potentially fair reason for dismissal in claims for unfair dismissal under the Employment Protection (Consolidation) Act (see below).

Medical conditions should be disclosed by the employee if they might have health and safety implications in the work concerned; any possible risks may then be appraised by the employer so that he can make arrangements to reduce or abolish the risks. It is, of course, important that in any pre-employment medical examination or questionnaire, any relevant questions are asked.

## Employment protection legislation

Employees have been given statutory protection from being unfairly dismissed and the relevant provisions can be found in the Employment Protection (Consolidation) Act 1978 (EPCA) and subsequent amendments.[5] Several aspects of these measures are important for those who develop illnesses or injuries while at work.

### Unfair dismissal

Employees have been given protection from unfair dismissal provided that they satisfy certain qualifying conditions (such as two years' continuous service as a general rule, and are below the Company's normal retirement age, etc.). Claims for unfair dismissal are heard by Industrial Tribunals.

The EPCA sets out five potentially fair reasons for dismissal—one being 'capability' which covers ill health. Lying about health at the pre-employment stage has been held by industrial tribunals to constitute another fair reason for dismissal, namely, 'some other substantial reason of a kind such as to justify the dismissal of an employee holding the position which that employee held'.[5] Thus, if a patient lost his current driving licence because of a medical condition or for any other reasons, he would not be able to continue driving at work and it would be illegal to continue to employ him as a driver.

Employers must advance factual evidence of the ill health preventing the individual from performing the jobs which they were employed to do, in order to justify the dismissal. Tribunals also have to be satisfied that the employer acted reasonably in treating that reason as sufficient for dismissal. The Tribunals have given guidance as to what constitutes reasonable conduct on the part of the employer in this regard (see below).

The mere fact that the individual is not prevented from performing all the duties, does not affect a decision to dismiss for ill health as long as the individual is unfit to perform some of the duties. This was stated in the case of *Shook* v. *London Borough of Ealing*.[6] Miss Shook was employed as a trainee residential care assistant who strained her back and was off work for some nine months. She was declared unfit to carry out her duties as a residential social worker because of the bending and lifting which was involved in her job and this was confirmed by both her GP and the Council's Medical Officer. She was eventually dismissed having been offered alternative posts which she had rejected.

She argued that her employers did not have any fair reason to dismiss her because she was not disabled from all her contractual duties since her contract actually contained a very wide flexibility and mobility clause and she worked in numerous posts within the Social Services Department of the Council.

The Court of Appeal ruled that the dismissal was fair and rejected this argument:

...The Tribunal were entitled to reject the submission that an employee is not incapacitated from performing...the work that they are employed to do unless he is incapacitated from performing every task which the employers are entitled by law to call upon him to discharge...

...However widely that contract was construed, her disabilities related to her performance of her duties thereunder, even though her performance of all of them may not have been affected...

## Medical evidence and medical reports

In assessing the fitness or unfitness for work and the prognosis as to the return date to work of an employee off sick, the Tribunals have made it clear that employers should not rely upon medical certificates alone. A full medical report should be sought by the employer or, if there is one, the occupational health physician or nurse. Employers are required to inform the doctor and the employee of the purpose of the medical report before asking the employee to submit to an examination.

In most cases, employers will state that the report is required in order to plan the work of the department and administer the sick pay scheme(s). Doctors should always ensure that they are clear as to why the employer is seeking such a report and write for clarification if necessary.

Employers without any occupational health personnel should inform the doctor from whom the report is requested about the reasons for their enquiry, the basic job functions of the individual and the length of the absence to date. The employer is required to obtain prior, written informed consent to do this from the employee. If the medical report is being sought from the employee's GP or own specialist, then the employer is required under the Access to Medical Reports Act 1988[7] to inform the employee of his rights under that Act (which include the right to see the report before it is sent to the employer and the right to refuse to allow the report to be sent to the employer).

Employees are now entitled to see their medical records (from 1 November 1991)—this includes occupational health records as well as the GP records and hospital records (Access to Health Records Act (1990).[8]

Employers may ask the specialist or GP a range of questions. Answers should be limited to the following list taken from the British Medical Association's model letter.[9]

1.  When is the likely date of return to work?

2.  Will there be any residual disability upon return to work?

3.  If so, will it be permanent or temporary?

4.  Will the employee be able to render regular and efficient service?

5.  If the answer is 'Yes' to question 2, what duties would you recommend that your patient does not do and for how long?

6.  Will your patient require continued treatment or medication upon his/her return to work?

### Conflicting medical advice

In some cases, employers receive conflicting medical opinions—the employee's own specialist or GP stating that the individual is unfit to return to work and the occupational health practitioner advising that the individual is fit to return to work.

In such a situation occupational health practitioners should be aware that the Tribunals have made it clear that employers are entitled to rely on the view of their Occupational Health Practitioner, unless:

(1)  the Occupational Health Practitioner has not personally examined the individual but has merely written a report on the basis of the medical notes;

(2)  the Occupational Health Practitioner's report is 'woolly' and indeterminate!

(3)  the continued employment of the individual would pose a serious threat of health and safety to the individual or others; and

(4)  the individual has been treated or is being treated by a specialist and no report has been obtained from or requested from that specialist.

The Tribunals have accepted that an unreasonable refusal by an individual to return to work following the advice of the Occupational Health Practitioner constitutes misconduct on the part of the employee. Here the reason for dismissal is refusing to obey a lawful and reasonable instruction.

### Absenteeism

Where an employee has taken excessive absences for persistent, short-term illnesses (normally unrelated), the Courts and Tribunals have ruled that the employer may have a fair reason for dismissal ['some other substantial reason of a kind such as to justify the dismissal of an employee holding the position which that employee held': section 57(1)(b) EPCA 1978].

However, the Tribunals have ruled in several cases—notably *International Sports Co Ltd* v. *Thomson; Walpole* v. *Rolls Royce Ltd;* and *Lynock* v. *Cereal Packaging Ltd*[10]—that the fairness of any such dismissal depends on the employer:

(i) examining the absence record objectively, assessing and investigating the underlying reasons for the absences with the individual, and measuring the amount and frequency of the absences against the Company or Department average; taking the absence record at face value will not be good enough;

(ii) warning the employee in a sympathetic, compassionate way and after attempting to understand the problems that the individual may be facing—these warnings should make clear that the continued absences are causing problems and that if the individual cannot attend work more regularly, even though the absences are caused by genuine symptoms, the employment may be terminated; and

(iii) giving the employee a disciplinary hearing and an opportunity to state his or her case and an appeal against any decision to dismiss.

Employers may ask a GP or company doctor to examine the individual to see whether there is any underlying medical problem which could explain all the absences. In many cases no such confirmation can be given since the GP may not have ever seen the patient during any of these short absences and the symptoms have normally resolved before the employee is sent to be examined. Nevertheless, it is good practice for employers to seek to confirm or otherwise whether there is an underlying medical problem in such cases.

## Confidentiality

It is not possible to cover the ethical questions such as the duty of confidentiality and medical ethics which are fully addressed in Appendix 6 and in *Law and medical ethics*.[11] Although there is no legal protection from the invasion of privacy, medical staff are under very strict ethical codes of conduct and can be severely disciplined by the General Medical Council for serious breaches of confidentiality and sued by the employee in question.

Employers are not entitled to require their staff to undergo medical examinations without obtaining, on each occasion, the informed written consent of the individual—this means ensuring that the employee understands the nature of the examination and tests and the reasons for them. Medical staff are best placed to ensure completion of the written consent forms.

Employers must also, on each occasion, obtain the employee's written, informed consent to disclosure of the results or outcome to the Company (a senior named individual).

*Failure to obtain these written consents will mean that no such medical examination or disclosure should take place.*

These and other ethical issues are dealt with in other publications[11] and the Faculty of Occupational Medicine's *Guidance on ethics for occupational physicians* (see Appendix 6).

## Disclosure of medical notes

As discussed above, employees are entitled under the Access to Medical Reports Act 1988 to see any medical report prepared by a medical practitioner who has or has had responsibility for their clinical care. There is considerable debate and confusion because of the ambiguity of the wording of the Act, whether occupational health practitioners' reports come within the ambit of the Act. It is clear that once an occupational health practitioner or a member of his or her staff has 'treated' an employee, the Act will apply to all subsequent medical reports.[12]

In a case of dismissal for refusing to return to work, the medical notes made by an occupational health practitioner may be ordered by the Court to be disclosed to the individual. This may include communications made by the occupational health practitioner to the employee's consultant, GP, and to the management of the company.

### Consultation with the employee

The Tribunals have ruled that in ill health dismissals, the employer should normally contact the employee, either by telephone or personally, ideally by visiting them at home by appointment. The purpose of this contact is to consult the employee about the incapacity, to discuss any possible return date, the continuation or otherwise of company benefits and State benefits, the employment of a temporary or permanent replacement, and the future employment or termination of employment. Consultation in this case takes the place of warnings which employees are entitled to receive in poor performance or misconduct cases. This was stated in a number of leading cases: *East Lindsey District Council* v. *Daubney, Spencer* v. *Paragon Wallpapers Ltd*; and *Williamson* v. *Alcan Foils*.[13]

There may, however, be exceptional cases where the tribunal views the lack of consultation as still rendering a subsequent dismissal fair. In one such case, *Eclipse Blinds Ltd* v. *Wright*,[14] the Managing Director received a very pessimistic medical opinion concerning the state of health of, and improbability of a return to work of the Company's receptionist, Mrs Wright, who had been off sick for some time with a bad back. The Managing Director felt it was not in her best interests to speak to her personally since Mrs Wright had no appreciation of the seriousness of her illness. The Managing Director decided instead to write to

Mrs Wright to inform her that a permanent replacement had been employed and that her services were to be terminated.

## Seeking suitable alternative employment

The Tribunals expect an employer to consider all alternatives other than dismissal and this includes looking for suitable alternative employment within the organization or with any associated employers. The duty also includes considering whether any modifications to the original job would be possible.

The leading cases cited above of *Daubney, Spencer* confirm that failure by the employer to seek alternative employment will normally render any dismissal for ill health unfair. This proposition has received judicial approval in the Court of Appeal in the case of *P* v. *Nottinghamshire County Council*[15] where Balcombe L J stated:

In an appropriate case and where the size and administrative resources of the undertaking permit, it may be unfair to dismiss an employee without the employer first considering whether the employee can be offered some other job notwithstanding that it may be clear that the employee cannot be allowed to continue in his original job ...

## Permanent health insurance benefits

Practitioners who advise employers offering long-term disability (LTD) or permanent health insurance (PHI) schemes as part of their contractual benefits ought to be aware that a failure to consider offering such benefits in an appropriate case could well be challenged in the common law courts as a breach of the contract of employment, i.e., breach of the implied obligations of good faith.

In a recent House of Lords case—*Scally* v. *Southern Health and Social Services Board*[16]—the House of Lords ruled that there was a positive duty on employers rather than their medical advisers to inform their staff of those benefits for which the employee must make an application. This includes the option of making additional voluntary contributions (AVCs) to the pension, claiming sick pay and PHI or LTD, maternity rights, etc. In the context of PHI and LTD schemes, it is essential for the management of any employer to inform any member of staff that they may be eligible for participation in such schemes.

Consideration of eligibility for an LTD scheme or PHI scheme may also be viewed by the industrial Tribunals as an important factor in any unfair dismissal case since the Tribunals could well decide that there was an alternative to dismissal which was not properly considered by the employer—thus rendering the dismissal unfair.

Company medical advisers should make themselves aware whether such benefits are offered so that they can advise effectively and appropriately.

If such a scheme exists, the doctor (whether GP or occupational health practitioner) ought to enquire of the employer whether the patient has been considered for such a scheme.

## Early retirement on medical grounds

In some cases where the employee is permanently incapacitated from (any) further full-time, permanent employment with the employer, the individual may be dismissed and given an early retirement pension. The common law courts have also indicated that the employer must act in good faith in deciding such cases—*Mihlenstedt* v. *Barclays Bank International.*[17]

It will be important for medical practitioners to read the exact wording of any pension scheme in this regard, particularly if a medical examination is to be performed in order to assess eligibility. It would be wise for medical practitioners to require a copy of the sick pay scheme, PHI scheme and Pension Fund Rules as they apply to Early Medical Pensions. In most cases, such potential retirees depend upon a recommendation from the Medical Adviser.

The liability of employers in such matters has been highlighted recently in the Court of Session (Scottish equivalent of the Court of Appeal), in the case of *Rutherford* v. *Radio Rentals.*[18] Here, the Court ruled that the failure by the employer to honour an insurance-based Accident Disablement Scheme, in a case which should have been successful, on the basis that the Insurance Company had refused the claim, was a breach of contract by the employer. The employers were deemed to owe money to the employee under the terms of his contract since the Scheme was incorporated, as a part of the employee's contract of employment. For further details on early retirement through ill health see Appendix 8.

### Management roles in sickness decisions

The Tribunals have emphasized that the option to dismiss an employee off sick and unable to work is a management decision and not a medical one. Doctors should therefore not allow themselves to be pressured into making such decisions for management. The doctor's role is to provide and interpret the medical information which managers will need, so that they can make decisions about the employee's position.

### Concealing medical condition(s)

Doctors should not advise their patients to conceal information about medical conditions such as mental illness, epilepsy, HIV or AIDS, alcoholism or drug addiction. Employees who are employed on the basis of false medical information given to the employer (or the occupational health team) can be fairly dismissed under the reason of 'some other substantial reason' [section 57(1)(b) EPCA 1978].[5] The

Employment Appeal Tribunal upheld the dismissal of an insurance salesman who lied about his long history of mental illness in *O'Brien* v. *Prudential Assurance Company Ltd.*[19] and an employee who lied about his drug addiction, despite the fact that he was being successfully treated in *Walton* v. *TAC Construction Ltd.*[20] However, a simple failure to disclose by an individual, because an appropriate question has not been asked, may not be viewed in the same way.

## European Union law

The influence of the European Union in occupational health has recently been highlighted by an interesting judgment in the European Court of Justice (ECJ).

In *Grimaldi* v. *Fond des Maladies Professionnelles* (1990), IRLR 400, the ECJ directed that Member States should take note of Recommendations made by the European Commission concerning prescribed diseases. In this case, the European Commission had recommended that Dupuytren's contracture be included in Member States' Prescribed Diseases. A Belgian workman developed the condition and successfully sued for the equivalent of the UK's industrial injury benefit, arguing that the Belgian Government ought to have followed the Recommendation and made Dupuytren's contracture a prescribed occupational disease.

Occupational health practitioners will need to keep up to date with potential legal changes in this field emanating from the European Union! (See also Appendix 7.)

## The Disabled Persons (Employment) Acts, 1944 and 1958

The main Act relating to the employment of people with disabilities was introduced in 1944, and amended in 1958. The 1944 Act aims to help people with disabilities to obtain and keep suitable jobs.[21] Most of its provisions are still in force. The main provisions are:

(1)   a definition of a disabled person for employment purposes;

(2)   the establishment of a register of disabled persons;

(3)   certain duties and obligations placed on employers under the Quota and Designated Employments Schemes; and

(4)   sheltered employment opportunities for severely disabled people.

## The register of disabled persons

The register was set up by the 1944 Act. Registration, which is voluntary, is open to employed as well as unemployed people with disabilities. Applicants for registration must meet a number of statutory eligibility conditions designed to ensure that they are in the labour market, but substantially handicapped by disablement in obtaining or keeping some form of employment (or self-employment) which would otherwise be suited to their age, experience, and qualifications. Medical evidence is usually, although not always, needed to help determine eligibility.

If an application for registration is accepted, the person is given a certificate of registration (the green card). Registration lasts usually for a maximum of 10 years, after which it may be renewed if the eligibility conditions are still being met.

## Advantages of registration

Being registered may make it easier to obtain and keep employment:

1. The 1944 Act places duties and obligations on employers relating to the employment of registered disabled people ('the Quota'—see below).

2. Vacancies for certain car park attendants and passenger electric lift attendants are reserved, under the Act, for registered disabled people ('designated employment').

3. Employment under the Sheltered Employment Programme is open only to severely disabled people who are registered.

4. Some kinds of special assistance from the Employment Service are only available to registered disabled people (see under 'Special schemes,' p. 38).

Despite these advantages, the majority of eligible people are not registered; registration is voluntary. The number who are registered has been declining for many years. Some do not know about the register; some do not regard themselves as disabled; some do not wish to be labelled; others see either no advantage to themselves, or think that being registered would put them at a disadvantage. The degree of advantage will vary between individuals.

## The Quota scheme

The 1944 Act places a duty on employers with 20 or more workers to employ a minimum proportion (usually 3 per cent of the workforce) of registered disabled people. When not meeting the Quota they have a further duty to engage suitable registered disabled people for vacancies. An employer with less than his quota of disabled persons must not engage other than a registered disabled person without first getting a permit, and must not discharge a registered disabled employee without reasonable cause.

However, as the number of registered disabled people has declined, it has become impossible for all employers to meet the Quota. The scheme is no longer working as originally intended. It has been the subject of several rounds of consultation in recent years. However, views on its future are mixed, and it remains unchanged.

## Current services for people with disabilities

Assistance provided through the Employment Department and its agency, the Employment Service, to help the employment of people with disabilities is based on the framework established by the Disabled Persons (Employment) Act 1944. However, it has been developed over time to reflect changes in labour market conditions, and to meet the vocational aspirations of disabled people. Developments have also taken account of the impact of improved medical techniques, and of advances in technology, on the employment capacity of people with disabilities.

A comprehensive range of assistance is now available to help people with disabilities to prepare for, select, obtain, develop in, and retain suitable employment. They have access to all the Department's employment and training programmes. In many of these, the eligibility conditions are relaxed for people with disabilities, and special assistance needed because of an individual's disability can often be made available. Most people with disabilities who are helped by the Employment Department now receive help through general or 'mainstream' programmes and services.

Disabled people who cannot be helped properly through mainstream services may receive specialist assistance through the Employment Service's Placement, Assessment and Counselling Teams (PACTS). These teams:

(1) help those people with disabilities who face particular difficulties in the labour market into open or sheltered employment or into self-employment, or to retain employment;

(2) promote, to employers, the value of people with disabilities and the range of employment services available for them.

PACTS are also responsible for administering the Quota Scheme and for maintaining the Disabled Persons Register. PACT members, known as Disability Employment Advisers (DEAs), working from local job centres provide a wide range of help and advice for people who have particular difficulties in finding or keeping work because of disability.

PACTs are supported by nine Ability Development Centres (ADCs) throughout the country which help to make sure that the service keeps up to date with the latest ways of assessing the kinds of work individual people with disabilities can do, and help to train people within the Employment Service as well as others.

Medical advice about clients is currently obtained, in confidence, from the Medical Advisers to the Benefit Agency, from hospital doctors if there has been recent hospital treatment, or from Employment Medical Advisers.

For help in finding or keeping employment, rehabilitation, or training, doctors should refer their patients to the nearest PACT by telephoning the local job centre. The schemes and services outlined below are available through the local job centres. Where specific medical advice is needed on health and work, patients may be referred directly to the Employment Medical Advisory Service; contact may be made by telephoning the nearest Health and Safety Executive office.

### Promoting good employment practice

The Employment Service works with employers to develop, on a voluntary basis, good practice in the employment of people with disabilities. This involves helping employers to draw up and implement policies for recruiting, integrating, and developing people with disabilities in the workforce, and for retaining employees who become disabled.

A Code of Good Practice on the Employment of Disabled People was first published in 1984 and revised in 1990. It is a non-statutory code which suggests objectives, and contains examples of good practice and advice—including advice on legal obligations. Its main focus is on encouraging the development of sound policy and practice in employing people with disabilities, whether they are registered as disabled or not.[22]

### Special schemes

A range of special provisions is available through PACTS to assist people with disabilities in their employment. This currently includes:

(1)   grants towards adaptations to premises and equipment;

(2)   provision of special aids or equipment needed to do the job;

(3)   financial assistance with fares to work for those unable to use public transport; and

(4)   financial aid for certain visually handicapped people towards the cost of a personal reader at work.

(*Note*: This range of help and the administrative arrangements were under review at the time of going to press.)

### Sheltered employment

The Sheltered Employment Programme provides job opportunities for around 20 700 people with severe disabilities who are unable to obtain or retain jobs in 'open' employment. Sheltered employment is provided by:

*Remploy*—a Government-supported company set up under the 1944 Act. Remploy employs around 8600 people with severe disabilities in 93 factories throughout the UK. Remploy is also currently developing the Interwork provision which allows disabled people to work in premises of outside companies (same integrated principle as the Sheltered Placement Scheme—see below).

*Sheltered workshops*—there are 124 sheltered workshops, run by local authorities and voluntary bodies, providing work for around 5100 people with severe disabilities.

*Sheltered Placement Scheme* (SPS)—provides opportunities for around 7000 people with severe disabilities to work, with appropriate support, alongside non-disabled colleagues in a wide range of occupations and locations. SPS workers receive the same wage as their non-disabled counterparts in host companies.

Further information can be obtained by contacting the Employment Service's Disability Employment Adviser at the local Placement, Assessment and Counselling Team (PACT).

## Employment rehabilitation

The Disability Employment Adviser (DEA) may offer a programme of employment rehabilitation to the client, as an aid to the completion of their resettlement action plan—if both parties agree it would help in preparing the client for work.

The Employment Rehabilitation Centres and Asset Centres which have been administered directly by the Employment Department (at various times by the Manpower Services Commission, Training Agency, and the Employment Service) and which have provided the bulk of employment rehabilitation nationally are being phased out gradually as part of the reorganization of the Employment Service's specialist disability services. The provision of employment rehabilitation is increasingly being transferred to agency contractors operating at local level. It is expected that, eventually, around 90 per cent will be delivered on a contract basis.

It is intended that employment rehabilitation should be flexible enough to provide individual programmes of support to those clients of DEAs who need extra help in coming to terms with the effects of their disability in the working environment, making decisions about their future career paths, and to be adequately prepared to pursue vocational training or job opportunities.

Referral for employment rehabilitation is dependent on the DEA having carried out an assessment of the client's potential, and it will ultimately be the DEA's decision whether or not to purchase employment rehabilitation on the client's behalf.

## Medical support to the employment rehabilitation services

People with disabilities seeking retraining or employment rehabilitation provide the specialist team at the job centre with a completed health questionnaire sometimes supported by additional confidential medical reports. The questionnaire helps the client and the specialist team (PACT) plan a course of action together. If the PACT team needs medical advice the questionnaire is referred to the Employment Medical Advisory Service (EMAS). The client may be interviewed, or examined by a member of the EMAS team and further medical evidence may be sought from the client's family doctor or consultant. These consultations focus on the client's concern about the disability, assessment of the residual functional abilities, and the appropriate choice of training or job. The medical information exchanged between EMAS and the clients' family doctor is subject to the usual ethical constraints of medical confidentiality and the requirement of current legislation on clients' access to medical information. The assessments carried out by PACT and EMAS teams are particularly useful in bringing together medical and vocational guidance to help clients comprehend their capabilities and consider the training and job options available to them.

## The Employment Medical Advisory Service (EMAS)

This service, set up under the EMAS Act of 1972, is now a part of the field Operations Division of the Health and Safety Executive (HSE) based at the offices of HSE throughout the UK. EMAS has about 100 specialist doctors and nurses who advise HSE and the public on occupational health aspects of work and on medical suitability for employment. This service is available to employers, employees, trade unions, family and hospital doctors and their patients, and young people seeking health guidance on choice of careers. EMAS also provides the medical support to the specialist disability services of the Employment Service Agency and assists them in the training of their staff and others who are engaged in rehabilitation activities.

The Health and Safety Executive publishes guidance on all aspects of health and safety at work, including advice on health aspects of job placement and rehabilitation (Guidance Note MS23[23]). People with disabilities can contact their nearest EMAS office. EMAS offices are listed in the telephone book under Health and Safety Executive.

## The Careers Service

The Employment and Training Act 1973[24] places a duty on Local Education Authorities (LEAs) to provide a careers guidance and placing service to people in full- or part-time education (other than universities). The Secretaries of State for Employment, Scotland and Wales carry central government responsibility and issue guidance when necessary for England, Scotland, and Wales, respectively. In Northern Ireland, the service is provided directly by central Government.

The Employment Department's Careers Service Branch (CSB) provides help and guidance to LEAs and collects from them statistical information of a general nature. Inspection and monitoring of the careers service is carried out by the Careers Service Inspectorate which is part of CSB. Careers Service Inspectors work closely with Inspectors of Schools from the Department of Education and Science. Similar arrangements apply in Scotland and Wales.

## Young people with disabilities

The School Medical Officer will notify the Employment Medical Adviser, the local Careers Officer, and the young person's medical practitioner, when a young person has a disability or medical condition which may affect suitability for some jobs.

Most LEAs organize their careers service to include Careers Officers who specialize in helping young people with disabilities.

Under the Factories Act 1961, employers are required to notify the Careers Officer within seven days of taking on a young person under the age of 18. If the Careers Officer thinks that the young person is in an occupation which may be hazardous or unsuitable they will contact EMAS and/or the employer and the young person.

# Training provision for young people and adults with disabilities

The Government, through the Department of Employment, funds training programmes for young people and unemployed adults, and a range of initiatives to encourage and develop training as an integral part of employers' business strategies.

Training and Enterprise Councils (TECs) in England and Wales and Local Enterprise Companies (LECs) in Scotland are responsible for the delivery of Government-funded training programmes. They must set out in their business plans how they intend to meet their obligation to people with special training needs, including those with disabilities. These plans form the basis of their contract with the Department. Vocational training for people with special training needs is provided through Youth Training (YT) and Employment Training (ET).

## Youth Training (YT)

Youth Training is designed to provide all young people joining the programme with the opportunity to achieve a National Vocational Qualification (NVQ) at or equivalent to NVQ level 2. All young people under 18 who are not in full-time education or employment are guaranteed a YT place. All young people with disabilities remain eligible for a guaranteed place on the programme beyond 18 if their availability for YT has been delayed by the effects of their disability or health problem. The Government's guarantee and extended guarantee for young people means that TECs have to give top budget priority to people with special needs including those with disabilities.

### Employment Training (ET)

Employment Training is designed to provide vocational training to people aged 18 to 59 inclusive who have been continuously unemployed for six months or more. Extended training programmes may be offered to people with disabilities where this will substantially enhance their chances of obtaining suitable employment. People aged between 18 and 24 inclusive, including those with disabilities, *and* who fall within the guarantee group are entitled to priority access. Additionally, people with disabilities aged 18 to 59 inclusive who are employed (regardless of length of any previous unemployment) form part of the target group and are entitled to priority terms of entry to ET, provided that TECs' obligation to the needs of the guarantee group are met.

Residential Training is also available for people with disabilities including the blind and the deaf who need the additional care available in a residential setting or for whom the residential environment is felt to be most helpful to their successful training. Fourteen residential colleges are funded centrally, providing around 1000 places. (For address details see Appendix 9.)

TECs and LECs are required to provide, where necessary, appropriate facilities and support to enable trainees who have disabilities to benefit from suitable training. These will, typically, take the form of:

- individualized training packages where existing contracted local provision is not appropriate in particular cases;
- adaptations to premises or equipment to meet the needs of a particular trainee;
- provision of special aids or specialized equipment to help with training;
- a personal readership service for blind trainees;
- a communication service for deaf trainees;
- part-time participation if a person's capacity to train full-time is limited by their medical condition.

This additional support is also available within Youth Training.

### Employment action

Employment Action (EA) is aimed at helping people with existing skills who, because of existing job shortages, cannot immediately obtain permanent work. It provides temporary work to help maintain skills, and offers additional help and support in finding permanent jobs. EA is delivered by TECs and LECs (see p. 41).

Places on EA are open to people who have been unemployed for at least six months. There are exceptions to this rule for people in special groups and people with disabilities can join EA after any period of unemployment as long as they are registered as disabled persons with the Employment Service.

While on EA, people receive their benefit equivalent plus a £10 supplement. They may also receive help with travel costs and be provided with protective clothing. At the end of their time on EA they are given a reference giving details of the work they have done whilst on EA.

## Students with disabilities

Skill:The National Bureau for Students with Disabilities is an independent organization which aims to develop opportunities in further, higher, and continuing education for students with disabilities. Its work covers the whole range of disability whether physical, sensory or learning difficulty.

Its activities include a number of specialist careers officers and learning support co-ordinators in colleges who have frequent contact with the Bureau. Membership is open to any institution, TEC/LEC, or individual with an interest in its work. The Bureau is a registered charity.

### Further and higher education

Following the Further and Higher Education Acts of 1992, a number of changes have taken place in post-compulsory education. The main effect for further education is that all Further Education Colleges and Sixth Form Colleges have become independent, and outside local education authority control since April 1993. In Higher Education, the distinction between Universities and Polytechnics has already disappeared, and the Council for National Academic Awards has been disbanded.

Potential students who have a disability should always let their preferred institutions know well in advance of their intended admission so that any special or additional provision needed might be discussed. Skill: The National Bureau for Students with Disabilities (see above), has produced a Guide to Higher Education for intending students going to university, and this includes details of facilities available and contact names. The choice of institution should be based on academic criteria, however, not on such matters as physical access most of which can be dealt with following or on acceptance (but in advance of admission).

### Selected references and further reading

1. *Paris* v. *Stepney Borough Council* (1951), All ER 42.
2. The Management of Health and Safety Regulations and Approved Code of Practice (1992) HMSO, London.
3. The Abbeystead disaster. *Hlth. and Safe. Inf. Bull.*, **149,** 5 May 1988. Published by Eclipse Publications.

4. Health and Safety at Work Act (1974). c37, HMSO, London.

5. Employment Protection (Consolidation) Act 1978 and Trade Union Reform and Employment Rights Act (1992). HMSO, London.

6. *Shook* v. *London Borough of Ealing* (1986), IRLR 46.

7. Access to Medical Reports Act (1988). HMSO, London.

8. Access to Health Records Act (1990). HMSO, London.

9. ACAS (Advisory Conciliation and Arbitration Service) (1987). *Discipline at work.* Advisory Handbook. ACAS.

10. *International Sports Co Ltd* v. *Thomson* (1980), IRLR 340. *Walpole* v. *Rolls Royce Ltd* (1980), IRLR 343. *Lynock* v. *Cereal Packaging Ltd* (1988), IRLR 510.

11. Mason, J.K. and McCall Smith, R.A. (1987). *Law and medical ethics*, (2nd edn). Butterworth, Kent. Kennedy, I and Grubb, A (1989). *Medical Law: Text and Materials.* Butterworth, Kent.

12. BMA (British Medical Association) (1988). *Advi.* (26 June 1989), BMA, London.

13. *East Lindsey District Council* v. *Daubney* (1977), IRLR 181; *Spencer* v. *Paragon Wallpapers Ltd* (1976), IRLR 373. *Williamson* v. *Alcan Foils* (unreported).

14. *Eclipse Blinds Ltd* v. *Wright* (1992), IRLR 133.

15. *P* v. *Nottinghamshire County Council* (1992), IRLR 362.

16. *Scally* v. *Southern Health and Social Services Board* (1991), IRLR 522.

17. *Mihlenstedt* v. *Barclays Bank International* (1989), IRLR 522.

18. *Rutherford* v. *Radio Rentals* (unreported).

19. *O'Brien* v. *Prudential Assurance Company Ltd* (1979), IRLR 140.

20. *Walton* v. *TAC Construction Ltd* (1981), IRLR 357.

21. Disabled Persons (Employment) Acts (1944) (1958) HMSO.

22. ES (Employment Service) (1990). *Code of good practice on the employment of disabled people*, (rev. edn). ES, Sheffield.

23. *Health aspects of job placement and rehabilitation* Health and Safety Executive. Guidance Note MS23 (1989). HMSO.

24. Employment and Training Act (1973). HMSO.

# 3

# Medication

*I.G. Rennie and L. Beeley*

## Introduction

Many people work while taking medication; in fact many can only work because of their medication. Additionally, many people have to take medication because of their work, e.g., those who travel regularly to malarious areas of the world.

The risks of side-effects and other consequences of taking medication must be balanced against the benefits of being at work or the health consequences of omitting the medication altogether. There are very few studies to help in making such an assessment.

Most people at work are not taking any medication. However, most treatment is prescribed by general practitioners and hospital doctors who, unfortunately, rarely have sufficient knowledge of their patients' work and working environment to assess the consequences of any incompatibility between medication and work.

Concern over the risks associated with alcohol has led to concern about other medication, particularly psychotropic drugs, impairing performance, skills, and memory and so placing those taking such drugs at risk.[1] The World Health Organization (1983) expressed further concern and gave advice and guidance on the subject in a booklet (*Drugs, driving and traffic safety*). Although this publication is concerned with drugs and driving, such advice is relevant not only to drivers of vehicles but also to those who fly aircraft, operate machinery, perform skilled tasks, or remain vigilant at a workstation.

## Prevalence of medication in society

Consumption of medication continues to rise in all developed countries. In 1963, in the United Kingdom, the average number of prescriptions per head on a National Health Service list was 4.6, whereas in 1991 it was estimated as being 8.1.[2] This figure, however, covers the entire population and the position regarding those at work has rarely been investigated. A study by Dunnell and Cartwright[3] indicated that 55 per cent of the sample population had taken or used some medication during the 24 hours before the interview, whereas a study by Rennie in 1984[4] indicated that 20 per cent of those interviewed in a factory population were taking medication, the difference doubtless due to the 'healthy worker effect'. The most common group of drugs taken by those in the latter study were beta-blockers, reflecting both the older average age and preponderance of men (88 per cent) in the study population.

The prevalence of medication within a working population will be dependent on a number of factors, in particular age and sex. Lader[5] found that psychotropic drugs were predominant in a female working population. In a predominantly male population cardiovascular drugs, especially beta-blockers will be more common. Both groups of drugs can affect performance adversely.

## Clinical aspects affecting work capacity

Unwanted effects of medication fall into two main groups; those which are predictable and usually dose-related, and those which are unpredictable and not usually dose-related (Rawlins).[6] In addition, unwanted effects may result from interactions with other drugs, with alcohol, and with other chemical substances which may be encountered at work. Of particular concern to the patient at work are effects on performance, especially for those who operate machinery, drive vehicles or fly aircraft, or whose sound judgement is imperative. Some drugs may produce particular problems for patients in specific jobs. Any doctor prescribing medication, or any occupational physician reviewing an individual returning to work, should consider whether there might be hazards to the patient from any drug effects, e.g., slowing of reaction time, drowsiness, or altered thermoregulatory systems. In addition, because of the wide individual variation that people can show, particularly in their reactions to psychoactive medication, any dangerous occupation should be avoided for at least a week after starting such therapy, and the situation can then be reviewed. These points will be considered in general terms initially, and then individual drug groups will be discussed.

## General effects of medication on performance

### Circadian rhythm

Changes in performance occur naturally as part of the circadian rhythm. Scores for most simple tasks rise during the day to a peak or plateau between 12.00 and 21.00 hours and fall to a minimum between 03.00 and 06.00 hours[7] correlating with body temperature. Scores for more complex tests may peak at other times of the day, depending on the particular components of psychomotor function required for the test, e.g., if short-term memory is the greatest component, the score will peak early in the day.

When a prolonged duty (e.g., of 12 hours) begins at noon, performance declines by between 10 and 15 per cent of control levels, but when the same work starts at midnight the decrease may be as much as 35 per cent. During the day, increased arousal partly compensates the effect of prolonged work, whereas at night the normal circadian decrease in alertness may add to the problem. Problems may occur in shiftwork, submarines, aircraft, and space flight, and any actions of drugs which affect performance may be additive in such situations.

There is also evidence that the absorption and elimination of some drugs are dependent on circadian rhythms as well as the pharmacological effect. For example, blood levels of *amitriptyline* are higher after a morning dose than after an evening dose and this is associated with greater sedative and anticholinergic effects[8] The mechanism is unknown, as is the relevance to shift-workers.

In patients on long-term corticosteroid treatment, suppression of the hypothalamic-pituitary-adrenal axis can be minimized by giving the steroid as a single daily dose in the morning, after the diurnal peak of adrenocorticotrophic hormone (ACTH) secretion which occurs just prior to waking in the morning. In long-term night-workers the diurnal rhythm is reversed, and the steroid should be given immediately on waking.

## Testing drugs to assess their effect on performance

This is complex and time consuming. Tests fall into two main categories; those that measure the effects of drugs on individual components of psychomotor function, and those which measure their effects on activities of everyday life, such as car driving. Assessing the effects of drugs on real-life activities has many problems but there is now much evidence that some laboratory tests of psychomotor function correlate well with, for example, real-life driving ability. The components of psychomotor function measured by laboratory tests include cognitive information-processing, short-term memory and learning, motor function, and activities involving sensory, central, and motor abilities. Such well-controlled psychopharmacological tests can now indicate with reasonable reliability those drugs which may affect regular activities such as driving and operating machinery.[9,10]

### Effects of environmental chemicals on drug response

Most drugs are inactivated by detoxication in the liver, and drug metabolism can be affected by factors which increase or reduce the activity of the hepatic enzyme systems responsible. Many environmental chemicals have been shown to be enzyme inducers and increase the rate of metabolism of many drugs in animals. They include polycyclic aromatic hydrocarbons and organochlorine and other pesticides. Studies of workers engaged in pesticide manufacture have demonstrated that enzyme induction occurs[11] but the practical importance of this is unknown.

*Effects on work capacity*

Drugs which primarily affect the central nervous system (CNS) and cause lethargy and drowsiness are all likely to reduce the work capacity. However, other drugs can affect the capacity to work and they include many commonly prescribed drugs, such as the beta-blockers.

*Effects on adaptation to extremes of temperature*

The human body temperature is maintained within +/– 0.5 °C of 36.6 °C despite wide ambient changes in association with the circadian rhythm which are individually consistent.[12] Drugs may affect the control of body temperature and place those taking them at risk if they are working in an inhospitable environment. Drugs may act on normal body temperature either by interfering directly with effector pathways or through the central control of temperature.

*Effector pathways. Sweating.* This provides coarse control of heat loss; it is under cholinergic control and hence may be diminished by drugs with anticholinergic (atropine-like) properties. Thus anti-Parkinsonism agents, antihistamines, tricyclic antidepressants, and neuroleptics, such as *chlorpromazine*, can cause heat intolerance. However, as most of these drugs cross the blood–brain barrier their effects on body temperature may involve central effects as well as peripheral mechanisms.

*Cutaneous blood flow.* This is responsible for fine control of heat loss, and drugs, e.g., the adrenergic neurone-blocking drugs, such as *bethanidine*, which act on the peripheral sympathetic nervous system; alpha-adrenoreceptor antagonists, such as *prazosin*; direct vasodilators, such as *hydralazine*; and calcium antagonists, such as *nifedipine*, may impair the vasomotor response to cold exposure. Normally, however, reflex mechanisms compensate for these effects.

The cutaneous vasoconstriction which occurs following administration of beta-adrenoreceptor antagonists does not affect body temperature but causes local signs and symptoms e.g., cold extremities, chilblains, Raynaud's phenomenon, and the development of ischaemic changes particularly in patients with pre-existing peripheral vascular disease. Those working in cold environments should be warned of potential side-effects, and the suitability of such work for employees requiring beta-blockers must be assessed.

*Central mechanisms.* Virtually all drugs with cerebral depressant properties may alter thermoregulation when given in sufficient doses. Individuals become poikilothermic, that is, their body temperature is dependent on their surroundings. Mechanisms are complex and not only is there suppression of hypothalamic control, but there may also be effects on the vasomotor centre producing disturbances in cutaneous blood flow. In therapeutic doses barbiturates, benzodiazepines, and neuroleptics may all impair temperature regulation. Tricyclic antidepressants and monoamine oxidase inhibitors may precipitate hyperthermia both singly and more commonly, in combination.

*Effects due to occupational exposure to CNS depressants*

Employees who work with solvents, e.g., in degreasing plants, printing, paint spraying, or with adhesives, and those who work in atmospheres where there may be a potential build-up of gases or fumes that can depress the CNS may be at risk if they take medications which also depress the CNS. Safe exposure levels at work are based on occupational exposure limits and these are derived from animal experiments and experiments on humans who are not on medication. The effects of such substances in the working environment may summate with any CNS depressant action of medication. (See also p. 128)

## Hypnotics and sedatives

These are all CNS depressants and most have been shown to impair psychomotor function, slow down responsiveness, and impair motor skills, co-ordination, and the responses concerned with self-preservation. The duration of effect after a single dose depends on the plasma half-life of the drug and on the dose given, but most hypnotics produce residual effects the following morning. Effects on psychomotor function persist during long-term administration although some tolerance occurs. They are potentiated by alcohol, and are more marked in elderly patients. Barbiturates have a greater effect on performance than benzodiazepines and should not now be used in patients who drive or operate machinery.

The individual benzodiazepines differ in their effects on psychomotor performance. When used as hypnotics, the short-acting drugs, such as *temazepam* and *lormetazepam*, are less likely than *nitrazepam* and *flurazepam* to produce effects the following morning. When used during the day as an anxiolytic *clobazam* appears to have less effect on performance than other benzodiazepines. However, all these drugs can affect performance in susceptible patients and differences between them are of degree only. Benzodiazepines have amnesic effects which are only partly secondary to the reduction in arousal produced by sedation. *Lorazepam* and *diazepam* severely affect performance of memory-based tests. Less is known about other benzodiazepines but some, e.g., *clobazam*, appear to have less effect on memory. Effects on memory are unlikely to produce problems when benzodiazepines are used as nocturnal hypnotics but the effects of daytime use on immediate memory could affect performance in a wide range of activities. *Temazepam*, because of its short activity time, is the only hypnotic approved by the Royal Air Force (RAF) for pilots.

Particular problems can arise when these drugs are stopped. Benzodiazepine withdrawal can produce a characteristic syndrome of anxiety, sleeplessness, perceptual disturbances, depersonalization, and general malaise. When severe, these effects can markedly impair work performance.

Barbiturates can interfere with central thermoregulation, and this may occasionally be a problem with benzodiazepines.

**Antipsychotics**

This group includes the phenothiazines, such as *chlorpromazine*; the butyrophenones, such as *haloperidol*; and similar drugs, such as *pimozide* and *fluspirilene*,
which are used mainly to treat schizophrenia and other psychotic illnesses.

Many of these drugs impair psychomotor performance and the degree to
which they do so probably depends on the amount of sedation they produce.
Thus *flupenthixol* and low doses of *sulpiride*, which have a predominantly
alerting effect, may have less effect on performance than the more sedative
phenothiazines such as *chlorpromazine*. Psychotic patients show impairment
of psychomotor function even without drugs and in some this will be improved by treatment. This needs to be considered when advising such patients
about the possible risks of working or driving while taking antipsychotic
medication. *Lithium* probably has little effect on performance, although impairment of some laboratory tests of psychomotor function has been
described.

The extrapyramidal side-effects of antipsychotic drugs, particularly tremor,
may interfere with precision work and affect driving. *Lithium* rarely produces
extrapyramidal effects but commonly produces tremor. Postural hypotension
may cause problems, particularly in hot environments. Interference with temperature regulation is more profound than with the hypnotic/sedative drugs. The
neuroleptics interfere both with hypothalamic temperature regulation and with
cholinergic control of sweating. Either hyperthermia or hypothermia can occur
when environmental temperatures are extreme.

**Antidepressants**

Many antidepressants produce sedation, especially when treatment is first
started, and this is markedly potentiated by alcohol. Psychomotor impairment
has been demonstrated and seems to be related to the sedative effect. Of the tricyclic antidepressants, *amitriptyline*, *doxepin*, and *trimipramine* are the most
sedative and *desipramine*, *nortriptyline*, *protriptyline*, and *clomipramine* the
least. *Mianserin* and *trazodone* are moderately sedative, but *viloxazine* does not
produce sedation; and monoamine oxidase inhibitors are usually stimulant but
*phenelzine* can sometimes be sedative. The newer serotonin re-uptake inhibitors,
such as *fluoxetine* and *paroxetine*, do not usually produce sedation and appear to
have little effect on performance. As tolerance develops to the sedative effects of
antidepressants, it seems sensible to advise patients not to drive or undertake
work which could be affected during the first few days of treatment with the
more sedative ones.

Tremor may be a problem in some types of work. Many antidepressants
produce blurring of near vision which may affect driving and the performance of
other tasks. Those with anticholinergic effects interfere with sweating and can

also affect central temperature regulation. All can produce postural hypotension, but this is more likely to occur with the monoamine oxidase inhibitors and with *imipramine* and *amitriptyline*, than with *nortriptyline* and some of the newer antidepressants, e.g., *mianserin*.

## Antihistamines and anticholinergic anti-emetics

The sedative effects of these are well known, as is the potentiating effect of alcohol. The effects vary, depending on individual susceptibility and the sedative properties of the individual drugs. Antihistamines that do not produce sedation, such as *astemizole* and *terfenadine*, should be used where driving cannot be avoided. Otherwise, patients should be warned that their ability to drive or operate machinery is likely to be impaired. *Hyoscine* is thought to have less effect on driving skills than most antihistamines and, although it produces some sedation, it is the anti-emetic of choice for drivers with travel sickness.

## Stimulants and appetite suppressants

Amphetamines and other stimulants increase risk-taking behaviour and can be expected to affect work performance and driving adversely, especially if combined with alcohol. *Fenfluramine* produces sedation but its effects on psychomotor function are unknown.

## Analgesics and anti-inflammatory drugs

The more powerful opioid analgesics, such as *morphine*, produce marked sedation, and patients requiring them should not drive or undertake work likely to be affected. Of the milder opioid analgesics *codeine* is known to affect driving-related skills and others, such as *dextropropoxyphene*, may also do so. Alcohol potentiates the effects of all these analgesics and even *dextropropoxyphene* is likely to be dangerous when combined with alcohol. *Phenylbutazone* and *indomethacin* have been reported to impair laboratory tests of driving-related skills. The effects of other anti-inflammatory analgesics are unknown.

## Anticonvulsants

Studies on cognitive function, both in normal volunteers and in patients on chronic anticonvulsant therapy, have shown impairment of concentration and sustained attention, and other aspects of psychomotor performance. Impairment is greater in patients on polytherapy than in those treated with a single drug, and there is some evidence that it is greater with *phenytoin* than with *carbamazepine*. The importance of these effects in patients well-controlled on long-term monotherapy is unknown. Driving must be stopped if treatment is changed (see p. 163).

Excessive doses of *phenytoin* and *carbamazepine* produce drowsiness, tremor, and ataxia. Particular care should be taken to keep blood levels within the therapeutic range for patients at work. *Sodium valproate* produces a troublesome tremor in some patients.

## Anaesthetics

As a general rule patients should not drive or operate machinery for 24 to 48 hours after anaesthesia for minor outpatient surgery, but this depends to some extent on the drug used, the duration of anaesthesia, and the response of the individual patient. Clear, written instructions should be provided for the patient at the time of discharge from the day surgery centre.

## Antihypertensive drugs

*Methyldopa*, *clonidine*, and *indoramin* produce sedation, and *methyldopa* has been shown to impair driving performance. Angiotensin converting enzyme (ACE) inhibitors do not usually have any central effects and do not appear to affect performance. Beta-blockers, especially the more lipophilic ones, such as *propranolol*, can affect psychomotor function but studies have shown that this returns to normal after three weeks administration. Air crew are permitted by the Civil Aviation Authority to take specified beta-blockers, but only after careful specialist evaluation and simulation testing. A period of ground duties should be undertaken first to allow stabilization and any habituation effects to occur.[13] (See also Appendix 2).

In a small proportion of patients beta-blockers have other side-effects which could impair work capacity. These include general fatigue, malaise, tiredness, and muscle fatigue which usually affects the limbs. Reduced exercise tolerance has been reported with all beta-blockers and there is no good evidence that the cardio-selective drugs are less likely than propranolol to produce it. For example, studies on the effect of beta-adrenoreceptor blockade on exercise tolerance in normal healthy men show that a fall in cardiac output, oxygen consumption, and endurance occurs with both *propranolol* and *metoprolol*. Both beta-blockers significantly increase the sense of fatigue during exercise compared to placebo, and a given workload appears harder. Many patients complain of lack of energy, fatigue, and aching muscles while taking these drugs. The exact mechanism is not entirely clear and several factors probably play a part. Beta-blockers reduce muscle blood flow and oxygen consumption by reducing cardiac output and partly by reducing beta-2-mediated vasodilation; they reduce the availability of substrates, such as glucose and fatty acids, necessary for muscle activity; and they may have an additional central effect on the perception of fatigue. Fatigue has been reported in about 5 per cent of patients on beta-blockers but minor unreported symptoms are probably more common, and it is important to be aware of the potential effect of these drugs on work capacity.

Beta-blockers can produce bronchospasm in susceptible people, and this should be considered when they are prescribed for such patients working in irritant atmospheres.

All antihypertensive drugs carry the risk of unexpected hypotension, and patients should therefore be advised not to drive or operate machinery at the beginning of treatment or when the dose is being increased. Particular care should be taken if the patient works in a hot environment. Most antihypertensive drugs affect cutaneous blood flow and can impair the vasomotor response to cold exposure (see p. 48). Diuretics increase the risk of dehydration at high temperatures and are not the antihypertensive of choice for patients working in a hot environment.

### Antidiabetic drugs

Psychomotor performance may be affected by even mild hypoglycaemia and insulin-dependent diabetics should not drive or operate machinery unless they are well controlled. They should carry sugar and be warned not to drive under conditions likely to be associated with hypoglycaemia (see Chapter 12, p. 224, 226).

### Anticoagulants

Consideration must be given to the suitability for employment of people taking anticoagulants. Usually the underlying condition is the limiting factor. Should bleeding occur, the guidelines given in the British National Formulary should be followed. It is advisable for employees taking such medication to carry anticoagulant treatment cards, or other means to indicate that they are receiving this treatment (see Chapter 17, p. 337).

## Other drugs

The muscle relaxants *baclofen* and *dantrolene* produce sedation and muscle weakness and make driving and operating machinery dangerous. Many other drugs produce sedation. They include *cyproheptadine, ketotifen, pizotifen, cyproterone, procarbazine, ciprofloxacin* and *thiabendazole*. Patients should be warned about the possible effects on driving and work when given these drugs, and that the effects are likely to be potentiated by alcohol. Mydriatic eye drops such as *homatropine, atropine,* and *cyclopentolate* paralyse accommodation and produce blurred vision. It should also be remembered that the effects of ototoxic drugs, such as *gentamicin* or *salicylates* will summate with any effects of noise on the middle ear.

## Malaria prophylaxis

The prospective traveller should consult his doctor, or a specialist in tropical diseases, who will determine the appropriate prophylactic drug and its dosage according to the area to be visited and the time to be spent away, also taking into consideration any drug contraindications. It is advisable to start chemotherapy a week before departure if the patient has not taken antimalarials before. The recommended prophylactic drug for malaria protection varies according to the type of malaria present in the area to be visited and the sensitivity of the parasites. The traveller's age and previous exposure to antimalarial drugs, the duration of stay and other conditions will need to be taken into account.

Drug prophylaxis should begin, at the latest, on the day of travel to the endemic area and continue for at least four weeks after returning. Whether drugs are taken daily or weekly, it is advisable to take them at the same time each day, or the same day each week. The correct dosage should be strictly observed. Whatever drug is taken it must be taken with unfailing regularity to be fully effective. Drugs should be taken with liquids after a meal in order to reduce the occurrence of nausea and vomiting or mild gastrointestinal upsets, particularly if *chloroquine* is used. (See Appendix 5 for advice regarding medical care of overseas employees.)

See Appendix 9 for agencies from which further information can be obtained.

## Conclusions and recommendations

Suggestions for advice to patients taking drugs which affect the CNS:

1. Do not exceed the stated dose.

2. Do not drive, fly, or operate machinery until the nature and extent of any side-effects are known.

3. Do not take any other medication or drugs while receiving this treatment unless they are prescribed for you.

General principles of prescribing for people at work:

1. Always enquire into the patient's occupation, and be aware of drug effects which can be hazardous in the working environment.

2. Make sure the patient understands what to expect and what action to take.

3. Be particularly careful with all drugs which act on the CNS and avoid polypharmacy if this is likely to have unintended additive effects.

4. Keep treatment regimes simple and avoid more than two daily doses, where possible, to increase compliance.

5. If a hypnotic is required, use one with a short duration of effect.

6. Avoid repeated unsupervised use of drugs; give a minimum of repeat prescriptions and supervise regularly.

7. Avoid the use of antihistamines in those who have to operate machinery, drive, or fly. Where they are essential, favour the more recently introduced, less-sedating agents.

8. Reserves of medication must be carried by those whose occupation takes them abroad for long periods of time, e.g., those on board ship. Reserves should also be available for emergency use for those working in isolated or dangerous situations where evacuation may be delayed.

## Special problems in specific occupations

**Flying** (see also Appendix 2)

All medication that affects performance is likely to be a hazard to aircrew. In addition, environmental factors, such as pressure, gravity, and temperature may all affect the performance of those flying, together with the potential effects of the medication. The Civil Aviation Authority (CAA) gives guidance to aircrew[15] and states that accidents and incidents have occurred as a result of pilots flying while medically unfit, and that the majority have been associated with minor ailments rather than overwhelming medical catastrophes. The following is an extract from the Civil Aviation Authority Aeronautical Information Circular—UK 90/1989, which gives guidance on 'Medication, flying and alcohol':

1. *Antibiotics*: apart from any potential effects of the antibiotics, the effects from the infection will almost always mean that the pilot is not fit to fly.

2. *Tranquillizers*, *antidepressants*, and *sedatives*: because of their effects on performance those who are required to fly must not take them.

3. *Stimulants*, e.g., *caffeine* and *amphetamine*: the use of such 'pep' pills whilst flying cannot be permitted.

4. *Antihistamines*: many cause drowsiness. In many cases the condition requiring treatment precludes flying and if treatment is necessary, expert advice should be sought.

5. *Drugs for the control of high blood pressure*: if the blood pressure is such that drugs are needed the pilot must be temporarily grounded. Any treatment instituted should be discussed with an expert in Aviation Medicine before return to flying.

6. *Analgesics*: the more potent analgesics may have marked effects on performance. In any case the pain for which they are being taken would indicate a condition which is a bar to flying.

7.  *Anaesthetics*: following local and general dental and other anaesthetics at least 24 hours should elapse before return to flying.

8.  *Other medication*: if there is any change in medication or dosage or if any other medication is taken, those flying are exhorted not to take such medication unless they are completely familiar with the effect on their own body. Those taking such medication should ask three questions:
    (i)   Do I really feel fit to fly?
    (ii)  Do I really need to take medicine at all?
    (iii) Have I given this particular medication a personal trial on the ground for at least 24 hours before flying to ensure it will not have any adverse effects whatsoever on my ability to fly?

In certain selected cases, aircrew who are under the care of cardiologists and consultants in aviation medicine may be allowed beta-blockers. Additionally, the use of *temazepam* as a hypnotic by aircrew in the RAF has been shown by Nicholson to have no residual effects on performance.[14] It is, however, most important that, before issuing hypnotics to aircrew, the cause for the requirement should be sought as this may be work-related and amenable to change, e.g., unusual work rosters.

Similar advice is given by the Civil Aviation Authority regarding medication and air traffic controllers in the Aeronautical Information Circular—UK 12/1991.[15]

The position regarding cabin crew is different, as these staff are unlicensed and each company sets its own health standards. However, Air Navigation Order 1989: Article 52: states 'It is an offence for a person to be on board an aircraft as a member of its Flight Crew if under the influence of alcohol or a drug to an extent which will impair his/her ability to perform his/her duties'.

The question of risks from medication to cabin crew is less relevant than their health status. The same applies to those travelling as passengers as part of their job.

**Merchant seamen** (see also Appendix 3)

The fitness of merchant seamen is determined more by the underlying condition than any medication. But it is doubtful if it is ever wise to commence seafaring if the loss of an essential drug could cause a rapid deterioration of health. Where medication is acceptable for serving seafarers, arrangements should be made for a reserve stock of the prescribed drugs to be held in a safe place, with the agreement of the ship's master.

**Diving** (see also Appendix 4)

Any medication that may affect performance will be a potential hazard to those who dive. Additionally, environmental temperature and pressure and the use of gas combinations, e.g., oxygen/helium, may cause further problems. Guidance is given on Form MAI from the Employment Medical Advisory Service (EMAS) on the medical examination of divers where it is stated in Note 3: 'The diver should be asked specifically for details of any current medication'. In general, it is the medical condition rather than the medication that is the bar to diving. Divers should, however, be asked specifically for details of any current medication.

The question of the effect and use of drugs in hyperbaric conditions is an interesting but practical problem for those who have to treat sick divers under pressure. Cox[16] lists drugs that have been used by divers; the depths to which they have been used; and whether there were any untoward effects.

**Offshore workers** (see also Appendix 4)

Guidance is given by the United Kingdom Offshore Operators Association in its 'Guidelines for Medical Aspects of Fitness for Offshore Work'. Referring to medicines it states the following require careful consideration:

- Individuals on anticoagulants, cytotoxic agents, insulin, anticonvulsants, immunosuppressants, and oral steroids are unacceptable.
- Individuals on psychotropic medication e.g., tranquillizers, antidepressants, narcotics, and hypnotics are unacceptable. A previous history of such treatment will require further consideration.
- Individuals taking medication have to ensure an adequate supply and report any adverse drug reaction to the Offshore Medic.

Those workers in the Norwegian and Dutch sectors of the North Sea will come within the legislation of those countries.

**Driving** (see also Appendix 1)

*Ordinary driving licences*

1. Section 5 of the Road Traffic Act, 1972: refers to 'Driving or being in charge under the influence of a drug'.

2. Poisons Rules (1972): requires a number of substances containing antihistamines to be labelled with the words 'Caution, may cause drowsiness, if affected do not drive or operate machinery'.

*Drivers of large goods vehicles (LGV), public service vehicles (PSV), and taxis*

Much stricter criteria have to be applied to professional than to private drivers. As a class they have to drive for longer hours, so that the risks of adverse drug reactions or interactions coinciding with a situation in which other road users could be injured by loss of control is far greater. Furthermore, it is not easy for a professional driver to stop if he is feeling unwell as a result of adverse effects of drugs.

Where there is a need for long-term medication, the issue of whether it is safe for vocational driving to continue may not arise as the driver will often be excluded from holding an LGV or PSV licence as a result of the medical condition requiring treatment. 'Medical Aspects of Fitness to Drive'[17] deals with the desirability or otherwise of LGV or PSV drivers being allowed to drive under treatment, and should be consulted where appropriate. In the case of short-term medication, the safest course is to give the driver a certificate for an initial period off work in any case where it is necessary for a drug to be given which might impair his driving ability. If treatment has to continue, a decision about returning to work can then be taken in the light of any adverse reactions which may have occurred in the initial stage of treatment.

As a general rule, the taking of drugs affecting the central nervous system and medication with insulin and hypotensive drugs (except diuretics and beta-blockers) is incompatible with vocational driving.

## Selected references and further reading

1.  Edwards, F. (1978). Risks at work from medication. *J. Roy. Coll. Phys.*, **12**, 219–29.
2.  Office of Health Economics (1992). *Compendium of health statistics*, (8th edn). Health Economics, Whitehall.
3.  Dunnell, K. and Cartwright, A. (1972). *Medicine takers, prescribers and hoarders*. Routledge & Kegan Paul, London and Boston.
4.  Rennie, I.G. (1985). *Accidents at work—risks from medication*. MFOM dissertation. Royal College of Physicians Faculty of Occupational Medicine, London.
5.  Lader, M. (1985). Benzodiazepines—long-term use and problems of withdrawal. *MIMS*, March, 1985.
6.  Rawlins, M.D. and Thompson, J.W. (1991). In *Textbook of adverse drug reactions*, (ed. D.M. Davies), (4th edn). Oxford University Press.
7.  Nicholson, A.M. and Stone, B.M. (1985). Disturbance of circadian rhythms and sleep. *Proc. Roy. Soc., Edinburgh*, **82BL**, 135–9.
8.  Nakano, S. (1982). Time of day effect on psychotherapeutic drug response and kinetics in man. In *Towards chronopharmacology. Advances in the Biosciences* (ed. R. Takahashi, F. Holberg, and C.A. Walker), Vol. 41, pp. 51–9.
9.  Hindmarch, I. (1980). Psychomotor function and psychoactive drugs. *Brit. J. Clin. Pharmacol.*, **10**, 189–209.
10. Broadbent, D.E. (1984). Performance and its measurement. *Brit. J. Clin. Pharmacol.*, **18**, 5S–9S. (see also the complete symposium report).
11. Hunter, J., Maxwell, J.D., and Stewart, D.A. (1972). Increased hepatic microsomal enzyme activity from occupational exposure to certain organochlorine pesticides. *Nature*, **237**, 399–401.
12. Blain, P.G. and Rawlins, M.D. (1981). Drug-induced body temperature changes. *Prescr. J.*, **21**, 204.
13. First European Workshop in Aviation Cardiology. (1992). *Eur. Heart J.* **13**, Suppl. H, 1–175.
14. Nicholson, A.N. (1984). Long periods of work and disturbed sleep. *Ergonomics*, **27**, 629–30.

15. CAA (Civil Aviation Authority) (1991). *Medication and air traffic control.* Aeronautical Information Circular, No. 12, CAA, Cheltenham, UK.
16. Cox, R.A.F. (ed.) (1987). *Offshore medicine; medical care of employees in the offshore oil industry*, (2nd edn). Springer Verlag, Berlin.
17. Raffle, P. A. B. *Medical aspects of fitness to drive* (4th edn). Medical Commission on Accident Prevention. HMSO, London.

# 4

# Hearing and vestibular disorders

*A. Sinclair and R.R.A. Coles*

## Hearing

## Introduction

Disorders of the ear can affect fitness for work in several ways: hearing difficulty, tinnitus, ear discharge, problems associated with barometric pressure changes, and balance disturbances.

### Hearing difficulty

This may be associated with obvious conditions such as disease of the middle ear or hearing disorder present since birth. In other cases the cause is uncertain. Often the affected person may be unaware that anything is wrong; for example, in hearing loss resulting from noise exposure the deterioration progresses gradually for a period of time before the impairment becomes evident. Hearing loss may not be compatible with particular tasks at work, such as where there is a requirement for good communication, where the safety of the sufferer or others may be compromised, or where there are exceptionally high levels of responsibility, e.g., radio operators and civil airline pilots. Fitness depends on interaction between the degree of disability and the auditory demands of the job. In severe or profound hearing loss, especially if congenital, speech production may also be impaired to such a degree that fitness for work may be adversely affected.

Hearing is vital for normal social and working communication. In contrast to a blind person whose disability is evident, the person with defective hearing has a hidden disability. His hearing aid, even if worn and visible, is usually regarded not as a sign of a major disability but as an appliance that restores normal hearing. This is not so, however, for the majority of hearing-aid users. The consequence is that when a hearing-impaired person fails to comprehend, he may be taken as mentally backward, and even ridiculed, or else he is shunned because of embarrassment and the time and effort involved in communication.

These attitudes often extend mistakenly towards the employability of hearing-impaired persons. The deaf, hard of hearing, and those with ear disorders need be excluded from only a minority of jobs. For further information on the impact of defective hearing on employability and the means of reducing its effect at work see Kettle and Massie,[1] ES Booklet EPWD 20,[2] and Appendix 9.

## Tinnitus

This is usually associated with hearing disorder and is present in approximately half of those with substantial hearing difficulties. Although the impairment of hearing will usually be the more significant factor regarding fitness for work, tinnitus may be associated with psychological upsets, including insomnia. These can be severe and incapacitating and can impair performance of jobs that are heavily dependent upon personal skills. Moreover, exacerbation of a troublesome tinnitus, from whatever cause, by exposure to noise at work, even when wearing hearing protectors, occasionally precludes further employment in a noisy environment: such exacerbations are usually, but not always, only temporary.

## Ear discharge

Most commonly this arises from a bacterial or fungal infection of the middle or external ear, but some forms of otitis externa are more akin to an eczematous dermatitis. It can affect fitness for work in several ways. These are considerations of appearance and of hygiene, and of ability to use hearing protectors or to use telephonic equipment. Not only does otitis media cause a conductive hearing loss, it can also result in a sensorineural loss. Hygiene considerations preclude work as a food-handler at all stages, from processing the raw food product to food retailing or catering: active or recurrent ear infections should be regarded as unacceptable in these industries.

## Barometric problems

Chronic or recurrent Eustachian tube insufficiency, or middle-ear disease, preclude people from certain occupations, notably flying and diving and work in compressed air. (See also Appendices 2 and 4.)

## Balance disorders

Vestibular disturbances are covered later in this chapter, and the non-vestibular disorders of balance in Chapter 7, but the possibility of their association with ear disorders, hearing defect, or tinnitus needs to be kept in mind when assessing fitness for work.

# Prevalence

As with most disabilities, the register of disabled persons gives very misleading statistics. In April 1992, the Employment Service identified 372 089 registered disabled persons aged between 16 and 64 years; of these, only 29 063 (about 0.1

per cent of the total population aged 16–64) were registered because of hearing impairment. The extent to which this is an underestimate is indicated by data from the National Study of Hearing (NSH), a nationwide epidemiological study in the United Kingdom. The prevalence of stated degrees of impairment ('hearing loss') as a function of age is given in Table 4.1. It should be noted that a 25 dB average hearing threshold level (HTL) in the better ear is just outside what is commonly regarded as the range of normal hearing; an HTL of 35 dB is the usual level at which otologists start to consider surgery or a hearing aid; an HTL of 45 dB is quite markedly hard-of-hearing; and an HTL of 65 dB is very handicapping in many listening conditions.*

Audiometric tests are useful as medical records before and during employment and as part of a hearing conservation programme, but they provide an incomplete indication of hearing disability. Data on the proportions of people experiencing various degrees of hearing difficulty, and ear discharge, are also available from the NSH and are shown in Table 4.2. It can be seen that hearing difficulties are common in the population at all ages and in both sexes, a factor which has to be taken into account in consideration of fitness for work.

**Table 4.1** Percentage of people in six age groups whose hearing threshold levels (averaged over 0.5, 1, 2, and 4 kHz) were at or over 25, 45, and 65 dB HL in the better ear[3]

| Age group | Percentage at or exceeding | | |
|---|---|---|---|
| | 25 dB HL | 45 dB HL | 65 dB HL |
| 17–30 | 1.8 | 0.2 | <0.1 |
| 31–40 | 2.8 | 1.1 | 0.7 |
| 41–50 | 8.2 | 1.7 | 0.3 |
| 51–60 | 18.9 | 4.0 | 0.9 |
| 61–70 | 36.8 | 7.4 | 2.3 |
| 71–80 | 60.2 | 17.6 | 4.0 |
| *Overall* | 16.1 | 3.9 | 1.1 |

---

* Pure-tone audiometry measures the hearing threshold level (HTL) at each of a range of test frequencies in each ear. The physical unit of measurement is decibels (hearing level), abbreviated to 'dB HL', except that the 'HL' should be omitted when the statement refers to HTL. The reference zero for dB HL is based on a standardized biological baseline of normal hearing in young persons, which varies with test frequency and with type of earphone and measuring coupler used for calibration.

The unit 'dB SPL' (sound pressure level) or 'dB(lin)' relates to an absolute physical measure of sound pressure of 20 μPa. The unit 'dB(A)' refers to the SPL after application of standardized A-weighting filters to reduce the influence of low and very high frequency components of a sound, thus giving a better representation of its potential for causing hearing damage, speech interference, reduced work performance, and annoyance.

**Table 4.2** Percentages in three age groups of males and females with various degrees of hearing difficulty and of ear disorder, sizes of samples shown in brackets (data from NSH; A.C. Davis 1985, personal communication).

| | Age group (years) and sex | | | | | |
| | 17–24 | | 25–44 | | 45–64 | |
| | M | F | M | F | M | F |
|---|---|---|---|---|---|---|
| *Difficulty in hearing* | | | | | | |
| *(better ear)* | (1980) | (2157) | (4038) | (4300) | (3734) | (4161) |
| None | 97 | 98 | 96 | 97 | 86 | 92 |
| Slight | 2 | 2 | 4 | 2 | 11 | 5 |
| Moderate | 0.4 | 0.1 | 0.5 | 0.4 | 2 | 2 |
| Great | 0.1 | 0.2 | 0.1 | 0.2 | 0.6 | 0.7 |
| Cannot hear at all | 0.1 | 0.0 | 0.1 | 0.2 | 0.2 | 0.5 |
| *Difficult to hear in a quiet room* | | | | | | |
| normal voice | (1674) | (1881) | (3291) | (3512) | (2937) | (3178) |
| | 1 | 2 | 2 | 2 | 7 | 5 |
| loud voice | (1664) | (1842) | (3457) | (3255) | (2837) | (3051) |
| | 1 | 1 | 1 | 1 | 3 | 3 |
| *Very difficult to* | (2859) | (3052) | (6030) | (6430) | (5709) | (6346) |
| *hear in noise* | 12 | 15 | 20 | 19 | 36 | 27 |
| *Discharging ear (ever)* | (2584) | (2761) | (5347) | (5762) | (5043) | (5617) |
| | 13 | 15 | 15 | 17 | 18 | 16 |
| *Hearing aid (ever)* | (2603) | (2774) | (5396) | (5827) | (5113) | (5722) |
| | 0.6 | 0.6 | 0.7 | 1 | 3 | 3 |
| *Registered disabled* | (295) | (341) | (748) | (778) | (778) | (894) |
| *(hearing impaired)* | 0.3 | 0.3 | 0.0 | 0.3 | 0.6 | 0.3 |

## Clinical aspects affecting work capacity

Hearing disorders will seldom lead to periods off work. Their impact is related more to working efficiency and safety, employers' responsibilities for the health of their employees, and sometimes to medicolegal problems. Tinnitus on the other hand quite often results in absences from work (see p. 61).

### Working efficiency and safety

Not only are there few jobs in which perfect hearing is essential, but a number of jobs can be done even by people with total or profound hearing impairment. For the majority of jobs it is sufficient that the applicant (wearing a hearing aid if appropriate) can hear what people say in the normal working environment and no special tests are therefore needed for pre-employment assessment. Where auditory requirements are more stringent, the needs for hearing, including the safety aspects, should be considered carefully to identify the real requirements.

Occasionally, in some quiet work environments it is essential to hear voices which may be soft, or spoken from a distance. For these, a simple clinical test for the hearing of speech (aided, if appropriate) is sufficient, e.g., voice tests carefully performed to a defined protocol (see pp. 75–8). Alternatively or additionally, correct identification of speech in a background of noise or of other voices may be needed. Here, the critical factors are the relative level of speech and noise (the signal-to-noise or S/N ratio), together with the individual's ability to detect one sound in the presence of another (frequency resolution) or immediately preceding or following another (temporal resolution). Both of these functions are likely to be impaired in cochlear hearing disorders. A practical test of hearing in the workplace itself is probably the most appropriate way to check the disabling effects of these and other forms of hearing dysfunction.

Most conductive hearing losses are due to middle-ear disorder and result only or mainly in loss of auditory sensitivity. Sensorineural hearing losses arising from cochlear damage (e.g., by noise exposure or associated with ageing) can impair both frequency and temporal resolution as well as causing loss of sensitivity. Pure-tone audiometry will detect loss of sensitivity for a range of pure tones and is a useful diagnostic and/or monitoring procedure, but it is a very imperfect indicator of speech identification ability and might therefore be considered to be unsuitable to define fitness for many kinds of work.

Some jobs have highly specific auditory requirements, e.g., the need to hear weak pure tones over a range of possible frequencies in radio operating, to detect changes in pitch or to identify the character of echoes in sonar operating. Many musicians need to have very good hearing, but others do not. The interactions between type of music and instrument played and the nature and degree of possible hearing disorder are so varied and complex that audiometric fitness standards cannot be specified. For these types of work, a practical test with the particular listening task is more appropriate. This is especially true with a trained operator, as his experience and skill in the job usually outweigh any potential disadvantage suggested by some auditory test unrelated to the task.

A more common requirement that can cause problems and thus affect employability is the need to hear warning signals or to detect the direction of their source. These sounds often occur in a background of high noise levels, when their detection is dependent primarily on the S/N ratio, although sensorineural hearing impairments make the task markedly more difficult, typically equivalent to a reduction of S/N ratio by 5–10 dB.

**Communication difficulties arising from hearing protection**

Earmuffs or earplugs may have to be worn in noisy occupations. Although these will reduce both signal and noise equally, they may also reduce the intrusiveness or attention-demanding properties of abnormal machinery sounds and warning signals. This is due to a general reduction of their apparent loudness particularly in hearing-impaired persons, and/or alteration of the spectrum of the noise reaching the ear with increased masking of high frequency signals by low frequency components, and/or a reduction in ability to directionalize their source.

The solution is to increase as far as possible the S/N ratio of the warning signals to a target of not less than 15 dB above its masked threshold,[4,5] and perhaps to alter the frequency spectrum of the warning signals. The 'design window' approach of Coleman and his colleagues[6] would at present seem to provide the most useful set of guidelines. In many cases the auditory signals should be supplemented by visual signals, especially when hearing-impaired persons are to be employed, whether in noise or not. Modifications to warning or communication systems may, if carried out for the safety of hearing-impaired workers, qualify for financial support from the Employment Service (Chapter 2) under certain circumstances.

In general, hearing protectors should provide adequate but not excessive attenuation. Although some have been developed to assist the hearing of speech and/or warning signals, they have inherent limitations. Amplitude-sensitive earplugs can protect against occasional explosive noises while interfering minimally with verbal communication, provided the intervals are quiet, a situation not often encountered in industry. Noise-attenuating communication headsets can be helpful, but may have reduced attenuation properties or be heavy and bulky. If cords are needed for signal-source connection, they are cumbersome; if cordless, using magnetic induction or radio systems, they are expensive and somewhat delicate.

## Rehabilitation

Hearing aids improve sensitivity, provided that there is some residual hearing to improve. They do nothing, however, for the reduction in the frequency and temporal resolving properties of the ear associated with sensorineural hearing loss, which is the most common form of hearing disorder in the general population. They also add their own distortions in greater or lesser degree. Thus, the benefit they provide falls far short of that given by spectacles for most forms of visual impairment. Because of these limitations, the fairest way to judge the employability of a hearing-aided person is to test his hearing ability in the listening conditions (aided or unaided, with or without lip-reading) that would be both permissible and appropriate in his intended working environment.

Most working conditions are compatible with wearing a hearing aid. However, only certain hearing aids are acceptable as intrinsically safe for use in coal mines or other places where there may be flammable atmospheres. Only particular models, and even batches within certain models, are safe; these change from time to time so it is important to check the latest version of Department of Health (DoH) information sheet B200 in its series 'Services for hearing-impaired people'. If in doubt, the Medical Devices Directorate of the DoH should be contacted (see Appendix 9). If the employee is dependent on a hearing aid, safety factors may need special consideration to allow for possible failure of the aid. A greater limitation on the use of hearing aids arises with work in high levels of noise, where an aid would be useless and would increase the noise hazard. On the other hand, communication in such conditions often depends largely on lip-reading and hand signals, which hearing-impaired persons understand usually better than those with normal hearing.

## Special work problems, restrictions or needs

### Defective hearing and accidents

It seems inherently probable that noise must sometimes contribute to accidents, from failure to hear shouts or warning signals. Nevertheless, serious accidents due to verbal communication failure arising from deafness or noise interference appear to be uncommon. On the other hand, some general statistical evidence relevant to this issue has recently become available (A.C. Davis, personal communication, 1993, data to be reported). In a lifestyle survey conducted by the Trent Regional Health Authority in 1992, there were over 6000 respondents to a postal questionnaire who were under the age of 50 years. Fifty-one of these possessed hearing aids: these people's reports indicated a sixfold increase in odds for accidental injury at work, but no increase in the home or on the road, as compared with those without hearing aids.

### Unsuitable work for people with hearing defects

The most critical types of work in this respect are those in which the actual task is an auditory one, such as in most forms of telephony, and where accurate hearing of speech and of other auditory signals is important. Exceptions can be made, particularly where the hearing-impaired person is already trained and experienced, or where there is some special connection with defective hearing, e.g., teachers of the deaf, social workers for the deaf. Major factors in defining acceptability include the degree of their expected responsibility for others, perhaps highest in passenger aircraft pilots, and the extent to which the impairment may undermine the public's confidence. These factors cannot be quantified. It is a matter for careful consideration by each employer as to whether or not it is essential to exclude people with defective hearing from certain jobs.

## Existing legislation and guidelines for employment

### Noise

The main employment problem related to hearing and the ear is that of noise exposure.

### *General legal background*

In 1981, the Health and Safety Commission reported that in British manufacturing industry alone about 600 000 individuals work in noise levels exceeding an equivalent continuous sound level of 90 dB(A), and over 2 million more are exposed to levels over 80 dB(A) (see footnote on p. 62 for definition). This followed two earlier publications, the Department of Employment's voluntary code of practice on noise in 1972 and the Health and Safety Executive's (HSE) discussion document on industrial audiometry in 1979. The more recent Noise at Work Regulations (1989) are concerned with protection from noise exposure, with limited hearing conservation measures now being required for equivalent continuous sound levels in excess of 85 dB(A). While these regulations permit the granting of exceptions from the requirement to use hearing protectors if their use increases the overall risk to the health and/or safety of the workers concerned, they do not include any guidelines on the employability of hearing-impaired persons. On the other hand, a new HSE guidance note on industrial audiometry is expected in 1993 and this will probably include advice on employability of hearing-impaired persons.

### *The extent of the problem*

It is difficult to obtain an accurate assessment of noise-induced hearing loss, since the prevalence will depend largely on noise levels and length of exposure. In one major manufacturing industry, however, which had performed audiometric screening for several years prior to the introduction of a full hearing conservation programme in 1988, one of us (A.S.) found evidence of noise damage in 40 per cent of the noise-exposed workforce, with 8 per cent reaching or exceeding a mean HTL of 25 dB averaged over 1, 2, and 3 kHz in at least one ear.

### *Current situation in industry*

Until the mid 1980s, the greater part of industry had been apathetic towards hearing conservation. Effective programmes had been limited largely to those organizations with comprehensive occupational health services, which only existed in about 15 per cent of firms. However, the situation is probably improving rapidly now since implementation of the Noise at Work Regulations in 1990, although hard facts remain difficult to obtain.

If hearing impairment does not involve substantial and unpreventable hazards to the health and safety of the individual or others, there is seldom any convincing reason for excluding the individual from employment in high levels of noise, but the employer should still provide him with properly selected and fitted hearing protectors, and keep him fully informed of the importance of wearing them and when to do so. With these precautions the individual is probably at little or no risk of developing further noise-induced hearing loss. The risk is probably one which, with due explanation and precautions, the individual is entitled to accept, either at pre-employment selection or in continuing employment.

The employer has a greater responsibility where the individual has only one functional ear (Chapter 2, p. 26), the other ear being totally or severely impaired. This is a not uncommon condition in the general population. The person is not always aware of it, sometimes even if the asymmetry is gross, and especially if it has been present since childhood. Such individuals may therefore have to be excluded from jobs where there is an inherent and not always preventable risk of damage to the remaining ear. In some working environments good directional hearing ability or ability to understand speech in a noisy environment may be particularly important and those with markedly asymmetrical hearing may not be able to cope in these respects. Great care is also needed in considering whether or not to employ persons with severely impaired hearing in conditions where there is a substantial risk of damage to the eyes.

Tinnitus can also present problems. It is often exacerbated by noise and/or stress at work, being much reduced after weekends or holidays. Hearing protection is advisable for persons with troublesome tinnitus when the noise level rises above about 80 dB(A) even for short periods. Even then, transfer to less noisy or stressful work has occasionally to be considered.

*Medicolegal considerations*

One of the arguments sometimes advanced for pre-employment audiometry is as a safeguard against possible claims, when the damage may in fact have been present before the employment began. The question then arises regarding the medicolegal risks of employing in noisy surroundings the considerable number of people who are likely to be revealed by audiometry as having some degree of hearing impairment (Table 4.1). However, providing the audiometry is followed by appropriate and properly conducted hearing conservation measures, including documented explanation to the employee about the hazards to hearing, the implications of hearing loss, and the means of preventing it, the medicolegal risk becomes very slight. The presence of pre-existing hearing impairment *per se* is not a valid argument against employment. Similar considerations apply to the use of serial monitoring audiometry and the action to be taken when hearing deterioration is detected.

*Assessment of fitness for work*

In the absence of guidelines, the position varies across industry. Many employers, particularly small firms, recruit staff without any medical screening.

Conversely, there are some who reject a potential employee if his pre-employment audiogram demonstrates a dip at or around 4 kHz. The majority of employers who perform audiometry do so to establish a baseline for the individual, particularly if he is to work in a noisy environment. Those employers who require routine pre-employment medical examinations may include audiometry. In fact, very few cases are encountered in general industry where the hearing loss causes a severe enough disability to preclude employment.

*Serial audiometry*

Periodic audiometric testing is generally considered to form part of a comprehensive hearing conservation programme. It is best conducted at intervals of 3–5 years, perhaps with shorter intervals in the initial years of noise exposure. Its main use is to detect deterioration in the hearing status of individuals or groups, and as an aid to their effective counselling. Safety indications for redeployment are restricted to those situations where hearing impairment puts the individual, the working group, or the plant at risk. Such instances are rarely encountered in general industry. Each case has to be assessed in the light of the particular job content and working conditions in order to reach an equitable decision.

## Existing employment regulations and standards

Where there are particular demands on hearing in relation to occupation, organizations develop their own internal standards. Examples are given below. In some cases there are detailed and specific regulations. More commonly, the decision is left to the occupational physician or the personnel officer, and the requirement is simply that of fitness for the job, informally and intuitively assessed.

*Flying (civil)*

The detailed requirements for professional pilots, engineers, and air traffic controllers are given in Appendix 2. Professional pilots rarely lose their licences from hearing loss because the aircraft radios and intercom systems function rather like hearing aids, amplifying the speech signal as required. Vertigo, however, does present a risk (see p. 85). The hearing standards are given in Table 4.3. These standards are likely to change when the Joint Aviation Authorities (JAA) implement harmonized standards within the European Community, probably in 1996 (see also footnote to Table 4.3).

*Armed services*

Medical fitness is expressed in terms of the PULHEEMS system (Chapter 1), in which 'H' refers to the Hearing acuity. Each quality is judged on a scale 1–8, where 1 is exceptionally good and 8 is unfit for service. Interpretation of PULHEEMS scales with respect to fitness for service tends to be stricter for recruits than for personnel already serving. The general entry standard is H2, but

**Table 4.3**   Hearing standards of the Civil Aviation Authority

| Audiogram | |
|---|---|
| Maximum HTL (dB) in either ear | Frequency (Hz) |
| 35 | 500 |
| 35 | 1000 |
| 35 | 2000 |
| 50 | 3000 |

This test is required every five years up to the age of 40, and thereafter every three years.

An applicant with a hearing loss greater than above must be able to hear an average conversational voice in a quiet room, using both ears, at a distance of 2 m from the examiner, with his or her back turned to the examiner. He or she must also pass a practical test in the air or in a suitable simulator.

*Note*: From about 1996 the harmonization of European Union flying licences will require that, at initial examination, the HTL shall not exceed 20 dB at 1000 Hz and 2000 Hz, and 35 dB at 3000 Hz.

**Table 4.4**        Audiometric standards in the armed services

| PULHEEMS H grade | Sum of HTLs (dB) | | General description |
|---|---|---|---|
| | 0.5, 1, and 2 kHz | 3, 4, and 6 kHz | |
| H1 | Not > 45 | Not > 45 | Good hearing |
| H2 | Not > 84 | Not > 123 | Acceptable practical hearing for service purposes |
| H3 | Not > 150 | Not > 210 | Impaired hearing; usually unfit for entry |
| H4/H8 | > 150 | > 210 | Very poor hearing; several restrictions on employability of serving personnel |

*Note*: The assessment is recorded as a two-digit number under H, the first digit for the right ear, the second for the left. The higher digit, representing the worse ear, will determine the individual's overall hearing category. The Royal Navy has a more stringent definition of H1, and certain branches within each service have particular requirements.

for aircrew is H1. These hearing standards are defined solely by audiometry. The audiometric standards are given in Table 4.4.

*Police*

The tests performed and their interpretation vary from one police force to another. In Nottinghamshire, for example, the screening test for hearing is based on pure-tone audiometry, with a preliminary upper HTL limit for new recruits of 30 dB in each ear and at each test frequency in the range 250 Hz to 8 kHz. This limit is only for general guidance however and, subject to ENT advice, may be relaxed in particular cases, especially with older recruits who may have worked previously in a noisy occupation. There is also periodic audiometric screening of serving officers who work in a potentially noise-hazardous environment, for example firearms instructors, motorcycle traffic officers, headphone users. The maximum acceptable HTL for such persons is 40 dB, again with flexibility in its application to individual cases.

*Fire service*

In 1970, the Home Office issued guidance (Godber Report[7]) on entry and periodic medical examinations. Different standards of fitness were required for recruits and for older men, who were recommended for reassessment every three years after the age of 40 years. The basic criterion was defined in a general way, typical of many occupations; that no man should engage in duties (operational fire-fighting in this case) who is not fit for those duties. While the definition is essentially circular and thus no more than a guideline, it had the merits of flexibility, adaptability, and of evident relevance.

The Godber Report was superseded in 1989 by the Report of the Joint Working Party of the Home Office on Medical Standards in Firefighters. With respect to hearing it comments as follows:

It is essential that firefighters should be able to hear instructions and signals, and good hearing is necessary. The whisper test combined with otoscopic examination and tuning fork tests can be used but audiometry is more accurate. A portable audiometer with ear muffs, used in a quiet room, would give sufficiently accurate readings capable of detecting significant hearing loss which could then be more fully assessed at an audiology clinic.

*Merchant navy* (see Appendix 3)

The General Council of British Shipping provides an audiometric testing service for shipping companies, but the standards of fitness vary according to individual company policy. Conditions leading to 'permanently unfit' categorization include impaired hearing sufficient to interfere with communication. A unilateral hearing defect is considered in relation to the particular job. Hearing aids are allowable in certain trades provided the aided hearing is sufficient for communication and safety: they are not allowed for engine-room, electrical, and radio personnel.

*British Rail*

The Board has issued guidelines on medical examinations and standards, but discretion is allowed in individual cases in respect of voice tests and, in the case of train drivers, a practical hearing test is carried out under operational conditions according to a defined protocol. With pure-tone audiometry there are stricter standards for new entrants than for periodic reviews of employees. For example, for entry to train crew and safety grades the HTLs must not exceed 20 dB averaged over 0.5, 1 and 2 kHz or 25 dB at 4 kHz, whereas this is relaxed to 30 dB at the periodic reviews carried out at ages 25, 30, 35, 40, 45, 50, 55, 57, 60, 62, 63, and 64 years. It is considered unsafe to employ a man who is dependent on a hearing aid to undertake 'footplate' duties on main lines, or in any grade which involves working on operating lines.

*British Steel*

One of the major problems encountered in heavy manufacturing industries, such as British Steel, is the potential effect of excessive noise on hearing. The main initiative has therefore been the implementation of a comprehensive hearing conservation programme which consists of a number of components, e.g., noise surveys and the identification of noise-hazard areas, engineering control, education and training in addition to screening audiometry, and the provision of personal protection. Audiometry is performed on all new employees to establish a baseline and is mandatory at three-yearly intervals for those employees working in noise-hazard areas. The incidence of cases where hearing loss is severe enough to act as a bar to employment, or where existing employees require redeployment, is minimal. A range of communication equipment is used: contact may be by means of personal radio, tannoy or visual signals. The basic criteria of auditory fitness for work are those described in detail above, i.e., ability to perform the job safely and competently, with each case considered individually. Accordingly, no specific hearing standards have been laid down.

*Driving* (see Appendix 1)

It is conceivable that defective hearing could result in failure to hear a warning sound and thus lead to an accident. However, 'There is no significant evidence that people with severe degrees of deafness have a higher accident rate than others. Deaf people qualify for an ordinary driving licence'.[8] Thus, defective hearing as such need not be declared in an application for a driving licence, or at onset of the condition in the case of the holder of a current ordinary driving licence. However, where it is symptomatic of some other disorder liable to affect fitness to drive, then that disorder must be notified to the Licensing Centre at Swansea.

For large goods (LGVs) and passenger carrying vehicle (PCVs) drivers the Department of Transport take the line that the new technology in computer systems enables profoundly deaf persons to communicate on the telephone and, as a consequence, as long as such persons can demonstrate their ability to use these systems, the Department has no objection to their driving heavy goods and passenger carrying vehicles.

The EC Directive on driver licensing states: 'driving licences shall not be issued to, or renewed for applicants or drivers in group 2 if their hearing is so deficient that it interferes with the proper charge of their duties'. [9]

The effect of this is that from the 1 July 1996 group 2 will include commercial mini-buses and goods vehicles between a metric weight of 3.5 and 7.5 metric tonnes laden weight, as well as the existing vehicles over 7.5 metric tonnes laden weight and other buses.

*Diving* (see Appendix 4)

*Ears.* The diver should be able to clear his ears. Complications of otitis media such as glue ear, deafness, perforation, and persistent discharge are causes for rejection. Mastoiditis would also debar. The following points should be covered during examination.

1. *Meati* should appear normal. If wax is present, it is not necessary to disturb it unless it is excessive or obstructing the canal. Acute or chronic otitis externa is a bar to diving. Exostoses are not harmful unless the canal is occluded, when the diver should be referred for their removal.

2. *The drum* should be seen: well-healed scars are acceptable. New entrants must demonstrate the ability to clear their ears. This may also be indicated after infection or barotrauma.

3. *Hearing.* The diver must be able to hear and understand normal conversation.

4. *Audiometric examination* must be carried out at each annual examination, using equipment covering the frequencies 250 Hz to 8 kHz and according to prescribed procedures. Particular attention should be given to divers who have only unilateral hearing, and the risks of further hearing damage should be discussed with the diver.

*Further education*

Certain universities specialize in supplementary provision for particular types of disability (Chapter 2, p. 43), for example, Durham, in the case of the hearing disabled. Many colleges of further education make special arrangements for technical courses in preparation for jobs not based on interpersonal communication, where prelingually hearing-impaired students are likely to be able to fulfil the job requirements. In considering deaf and hard-of-hearing students, particularly for lecture-based curricula, proper account should be taken of the extra support which the teaching staff (who should be consulted over admissions) may need to give, and to the possible need for supplementary aids, such as a microphone and an induction loop, radio or infrared transmission system, to overcome poor room acoustics. An audiological assessment prior to admission, or assessment by an educationalist with relevant experience, would be valuable.

## Conclusions and recommendations

Normal hearing is difficult to define in terms of either normal function or lack of perceived disability, especially as any definition is essentially arbitrary and may be ambiguous as to whether or not 'normal for age' is intended. There is wide individual variation in the degree to which a hearing impairment causes measurable hearing disability, and to which it is perceived by the person affected. Moreover, the effect of a disability in the context of fitness for work depends greatly on the particular job requirements and working environment. These difficulties have to be seen in relation to the quite high prevalence of measurable hearing impairments (Table 4.1) and of reported hearing difficulties (Table 4.2) in the general adult population.

Totally normal hearing, implying a stringent audiometric definition, is truly necessary in only very few jobs. But there are a number of occupations in which more than a minor impairment or disability, or having monaural hearing, is not acceptable for a variety of reasons. These include high levels of responsibility to others, need for efficient and easy communication, particular listening tasks, and safety with respect to hearing warning signals, especially when having to wear hearing protectors. The hearing requirements of each job have to be considered carefully when setting standards for entry or for continued employment, but care is needed to counteract natural or traditional prejudices against employing hard-of-hearing or deaf persons. The problems that their hearing difficulties cause can be much less than are widely imagined, and can often be reduced or abolished by suitable modifications in equipment and/or in work and safety procedures.

For the majority of jobs, actual tests of hearing are unnecessary, other than a simple observation of the applicant's or employee's hearing ability at interview. This can be done, as may be applicable, with or without the interviewee wearing a hearing aid if he has one, and with or without lip-reading (being able to see the interviewer's face). This is preferably coupled with some form of health declaration and statement of any disability. For those already employed, there may also be evidence regarding the importance or otherwise of any problems due to hearing difficulties that may have occurred with the particular employee and job.

Where the job requires a more definite degree of hearing ability, or minimum of disability, a test of ability to hear speech would probably be sufficient in most cases. Such tests are discussed in the next section. The choice depends on the nature and environment of the work, particularly whether or not there is need to hear speech in a background of noise. Audiometry is less relevant as a test of communication ability, relatively costly, and also raises problems of correct interpretation and subsequent management. It is probably best reserved for testing those in whom particularly good hearing is required and when speech tests are insufficiently sensitive to detect minor impairments of potential significance, or where a medicolegal baseline or rejection criterion is desired, or where the test has to form the baseline for periodic monitoring in support of a hearing conservation programme.

## TESTS OF HEARING FOR ASSESSMENT OF FITNESS FOR WORK

A wide variety of hearing tests has been or could be used for assessment of auditory fitness. Those outlined below should meet most situations. In selecting a test, it is advisable first to define clearly the objective(s) of the test and obtain the agreement of the involved parties to this definition. It should then be a relatively simple matter to choose which test or tests are the most suitable. The final selection may also be influenced by financial, administrative, and space considerations, and by the acoustics of the proposed test environment.

### Tests of hearing speech in a quiet background: voice tests

Free-field live-voice testing, widely used in clinical and occupational assessment of hearing ability, gives both a quantitative method of assessing hearing and one which has obvious practical relevance. It requires no instrumentation. It has, however, fallen into some disrepute in recent decades due to inadequate test protocols, calibration, and interpretative criteria, as well as appearing to be overtaken in accuracy by audiometry. The principal deficiencies in live-voice tests have been:

(1)  substantial inter-examiner and intra-examiner variability in voice levels and clarity;

(2)  tendency to raise the voice level when the ambient noise level rises; or

(3)  when distance from the subject increases;

(4)  lack of a standard technique or sufficiently detailed test protocol;

(5)  ambient noise;

(6)  too small a test space; and

(7)  too narrow and reverberant a test space.

A major contribution to restoring confidence in voice tests has been made by Swan *et al.*[10] He showed that deficiency (1) need not be a cause of major concern given suitable interpretative criteria, and deficiencies (3), (6), and (7) can be obviated by using the near field only. He argues that deficiency (2) is rarely a problem and (5) should not be for most medical examination rooms. He has also shown how the non-test ear can be efficiently, easily, and inexpensively masked. As a consequence, it is hoped that the recommendations below will meet the remaining need for a detailed protocol for conducting and interpreting the tests.

### Test protocol for voice tests

The examiner positions himself in front of the subject at a nominal distance of 60 cm between his mouth and subject's ears. He speaks the test material clearly in a whispered voice after full expiration (WV), conversational voice (CV), or loud voice (LV). The test material consists of trios of words: a numeral, a letter, a numeral (e.g., 5B6). Different combinations of numerals and letters must be used in each trio. Two trios are used for each type of voice, and the subject is considered to have passed that voice test when he has repeated correctly at least three of the possible total of six numerals and letters. If fewer than three are repeated correctly, the next (louder) type of voice is used, and so on. When required, masking of the non-test ear is accomplished by pressing a finger on the tragus of the non-test ear and moving the skin over the cartilage to and fro, thus producing a continuous noise in the ear.

The hearing requirements of the job will define the other test details as follows:

(1)  whether each ear is to be tested separately with masking of the non-test ear in order to detect monaural disorders, or whether the ears are to be tested together;

(2)  whether the subject's hearing aid may be worn, which in turn depends on whether it is possible and permissible at work; and

(3)  whether the subject can make use of lip-reading (told to watch the examiner's face) or not (told to shut his eyes), which also depends on whether lip-reading is always or normally possible at work.

Swan related the results of response to such voice tests to the audiometric thresholds of the large number of clinical patients included in his study, both retrospectively and prospectively. For test distances nominally at 60 cm and for hearing by a single ear without hearing aid or lip-reading, he established the approximate equivalents shown in Table 4.5, which include the effects of inter-clinician variability in voice levels.

Since voice levels can vary considerably between examiners and also between occasions with the same examiner, the best practice would require the examiner to calibrate his own voice levels and clarity for the test materials and in the test environment, both initially and at intervals. They can then be compared with, or adjusted to, the mean voice sound pressure levels measured by Swan, which were 57, 71, and 91 dB(A) for WV, CV, and LV, respectively when measured at a distance of 60 cm from the clinician's mouth with a sound-level meter set to the fast response. For such self-calibration of voice levels an inexpensive non-precision sound-level meter would be adequate.

Where the test is conducted binaurally, with or without a hearing aid, and with or without help from lip-reading, the result of the voice tests can be expressed in functional

**Table 4.5**  Relationship between voice test results and pure-tone Hearing Threshold Levels (after Browning *et al.*[10])

| Grade | Voice test result | Approximate equivalent HTL (0.5, 1, and 2 kHz average) |
| --- | --- | --- |
| 1 | Pass WV | Less than 30 dB |
| 2 | Fail WV, pass CV | 20–60 dB |
| 3 | Fail CV, pass LV | Over 45 dB, probably over 60 dB |

*Note*: WV, whispered voice after full expiration; CV, conversational voice; LV, loud voice.

terms equivalent as above to unaided monaural listening. Grade 1 hearing would be quite adequate for nearly all jobs; Grade 2 for all jobs, other than those in which there is an operational or safety requirement for good hearing *per se* or possibly when wearing ear protection and/or working in noise. Grade 3 applicants should be carefully considered in relation to the actual hearing requirements of the jobs concerned and not be excluded unnecessarily.

**Finally, it is recommended that where audiometry is to be carried out, this should not replace voice tests but supplement them. For each subject, the results of voice tests can provide a very useful check on the apparent hearing ability as measured with an audiometer; and they also give information on another often more relevant dimension of hearing ability.**

**Test of ability to understand speech in noise**

In noisy conditions, someone with a substantial loss of hearing sensitivity only (such as caused by conductive hearing loss) would be at no disadvantage relative to persons with normal hearing and even at some advantage, as they often hear better in noise than in quiet, an observation resulting from the fact that those with normal hearing raise their voice levels in noise. This well-known diagnostic feature (paracusis Willisii) suggests that the patient's hearing loss is probably of conductive type.

In contrast, persons with sensorineural hearing loss have particular difficulty in hearing in a background of noise. Lip-reading and signing is a help but cannot always be relied on, although workers in high levels of noise tend to learn from experience how to make maximal use of their hearing. These factors, together with a wide range of individual variability in the relationship between hearing sensitivity (as measured by voice tests or pure-tone audiometry) and ability to identify correctly speech sounds in noise, may make it desirable to have a test of the latter. Ideally, this should be based on samples of the sort of speech to be heard under the listening conditions to be expected, or with the communication equipment likely to be used, and in the actual noise background. Unfortunately, this is usually impracticable.

A general purpose test of hearing speech in noise would have rather limited face-validity, and there is also no such test available in standard clinical use. Thus it may be better, and certainly much simpler, to use the sort of voice and whisper tests outlined above and just interpret them more stringently where the working environment requires accurate vocal communication in poor listening conditions. Alternatively, if the auditory requirement is very strict, a practical test of hearing ability may be arranged in the actual working environment and with the sort of messages that need to be heard.

**Pure-tone audiometry**

In the present context, the purposes of audiometry are to obtain a frequency-specific and a more precise and diagnostic measurement of hearing ability than is provided by speech tests, although its results will usually have less practical relevance to defining fitness for work than voice tests. It also has many disadvantages, needing costly and carefully calibrated equipment, trained operators, and (for low frequencies) particularly good acoustic conditions. The latter will require an acoustic booth which takes up more space and is heavy and expensive. Recommended techniques and maximum ambient noise levels for audiometry have been included in international and national[11] standards. Despite the basic precision of the stimulus and measurement technique in audiometry, its sources of imprecision are often overlooked. Not everyone performs well at audiometry and it is not always easy to detect poor performers. There is a considerable degree of test/retest variability, which may be due to several factors. Substantial uncertainties in interpretation of audiograms may lead also to mismanagement in terms of initial or continuing fitness for work. Audiometry is a two-edged tool and one not to be embarked on without careful consideration.

Further guidance on industrial audiometry equipment and techniques and interpretation of results is available from two booklets specially written for the purpose.[12,13] There is also a useful standardization of technique described for manually performed audiometry.[14] However, automatic self-recording audiometry is preferred to manual audiometry in most industries, particularly where there are large numbers to be tested or the audiometrician's skill is uncertain.

# Balance

## Principal disorders

Dizziness and giddiness describe symptoms encompassing a wide variety of experiences. They may result from disorders of the vestibular, neurological, ophthalmic, cardiovascular, or orthopaedic systems, or they may be of psychological origin, or some combination of these. Their cause, and even the likely system of origin, is often difficult or impossible to define. Distinction between central vestibular and general neurological (including psychological and vasovagal) disorders is often arbitrary, or unwarranted when both forms of disorder are present as is not uncommon. On the other hand, differentiation between peripheral (end-organ and 8th cranial nerve) and central, neural origin is usually possible and helps to define the type of disorder, its likely prognosis, and appropriate management. Vertigo is best defined as an hallucination of movement, its occurrence usually meaning a peripheral or central disorder of the vestibular system. Two important aspects of vestibular physiology explain most of the symptoms, signs, and prognosis of peripheral vestibular disorders as follows.

First, the vestibular end-organs have a resting rate of nerve discharge: stimuli can either increase or decrease the firing rate. The end-organs of the semicircular canals on the two sides of the head are paired, and the afferent inputs to the central nervous system from each side act in opposition. Most, but probably not all, disorders of the *peripheral vestibular system* cause a reduction in the resting rate in the corresponding part of the 8th cranial nerve. In such cases, the left/right imbalance so caused results in the eyes and body being reflexly deviated towards the side of the lesion. This is often experienced as a falling, or imbalance, to that side, and seen as the slow phase of nystagmus to that side. The vertigo or sense of rotation and the fast phase of nystagmus will go in the opposite direction, to the unaffected side, in such a case.

Secondly, the *central vestibular system* has the great ability to compensate for a chronic imbalance in the neural tonus coming from the two sides, or to habituate or adapt to frequently repeated or constant stimulation, such as 'getting your sea legs' in habituation to motion sickness. Habituation and compensation are such that the acute disturbance of a severe unilateral vestibular failure is essentially self-limiting, especially in young patients. Over a few weeks, the sufferer passes from intolerable vertigo with nausea and vomiting, through to no vertigo while keeping still but subject to vertigo with movement, to some imbalance and only momentary vertigo accompanying major rotational movements of the head or body. **If symptoms of dizziness last continuously for longer than 2 or 3 weeks, the cause is not vestibular.**

## Stimulation by sound

The cochlea responds readily to faint acoustic stimuli and yet is susceptible to damage over the long term by excessive noise levels. In contrast, the vestibular part of the internal ear, whose perilymph and endolymph are in direct continuity with the corresponding fluids in the cochlea, is little affected. The explanation lies in the cochlea's microstructure which is so uniquely responsive to mechano-acoustic stimulation. On the other hand, the organization of the vestibular labyrinth is such that the cupulae or maculae are much less likely to respond to rapid to-and-fro stimulation arising from sound at ordinary levels. Nevertheless, the human vestibular system is not totally unresponsive to acoustic stimulation, in several ways.

Even in health, very high noise levels, at and above about 135 dB sound pressure level (SPL), such as experienced by those very close to powerful jet engines running at high power, can cause vertigo and nausea together with other unpleasant symptoms, such as fluttering of the cheeks, chest, and abdomen, and heating of hairy surfaces and skin-folds. The saccule may also function as a receptor for low frequency acoustic signals.

When a pathological disorder of the internal ear is present, however, levels of sound in the region of 110 to 120 dB SPL may cause a form of vertigo known clinically as the Tullio effect. The 'sono-ocular' test takes advantage of this: if such stimuli cause nystagmus in the absence of visual fixation, this is taken as evidence of internal-ear pathology. The mechanism is uncertain. Its importance in the industrial context is that industrial noise seldom stimulates giddiness unless there is some pre-existing disorder of the internal ear.

The potentially damaging effects of noise exposure on the cochlea are now recognized without question. Noise-induced damage to the vestibular part of the internal ear is less well documented, although evidence relating to this is accumulating. Noise-induced vestibular disorders exist, but whether or not these (apart from the Tullio phenomenon) can be produced by the acoustic conditions of civilian industry has yet to be established. Further epidemiological and clinical research is required. The importance of this is not so much to identify a possible new form of occupational disease or group of diseases, but to warn that signs or symptoms of peripheral vestibular disorder would not necessarily imply that an accompanying disorder of the cochlea is likely to be of constitutional origin. Not only is it perfectly possible for coincident vestibular and cochlear disorders to have different aetiologies, it seems possible that the vestibular disorder itself might sometimes be due to damage by noise.[15]

Although there may be very reasonable anxieties about the employability of people with dizziness in certain jobs, there are liable to be additional prejudices for the following reasons:

1.  Vestibular disorders rarely yield unambiguous features in the overt behaviour of the person affected, and even when evident there may be suspicion of functional origin or overlay.

2.  The disorders are seldom diagnosed with any more precision than vertigo (which is a symptom, not a cause or disease state), are often without any reliable treatment, and may have a very uncertain prognosis.

## Prevalence

### Hinchcliffe's study[16]

Two random samples of rural populations, in the Vale of Glamorgan and in mid Annandale (Dumfries and Galloway), were studied in 1957 and 1958 respectively. The target number was 800 subjects, divided equally between males and females and between the two locations; 90 per cent and 95 per cent of the Welsh and Scottish samples, respectively, were actually examined. The prevalence of a history (past or present) of dizziness and giddiness as a function of age is shown in Table 4.6: overall it was 23 per cent. Most of the episodes of vertigo were transient and not troublesome, but 3 per cent of the whole sample had experienced recurrent sustained vertigo with or without other symptoms over a period of at least one

**Table 4.6**   Prevalence of history (past or present) of dizziness or giddiness according to age group (after Hinchcliffe[16])

| Age group | History of dizziness or giddiness (percentage of each age group) |
|-----------|------------------------------------------------------------------|
| 18–24 | 17 |
| 25–34 | 20 |
| 35–44 | 19 |
| 45–54 | 23 |
| 55–64 | 35 |
| 65–74 | 29 |

year. Hinchcliffe considered that the major basis of this was probably endolymphatic hydrops and that in about one-third of these (1 per cent) a diagnosis of Ménière's disorder would be appropriate. He surmised further that the bulk of vertiginous histories, especially the episodes of transient vertigo, may have been arteriosclerotic in origin in the older individuals, but not in the younger ones.

## The National Study of Hearing

This has already been referred to in the previous section. In a postal questionnaire to a random sample from the electoral register, an opportunity was taken to add a question (C5) on vestibular-type disorders: 'Have you ever suffered from attacks of giddiness, dizziness, unsteadiness, or light-headedness?' Two-thirds of recipients responded to this question: 41 per cent of these answered 'Yes'. A higher proportion of women than of men responders admitted such a history (Table 4.7). A feature of both studies was that there was little age dependence in the prevalence of dizziness. This might be an artefact, due to age differences in awareness or memory, or to increasing expectancy and tolerance (and therefore non-reporting) of balance disturbances with ageing, akin to that which occurs with hearing difficulties. In contrast, several studies have shown a considerably increased prevalence of vertigo-like symptoms after retirement age. Thus, giddiness and similar symptoms appear to occur quite frequently throughout the working age range. The possible occupational significance of this is indicated below.

A further questionnaire was sent to 1720 people in a subset of 'Yes' responders. Non-responders to this were not followed up, and only 657 (38 per cent) responded. Major biases may thus have occurred if only those with more troublesome symptoms bothered to reply, exaggerating any prevalence estimates

**Table 4.7**  Prevalence of history (past or present) of giddiness, dizziness, unsteadiness, or lightheadedness according to location, sex, and age group

|  | Percentage of responders to question C5 who answered 'Yes' | | | |
| --- | --- | --- | --- | --- |
|  | Cardiff | Glasgow | Nottingham | Southampton |
| *Sex* | | | | |
| Males | 34 | 34 | 36 | 33 |
| Females | 47 | 43 | 50 | 45 |
| *Age group* | | | | |
| 17–40 | 39 | 37 | 41 | 38 |
| 41–60 | 43 | 40 | 46 | 42 |
| Over 60 | 43 | 41 | 45 | 40 |

*Note*: Answers to question C5, in Phase III of the National Study of Hearing, MRC Institute of Hearing Research. Total postal questionnaire sample, $n = 25\ 642$; 18 677 responded. Total responding to question C5, $n = 16\ 964$.

derived from answers to the further questions by up to threefold. Nevertheless, some of the results are interesting, given due caution in their interpretation.

Only 13 per cent of these further respondents said their dizzy symptoms caused moderate or severe restriction of their current activities. In the context of fitness for work, this suggests that perhaps 2–5 per cent of people of working age experience intermittent disturbance of their working ability from this cause.

The episodes reported were very transient 'a few seconds' in 55 per cent of the further respondents, and fairly infrequent 'less than once a month' in 43 per cent. Responders were asked about associations with other factors. These included physical events—such as transport, 10 per cent; faints or near-faints, 23 per cent; physical strain, 32 per cent; or psychological factors such as heights, 29 per cent; open spaces, 5 per cent; enclosed spaces, 15 per cent; mental strain, 30 per cent; strong emotion, 21 per cent; anxiety, 37 per cent; when tired, 46 per cent. Episodes were brought on by various activities, notably getting up from a bed or chair, 53 per cent; straightening up after bending down, 62 per cent; looking down or bending down, 41 per cent; looking around or making a sudden turn, 51 per cent.

## Clinical aspects affecting work capacity

### Relation to fitness for particular types of work

Fitness for work in those suffering from dizziness has to be judged in two ways. First, those with acute disorienting episodes coming on without warning may be a potential danger to themselves or to others in some types of work (see below). Secondly, those who have due warning, whose episodes are not dangerously disorienting, or who do not work in hazardous situations but are liable to recurrent and unpredictable absences from work on account of dizziness, may be unsuitable for jobs which are dependent on a specific individual.

These sorts of disorder may sometimes lead to premature retirement, especially where the disabling effects are recurrent or prolonged and there seems no reasonable prospect of an acceptable degree of recovery or rehabilitation. *Per se* they seldom lead to death, although occasionally death or serious injury results from accidents due to acute and unexpected disorientation. In some cases, however, dizziness is a manifestation of a more serious underlying disorder, such as cardiovascular disease, cerebral tumour, or multiple sclerosis, which itself may have serious implications for work ability and life expectancy.

### Treatment and rehabilitation

In the acute phase, the management of vestibular symptoms should be based upon vestibular suppressive drugs. In the chronic phase, vestibular rehabilitation should be based upon Cawthorne and Cooksey's head and balance exercises. Dizziness may nevertheless lead to prolonged or frequent absences from work.

Additionally, sedative side-effects occur with many of the vestibular suppressive drugs used, such as *cinnarizine* and *prochlorperazine*. This is especially true of drugs used to prevent motion sickness, such as *hyoscine*, and those with antihistamine-like properties, e.g., *meclozine, dimenhydrinate*, and *promethazine*. Treatment with drugs of this sort has clear implications for work efficiency and safety, and especially for safety in driving road, rail, air, or factory vehicles, or if combined with alcohol. Special warning has also been given on the treatment of unsteadiness in older people with phenothiazines, such as *prochlorperazine*; this tends to aggravate postural falls in blood pressure and, if continued for long periods, may result in Parkinsonism. Because of these side-effects, vestibular suppressive drugs should be phased out as soon as possible and replaced by a programme of vestibular rehabilitation.

## Special work problems, restrictions or needs

The disadvantages to the employer of workers with recurrent or prolonged periods of illness and the possible side-effects of treatment have been mentioned above. They are not specific to any particular job, but there are certain kinds of work in which an acute attack of vertigo or imbalance could be very dangerous. These are outlined below.

### Work on or near potentially hazardous machinery

The degree of the hazard will depend on the size, nature, and power of the machine, and the extent to which the dangerous parts are shielded. Each individual has to be considered separately, particularly the ways in which the disorder might affect him and whether he is likely to experience warning symptoms of an impending attack and can then take appropriate avoiding action.

### Work at heights

Much the same considerations apply as with work near moving machinery. Some patients' attacks may be related to or induced by heights.

### Work in other potentially dangerous environments

Such as those involving molten metal, caustic acids or alkalis, and working in isolation or near deep water.

### Work in moving environments

The likelihood of motion sickness is increased by most forms of vestibular disorder. Preventive drugs may be used, but due thought must be given beforehand to the potential side-effects and their influence on work safety and efficiency. Probably the best solution, if possible, is to give the affected worker a conditional trial in the actual environment in question.

### Diving (see Appendix 4)

Chronic or recurrent vestibular disturbances are usually incompatible with work or sport as a diver, especially scuba diving. This is because spatial orientation depends on three main factors: vestibular, pressure sense coupled with proprioceptive input, and visual. Underwater surroundings may be dark or murky, reducing or removing the visual input; there is also a much reduced pressure sense even when the diver is on the bottom, as he has a similar specific gravity to that of his environment. Orientation sense then depends heavily on the vestibular system; if that is deficient or disturbed, the diver's predicament can be highly dangerous.

### Jobs with high levels of responsibility for the safety of others

Sudden onset of acute vestibular impairment while in control of a vehicle can give the operator a false impression that the vehicle has veered from its correct direction. This can lead to unnecessary corrective action which could cause an accident. Acute vertigo can also cause a reflex response which could cause the driver to pull the vehicle out of its correct direction without him initially being aware of it. Persons subject to vestibular or similar disturbances are not fit to be in control of vehicles on roads, work sites or farms, or in the air, until they are fully recovered and have had no attacks for a long period, perhaps for a year or even longer.

## Existing legislation and guidelines for employment

### Medical examination

Unlike hearing, vestibular function cannot be measured quickly and easily. Therefore, vestibular function tests have not been a subject for standardization for employment purposes. If carried out at all, which is unusual, they are limited to simple clinical tests, such as the Romberg test or heel–toe walking in a straight line. This may be supplemented by direct observation of the eyes to check that there is no nystagmus. These procedures will only detect substantial disturbances of balance, or nystagmus due to central, or to recent and severe peripheral, vestibular disorders. Usually the history of severity, duration, frequency, nature, and effects of vestibular episodes is more important.

### Regulations

Some examples from particular occupations follow.

*Driving* (see also Appendix 1)

The Licensing Centre must be informed by the licence holder or applicant with such a disability. Persons who are liable to sudden disabling attacks of giddiness or fainting are banned from holding any motor vehicle driving licence. In the case of attacks of vertebrobasilar artery insufficiency, a person is advised to stop driving and report the condition. After a first episode, the ordinary driving licence is revoked for at least three months. In recurrent cases, driving can be resumed if there have been no episodes for a period of at least six months. In the case of vocational drivers, a single transient ischaemic episode is a permanent bar.

Ménière's disorder, vestibular neuronitis, and positional vertigo are normally regarded as a bar to ordinary motor vehicle driving until they have been adequately controlled for a reasonable period of time as a result of treatment, or by spontaneous remission. Normally, any person with a persisting vestibular disorder is regarded as unfit to drive vocationally (passenger carrying vehicles, large goods vehicles, and taxis).

*Flying* (see also Appendix 2)

The criteria are whether the licence holder may become incapacitated while in control of an aircraft and whether he or she can function effectively. Clearly, vertigo or imbalance arising from Ménière's disorder, vestibular neuronitis, or positional vertigo would not be compatible with flying. More borderline or uncertain conditions will occur, and the question of fitness for flying is finally decided by the Civil Aviation Authority following examination by a doctor specially qualified in aviation medicine.

*Merchant navy* (see also Appendix 3)

Ménière's disease is the only vestibular disorder specified in the Department of Transport regulations on medical fitness of seafarers: it implies permanent unfitness, as do transient ischaemic attacks, which often present as episodes of dizziness.

*Diving* (see also Appendix 4)

Fitness to dive is covered by statutory medical standards. With few exceptions, disorders of balance constitute an absolute bar to working as a commercial diver.

*Armed forces*

The degree to which a vestibular disorder will affect the 'P' (physical) assessment in the PULHEEMS system depends on its nature, severity, and effects. The interpretation of the P assessment in terms of fitness for service depends on the particular branch of service, and is closely related to the actual requirements of the job and the limitations which physical disorders would place on its performance.

*Police, fire, and other public services*

In general, there are no specific regulations. Certification of fitness would depend on a non-specialist medical opinion on whether the vestibular symptoms were likely to incapacitate the individual for operational duty. For firemen, the latter may involve work up ladders or with minimal visibility from smoke, and so a more stringent criterion needs to be applied. Indeed, the Home Office guidelines in 1970 specified 'evidence of labyrinthine disturbance, a history of vertigo or any condition which would impair a candidate's sense of balance' as rendering a recruit unsuitable.

*General industry*

Where pre-employment screening is performed, unless there are requirements specifically related to the work, any enquiry will probably be limited to the general question: 'Do you suffer from fits, faints, blackouts, or dizzy attacks?' If the individual admits to the last, experience in industry supports the data obtained from the National Study of Hearing that it rarely interferes with work (see pp. 81–2). Where the severity is sufficient to cause problems, the potential employer tends to err on the side of caution, sometimes to the detriment of the individual. Occupational physicians tend to be more liberal. This unsatisfactory situation arises from the difficulties in diagnosis and uncertainties in prognosis mentioned earlier.

Similar problems are encountered with existing employees. If an employee develops disabling vertigo, the employer must then consider the safety of the individual and the group with whom he works. Accordingly, restrictions on driving, work at heights or near moving machinery are common which, together with the uncertainties regarding regular attendance at work, must raise questions of employability. In such cases, as much information as possible on the aetiology, treatment, and prognosis should be obtained and considered against the job requirements before any decision is made.

## Conclusions and recommendations

Vestibular disorders, and those masquerading as or confused with them, are common in men and women of all ages. Most are transient and probably of vascular (including vasovagal) origin. Few have substantial implications for fitness for work, although in many instances they will lead to absences from work. By and large, they are difficult to diagnose; in most, prognosis and treatment are also difficult.

Real work limitations may be applicable if there is liability to acute episodes of vertigo or imbalance, especially if these are unpredictable. Limitations have to be considered where the work is near unguarded moving machinery, at heights, involves driving or exposure to motion (as in ships), or is in certain jobs with a high level of responsibility or potential risk to others. Such episodes are generally incompatible with diving, or flying as aircrew, either commercially or for sport.

## Selected references and further reading

1. Kettle, M. and Massie, B. (ed.) (1986). *Employers' guide to disabilities*, (2nd edn), pp. 19–23. Woodhead-Faulkner, Cambridge.
2. ES (Employment Service)(1988). *Deaf and hearing impaired*. Booklet, EPWD 20. ES, Sheffield.
3. Davis, A.C. (1989). The prevalence of hearing impairment and reported hearing disability among adults in Great Britain. *Int. J. Epidemiol.* **18**, 911–17.
4. Acton, W.I. and Wilkins, P.A. (1982). Can noise cause accidents? *Occup. Safe. Hlth.*, **12**, 14–16.
5. Wilkins, P.A. and Martin, A.M. (1985). The role of acoustical characteristics in the perception of warning sounds and the effects of wearing hearing protection. *J. Sound Vib.*, **100**, 181–90.
6. Coleman, G.J. *et al.* (1984). *Communications in noisy environments*. Report TM/84/1. Institute of Occupational Medicine, Edinburgh.
7. Sir George Godber, Chief Medical Officer of the Home Office (1970). Report of the Committee to Review the Medical Standards for the Fire Service. Home Office, London.
8. Raffle, A. (ed.) (1985). *Medical aspects of fitness to drive: a guide for medical practitioners*, (4th edn). Medical Commission on Accident Prevention, London.
9. Taylor, J. Chief Medical Adviser, Department of Transport, (personal communication).
10. Browning, G.G., Swan, I.R.C., and Chew, K.K. (1989). Clinical role of informal tests of hearing. *J. Laryngol. Otol.*, **103**, 7–11.
11. BSI (British Standards Institution) (1986). *Pure tone air conduction threshold audiometry for hearing conservation purposes*. BS 6655. BSI, London.
12. Bryan, M.E. and Tempest, W. (1976). *Industrial audiometry*. Werth, London.
13. Bryan, M.E. and Tempest, W. (1978). *Examples of industrial audiograms*. Werth, London.
14. Anon. (1981). Recommended procedures for pure-tone audiometry using a manually operated instrument, (Joint recommendations by the British Society of Audiology and the British Association of Otolaryngologists). *Brit. J.* Aud., **15**, 213–6; *J. Laryngol. Otol.*, **95**, 757–61.
15. Hinchcliffe, R., Coles, R.R.A , and King, P.F. (1992). Occupational noise-induced vestibular malfunction? *Brit. J. Indust. Med.*, **49**, 63–5.
16. Hinchcliffe, R. (1961). Prevalence of the commoner ear, nose and throat conditions in the adult rural population of Great Britain: a study by direct examination of two random samples. *Brit. J. Prev. Soc. Med.*, **15**,128–40.

# 5

# Visual and ocular disorders

*P.A.M. Diamond and C.G.F. Munton*

## Introduction

Vision is necessary for most types of work, although there are some jobs which can be performed with a low degree of visual acuity, and even with total blindness, if Braille and a keyboard is an option, or a computer with audible output. A consideration of visual acuity is of primary importance when deciding whether on ocular grounds any particular work can be undertaken. The use of spectacles and contact lenses may improve visual acuity, but there are some occupations where the use of either of these aids is not possible.[1] The extent of the visual fields, problems of binocularity and double vision and the integrity of colour vision also influence decisions about suitable work. The eye should always be guarded against damage from the work process with appropriate eye protection and visual equipment.

## Prevalence

In both men and women all degrees of visual acuity occur at any age, although serious defects are more common in later life. Other ophthalmic defects, such as monocularity, visual field defects, and imbalance of the eyes, also occur in both sexes and throughout life. Ocular injuries may cause serious visual defects.

It is estimated that there are 126 828 people in the British Isles who are registered as blind and 79 048 who are registered as partially sighted.[2]

## Clinical aspects affecting work capacity

There are varying degrees of visual defect. Some people on the register of blind persons have no sight, but it contains others who have enough vision to walk about independently, even though they experience some difficulty and are unable to read, or recognize others at a distance.[3] Certain types of work can only be undertaken by those with normal visual function, but people with poor vision, or even none, will often be able to do some work. A period of training may be required when visual function has been damaged but thereafter there is no reason why the standard of work should not be satisfactory and done, at home if necessary, without interruption.

People with defective vision which cannot be improved with spectacles may be helped by low vision aids. The simplest of these is a hand held magnifying glass of about 12 dioptres which helps a person with low visual acuity to read, but it is an inefficient method. Desk- or chest-mounted magnifiers free the hands for some tasks. Some low vision aids are small telescopes, with compound lenses fitted into spectacle frames, and can improve near or distant vision. These aids give considerable magnification, but the reduced visual field is a disadvantage. They may, however, enable people with severely defective vision, not amounting to blindness, to carry on with some close work. Recent advances in electronic scanning and machine vision enable the visually handicapped to read and visualize information, and even to inspect engineered parts.

The definition of a blind person for registration purposes is one in whom there is insufficient sight to carry out work for which sight is essential; for practical purposes this is considered to be a corrected visual acuity of 3/60 or less in each eye. This is an inability to read the top letter of the standard sight-testing chart at a greater distance than 3 metres. Severe visual field defects, even in the presence of good visual acuity, may be sufficient to prevent independent activity in daily life.

Many conditions cause visual field defects. Vascular lesions of the nervous system can result in hemianopia (loss of half the visual field) and may be bilateral, complete, or partial. Homonymous hemianopia causes some difficulty in walking, since the same side of the vision is absent in each eye. A complete quadrant homonymous defect, upper or lower, is a bar to driving, since traffic information and hazards exist in both upper and lower areas of field.[4,5] Bitemporal hemianopia occurs in disease of the pituitary gland and results in defective vision on both sides although the vision straight ahead is satisfactory. Bitemporal hemianopia precludes the driving of any vehicle and also the performance of any work where safety would be compromised by lateral field loss. In retinitis pigmentosa, or pigmentary degeneration of the retina, all the peripheral field of vision is lost so that only the 5–10 degrees of central vision persists. This is known as tunnel vision, causes considerable, often progressive, disability and should be considered to be a bar to all driving. Additionally, night vision may be severely compromised. It also affects the capacity to do many other tasks safely and effectively. A similar condition occurs in advanced chronic simple glaucoma (see below), and should be similarly regarded.

Blind persons receive instruction through the Royal National Institute for the Blind (RNIB). Braille or Moon and keyboard skills are taught, together with instruction in how to walk about independently using a stick, usually coloured white, which indicates a significant visual handicap. The long-cane technique, and devices using ultrasound, allow even more independence. Training in personal life-skills is undertaken soon after the sight is damaged. Blindness associated with deafness causes additional problems.

Blindness has many causes. Congenital defects and trauma are the usual causes in the young, while acquired defects such as cataract, glaucoma, and macular degeneration damage sight in older age groups. Increasingly, the results of trauma can be treated to prevent loss of sight. Cataract can be surgically treated in almost all people, sometimes as day cases. It is essential that glaucoma is treated early to limit further damage. Macular degeneration, which damages central vision, is fairly common in the elderly and is in many cases untreatable. Some cases can be halted by laser treatment, but the condition cannot be cured. Diabetes is the most common cause of blindness in the Western world and accounts for 7–8 per cent of all registrations.

## Special work problems

The main difficulty for those who have defective vision is that they are more liable to have accidents in hazardous situations. People with defective vision, restricted visual fields, or imbalance of the eyes with resulting diplopia should not work on ladders or scaffolding where they will fall if they overstep the boundaries, and they should not work among moving machinery where they might also suffer injury. People with seriously defective visual function must be barred from driving vehicles not only on the public highway, but also as heavy plant operators on construction sites and industrial and other locations. They should not operate cranes, hoists, or fork-lift trucks. They cannot be employed in the armed services, the police or the emergency services.

It is particularly important that young people with ocular problems should receive informed advice about a suitable career after their visual state has been assessed. It is essential that their lifetime visual prognosis should be considered when a decision is being made about their employment. Candidates for the armed services, the police force, the mercantile marine (see Appendix 3), and aircrew (see Appendix 2) undergo full medical examination on entry, and careful examinations are undertaken for train and bus drivers. Normal vision and ocular function is required in all people who propose to spend their lives in transport or in occupations where driving is an essential component, and it is necessary that they can be given reasonable assurance that their ocular function (with correction, if necessary and if allowed) will remain at a satisfactory level for their expected workspan.

### Normal vision

The majority of the population falls into this category. The visual acuity is normal (6/6 in each eye), with or without optical help; the visual fields are full, the balance between the two eyes is normal, and colour perception is satisfactory. Such people can in general undertake any occupation, although the wearing of contact lenses or spectacles may, exceptionally, result in some difficulty. Special visual standards are required for aircraft pilots (see Appendix 2), for navigators of ships at sea (see Appendix 3), and for drivers of trains and public carriage and large goods vehicles. Officers in the police force and members of the fire and rescue services must also have a high standard of visual acuity. People who wear breathing apparatus must not require spectacles as these will prevent a gas tight fit and can allow the ingress of toxic fumes and gases.[6] Members of the armed services are required to achieve defined visual standards which differ according to the duties to be undertaken.

All workers in occupations with rigorous visual requirements must have regular examinations to ascertain that they have not fallen below the necessary standards. Serious visual defects, such as the loss of an eye, will often lead to dismissal from their occupation.

**Intermediate vision**

This group comprises those who have defective sight (less than 6/6 in each eye) but who are not in the blind or partially sighted categories. Many can achieve satisfactory visual acuity with spectacles or contact lenses, but others have some degree of subnormal vision even with optical help. Some have mild defects of visual fields, ocular muscle balance, or colour vision. People in this group are ocularly fit for all occupations except those requiring the highest visual standards. They can undertake clerical work, most manufacturing and servicing tasks, and all professional occupations, and are usually fit to drive private cars. Those with marked defects of the visual fields (see above) must be regarded as being at risk if they work at heights or among moving machinery. Crane operators, fork-lift truck drivers, and drivers of electric trucks within stores or on work sites all require good peripheral vision both for driving itself and for the control and manipulation of the loads they carry. Difficulty with the task may indicate that further investigation may be needed, particularly of stereoscopic vision. Double vision should disqualify from work in all hazardous situations, and from vocational driving. In less exacting tasks the disability can be overcome by retraining and covering one eye.

**Aphakia and pseudophakia**

In aphakia the lens of the eye is absent, usually as the result of a cataract operation to remove an opaque lens. Such cataracts are commonly of the senile type but they can occur after trauma or as a secondary consequence of some eye diseases. Removal of the lens alters the optical properties of that eye so that in most cases satisfactory vision can be obtained only by the use of strong convex spectacle lenses. These magnify the image seen in the operated eye, so that if only one eye has been operated on, fusion of the images of the two eyes is not possible and double vision may result. People who are aphakic in one eye and who have no implanted lens or contact lens are functionally monocular. Even in bilateral aphakia the spectacle optics may produce severe spherical aberration, so that linear objects are curved and visual space is distorted, which can make walking difficult. Additionally, the optical defect causes the 'jack-in-the-box' phenomenon, where peripheral objects (such as a pedestrian crossing the path) disappear at the outer lens zone, and reappear in the central zone magnified and with alarming suddenness. All these problems (unilateral aphakia, spherical aberration, and 'jack-in-the-box') can be overcome very successfully by the use of a contact lens or by an intraocular lens implant at the time of operation (pseudophakia).

## Monocularity

Monocular vision results not only from the removal of an eye but a similar state will exist if the vision of one eye is very defective. This causes difficulty in the estimation of distance, although this improves with learning, and the visual field is reduced. An eye may have to be removed because of injury, because of severe and continuous pain, or as the result of malignancy. Damage to the vascular supply of an eye by embolus or thrombosis may cause loss of vision, as will the chronic inflammation of uveitis in some patients.

People who are monocular are at increased risk if they work in hazardous jobs, such as on scaffolding or moving machinery. They are excluded from work as pilots of ships and as drivers of trains, large goods vehicles (LGV), and public carriage vehicles (PCV).[7] A minimal level of binocularity is required for all new entrants requiring licences for large goods and public carrying vehicle licences. LGV and PCV drivers who become monocular are required to surrender their licences, while such drivers who have had cataract surgery with an intraocular implant or contact lens are allowed to continue two months after the surgery, provided they fulfil the necessary minimum binocular visual standard, and are subject to annual checks.[8]

## Injuries

Perforation can occur when the eye is struck by some pointed object. Injury commonly occurs from the use of a hammer and chisel. When the intraocular foreign body is a chip of metal from the hammer which is usually made of hard but brittle steel, damage to the lens and retina is a common result. Heavy blows on the eye with a blunt object may rupture the eyeball, which necessitates removal of the eye. Lesser blows, as from a fist, may cause a traumatic cataract or retinal haemorrhage and detachment. These do not usually result in removal of the eye, but a cataract may require removal of the lens (see Aphakia, p. 91).

## Eye protection

Eyes should always be protected from high velocity particles, dust, irritant fumes, gases, radiation, and chemical splashing. Safety spectacles, or goggles where a complete seal is required can be supplied with correcting lenses[9] and manufactured from toughened glass or plastic lenses to British Standard specification. Spectacles cannot be worn satisfactorily under goggles or breathing apparatus.[6] Protection is particularly important where there is effective vision in only one eye, since this is doubly valuable, and monocular workers must be warned about occupational hazards. Monocular vision, however, has a considerable effect on employer liability[10] and a skilled craftsman who loses the sight in one eye may be moved to a less hazardous occupation. People who have a squint in early life may have an amblyopic, or lazy, eye which renders them virtually monocular. Such people, together with the monocular group, should be advised not to enter occupations which may create a high risk to the remaining eye.

## Conditions causing sudden variation of vision

Sudden variation of vision is unusual but may cause difficulty, especially in exacting work. It may occur in migraine, sometimes associated with a sensation of flashes of light. Spasm of the central vessels of the retina may cause blurred vision which is usually transitory. Blood sugar variations in diabetics who are unstable or undergoing stabilization, and medication which affects accommodation are more common iatrogenic causes. The onset of cataract or glaucoma may cause similar variation.

## Colour perception

Defective colour vision is inherited in the majority of cases, occurring in 8.0 per cent of men and about 0.2 per cent of women. There are different types of defect, but for practical purposes the problem is identification of red and green. Acquired defects are rare, but do exist, and may be permanent. They may be temporary in various ocular diseases such as tobacco amblyopia, toxic amblyopia due to medication, and lens opacities. Where good colour perception is necessary for safety reasons, therefore, periodic re-examination is necessary. Prolonged work with display screen equipment may produce a perceived transient colour shift, which is complementary to the colour of the screen.

Only a very small proportion of occupations require perfect colour discrimination; a few others present some difficulties but are not necessarily precluded. Pre-employment rejection of those with defective colour vision will eliminate up to 8.0 per cent of male applicants, depending on the tests used. Colour vision assessment is only necessary if normal colour vision is essential for the job in question. Further investigations to diagnose the type and severity of the colour defect are best left to specialists.

## Methods of colour vision testing

Conditions for all tests are exacting, and findings will be useless if these are not followed. Equipment must be clean, and not left on the window sill to collect dust and fade in the sun. The most practical acceptable ambient illumination is ordinary daylight through a north-aspect window. Artificial illumination standards must be precise, and variations in the colour of light are not acceptable. The subject should wear corrective lenses (not tinted) if necessary, to enable him to define the characters. There needs to be a good understanding between the tester and subject; the procedures are complex.

*Pseudo-isochromatic tests*, such as the *Ishihara plates* or the *City University* test, are the most commonly used. It is not unknown, however, for pre-employment applicants to memorize the characters and plate numbers, and rapid random replies should be sought. *Matching tests* are the oldest type of colour vision examination. The *Holmgren wool test*, which requires the subject to match colours of various skeins of wool, was used in the railway industry until other more sophisticated techniques were developed. Modern matching tests, such as the *Farnsworth–Munsell 100 Hue test*, detect more subtle defects. *Lantern tests* rely on transmitted light through filters. Ambient illumination is less critical, and lanterns more easily simulate signals for testing for navigation and transport purposes.[11] Often they use only the relevant signal colours, but they may include any colours in the range. Well-known lanterns are the *Giles–Archer*, *Holmes–Wright*, and *Edridge–Green*. Practice and custom usually decree which is used in any occupation or industry: for instance, the railway industry currently uses the *Edridge–Green Lantern* as an ancillary test to the *Ishihara plates*. The anomaloscope is a highly specialized diagnostic instrument which has no place in occupational screening procedures. A good comprehensive review of tests for colour vision with recommended lighting standards, etc., can be found in *Defective colour vision* by Fletcher and Voke.[12]

### Occupations requiring normal colour perception

These fall into three categories, which are discussed below.

*Transport, navigation, and the armed services*

For these occupations, the need is to interpret colour signals without error, both in operating tasks and in the installation, maintenance, and testing of these signals. There is usually no positional reference, and the signal may be at a great distance and weather conditions adverse, with fog, rain, or bright sunshine. Testing procedures evolved because accidents on the railways and in navigation were attributed to incorrect colour perception. Driving on the road, however, does not require colour perception because road traffic signals can be interpreted by the relative position of the lights. These are of a standard high intensity, but other red lights of low intensity may be difficult to distinguish. There is no statistical indication that drivers with defective colour perception have more traffic accidents than those with normal vision,[13] and such people probably learn to compensate for their defect, making them more vigilant. Drivers of public carriage and large goods vehicles undergo intensive training; in London Buses prospective bus drivers spend 10 days driving with an experienced instructor, and are expected to achieve a high standard of driving performance. This tends to eliminate bus drivers who do not compensate for defective colour perception.

## Occupations using colour coding for safety and technical purposes

Colour differentiation is used for hazard warning systems, cables and wiring, coding of pipes, etc. In the concept of British Standard colour coding,[14] those with defective colour vision have not been sufficiently considered. Coding may have to be done under dirty and poorly lit conditions by people who are not aware that they have a problem. The best solution is a practical test, e.g., wiring or gas cylinder codes. Other features which supplement the colour code (as in the pin index used with medical gas cylinders) are useful. Chemical analysis and medical diagnosis (clinical and technical) may present difficulties, such as with urinalysis and, indeed, with colour vision screening itself. These problems may be reduced by screening at school so that appropriate career advice can be offered to the very small number of affected children who are unable to follow these colour-critical occupations.

## Occupations commercially dependent on sophisticated colour selection

Examples range from fruit picking to ticket collection, but are mainly concerned with dyeing, textiles, paper, and printing. Employers in these industries may not consider formal colour vision screening until an expensive mistake has been made. Trade tests are useful, and for some less exacting tasks colour filters may help. Coloured pens can be labelled; this helped a clerk to avoid writing in green on accounts sheets, the colour reserved exclusively for audit checks within his firm. With more artistic vocations, there will be a degree of self-selection.

## Visual fatigue at work

This condition does not ordinarily occur in people who have normal vision, who have satisfactory balance between the two eyes, and where there is adequate illumination. A person will seek relief from any exacting visual task by attempting to focus on infinity or looking out of the window; this can be assisted by altering the desk position or with the help of a picture or mirror.

## Display screen equipment

Rapid expansion in the use of display screen equipment (DSE) has aroused concern about the ability of the eyes to cope.[15,16] There is no evidence that working with DSE can harm eyesight. Partially sighted persons need not be excluded from this type of work. They can be helped by using DSEs with enlarged text; and the Disability Employment Adviser can provide low-vision aids if they

are necessary. Headaches attributed to eyestrain are usually caused by ergonomic problems, with consequent awkward posture and muscular strain (see
also Chapter 10, p. 194). Equipment should be properly maintained to avoid
flicker, glare, and reflection, and have sufficient flexibility in positioning of
screen, keyboard, and source documents to enable the operator to adjust them to
his or her particular visual requirements. Middle-aged and elderly people may
experience difficulty because their ordinary reading glasses do not correspond
with the distance at which they need to carry out their DSE work. They may be
more comfortable with working glasses, with focus adjusted for the screen distance, and any associated paper text. Bifocal spectacles may not be as conve-
nient. Excessive heat generated by electronic equipment in a confined or
overcrowded space with inadequate ventilation may exacerbate dryness or sore-
ness of the eyes.[15]

### Limitations of spectacles and contact lenses at work

Some circumstances can pose problems for persons who have to wear spectacles
or contact lenses at work. Protective clothing, such as safety helmets, welding
visors, and ear defenders can make spectacle-wearing and even the use of
contact lenses uncomfortable. In such cases goggles should be provided with
correcting lenses.

Spectacles with flat temple pieces improve compatibility with certain items of
personal protection, such as earmuffs or respirators, but when worn with self-
contained positive pressure breathing apparatus may still allow ingress of toxic
fumes.[6] The wearing of tinted spectacles or lenses reduces visibility, especially
in dull weather and at night. Reactive lenses do not change sufficiently quickly
to cope with sudden changes of illumination such as driving through road
tunnels, or passing headlights, and their use should be limited. Drivers may have
to perform exacting manoeuvres, such as reversing, even when spectacles have
become dislodged by accident. For this reason large goods and public carriage
vehicle drivers must have an unaided visual acuity in each eye of at least 3/60.
For further details on visual standards and driving, particularly vocational
driving, see Cross 1985[7; 5, 8] (see also Appendix 1).

Contact lenses may be useful in occupations where spectacles may become
misted, in aphakia, and where distortion occurs when looking through the marginal parts of the spectacle lenses. While hard acrylic contact lenses are still
widely in use, particulary the microlens type, there is a trend towards soft water
permeable and high oxygen permeable contact lenses, both hard and soft. Some
of these lenses allow longer periods of wear but the soft lenses are less applicable where there is high astigmatism of the cornea, as the contact lens may mould
to the astigmatism. Contact lenses help in aphakia where they overcome the
magnification problem of aphakic glasses. Intraocular lenses have recently
largely overcome this problem. Some occupations are associated with the production of dust and particles which may cause irritation when trapped under

contact lenses. Usually, the particle cannot be removed without removal of the lens, and headache or conjunctivitis may persist. This is a hazard in dirty and dusty environments, such as railway track work, mining, and work with rescue teams, and requires constant vigilance. There are many dangers when using all types of contact lenses, particularly where bacteria or fungal spores are in the air. This applies especially to the soft water permeable contact lenses, for example in high-speed lathe and machine work, where a slurry of oil/water mulch may be in use to cool the cutting tools and where a fine aerosol of the slurry arising from the process can be deposited on the contact lenses. These aerosols can contain large numbers of bacteria with obvious hazard. Ultraviolet and infrared rays are partly filtered by contact lenses. People who wear contact lenses at work must be identified because there are certain occupations in which they should not work, and in some cases protective measures may be required. There has been a recurrent and unsubstantiated myth that contact lenses can be welded to the cornea by ultraviolet exposure in occupations such as arc welding; this does not occur but the ultraviolet component of electric arc welding can cause corneal epithelial loss, with or without contact lens wear.[17]

Cosmetic considerations are the motivating factor for many people who wear contact lenses, but there is also no doubt that they give better optical correction where myopia exceeds 5 dioptres. They are useful in irregular astigmatism. Oxygen is absorbed by the cornea, and those contact lenses which are not gas permeable may inhibit this absorption with resulting discomfort. Soft contact lenses may absorb fumes and this can cause irritation. Working in extreme cold, as in cold stores, can cause discomfort in people who wear soft contact lenses. Contact lenses may therefore be helpful at work but there are certain disadvantages which must be considered. Individual tolerance is variable and is affected by sensitivity to lens care solutions, by photophobia, and by personal lens hygiene. The carrying of a spare pair of spectacles may be essential in some occupations, such as offshore workers.

### Conditions of work which may be detrimental to vision

Contrary to popular opinion, the intensive use of the eyes either for distance vision or close work does not result in damage to the vision of healthy eyes. The presence of dust may cause irritation and diminished corneal sensation may sometimes occur in workers in dusty occupations. This may be reduced by wearing protective goggles but the best solution is a change of occupation.

Corneal ulcers have many causes. They are usually treatable but tend to recur which may restrict affected workers in dusty atmospheres.

Workers under constant fluorescent lighting may complain of some discomfort but there is no evidence that this illumination damages the sight. Flicker is a more severe problem which can be avoided by timely replacement of tubes or by the use of electronic high frequency fluorescent lighting, to avoid strobic effects. The use of tinted lenses in spectacles may minimize the symptoms.

### Non-ionizing radiation

Ultraviolet light may cause superficial corneal lesions associated with gross discomfort, and workers who are exposed to this form of radiation should wear appropriate goggles to British Standard specifications.[9] Similar corneal lesions may occur with electric flashes from short circuits, arc lights, and welding. Infrared rays can cause lens opacity. Heat, from furnaces and in the glassblowing industry, can also cause lens opacity and it is essential that ocular protection by filtered goggles or visors is provided. High-output pulsed and cutting laser devices pose a specific hazard for workers.[18] Protective goggles of appropriate wavelength absorption designed specifically for work with lasers should be worn, and the working head of the laser should be enclosed. The goggles should be checked regularly for wear or damage, and must not bleach under high laser irradiation. Such bleaching could otherwise allow a sudden and unpredictable transmission of high laser irradiation through to the eye with consequent hazard. Stringent safety precautions should always be enforced and practised in work with lasers or with microwaves.

### Ionizing radiation

Ionizing radiation which results from exposure to radionuclides and X-rays can cause cataract, and workers in radiology departments should always be provided with eye protection, such as leaded glass.

### Ocular problems in older workers

It is inevitable that some older workers will suffer a degree of visual disability and this cannot be foreseen in any individual. Cataract, macular degeneration, and glaucoma may occur in later life without any indication of these conditions being present in earlier years. If visual acuity is reduced as a result of these diseases, treatment must be undertaken according to the current clinical findings. Cataract can be treated surgically sometimes as a day case, and this may enable patients to continue at work. Early macular degeneration can often be controlled by laser therapy. But, for some people, premature retirement may be necessary. Experience may override the disability, and it is not always appropriate to apply the same strict visual standards to older long-term employees. Good illumination is necessary for the maximum degree of close work by older people; intermediate range spectacles may be required. For demanding work a period of adaptation may be required for bifocal or varifocal glasses.

### The anaesthetic cornea

The cornea is normally a very sensitive part of the eyeball and, with the corneal reflex, reacts immediately to injury and to the presence of a foreign body.

Corneal sensitivity declines in later life but the cornea still reacts even to minor trauma. Complete corneal anaesthesia is the result of injury or disease of the trigeminal nerve. It usually requires treatment by tarsorrhaphy which effectively produces monocular vision with all its consequences (see above). More recently, the use of a bandage soft contact lens instead of tarsorrhaphy has enabled binocular vision to be retained. Bandage lenses are very thin soft and highly permeable contact lenses used for therapeutic purposes only. They are used both as a mechanical cover and occasionally as a slow release store for antibiotic and other drug therapy.

## Some common eye diseases and their effects

A number of common eye diseases cause difficulty at work, and are discussed below.

### Conjunctivitis

This condition is characterized by discomfort rather than pain, and by a discharge from the eyes which may be muco-purulent. It yields rapidly to treatment with antibiotic drops. It may be associated with ulceration of the cornea and with inflammation of the eyelid margins (blepharitis). This latter condition is the result of inflammation of the glands at the margin of the eyelids and responds to the same treatment. Watering of the eyes due to obstruction of the nasolacrimal ducts may cause annoyance at work but can be treated by simple surgery.

### Uveitis

This is an inflammation of the uveal tract. A part or the whole of the uvea, which is responsible for the nourishment and focusing of the eye, may be affected. It occurs in all states of severity from the mild form, causing only a slight blurring of vision, to the acute state where there is severe pain and serious visual defect. The condition usually responds to treatment with local or systemic steroid preparations but a long period of therapy may be necessary and uveitis can be a recurrent condition. It is sometimes associated with secondary glaucoma, complicated cataract, and rarely with the loss of sight of the eye. It may occasionally cause severe disablement and inability to continue in employment. Early treatment is therefore important. Ophthalmic *Herpes zoster* may cause uveitis, but this can usually be treated and does not usually recur.

### Glaucoma

In this condition the pressure in the eyeball is higher than normal. It occurs in two common forms. The acute form causes sudden severe pain and visual defect, and may be preceded by premonitory attacks with brow ache and haloes round lights at night. When treated immediately long-term results are good. The chronic form, which usually occurs in later life, may cause a serious degree of visual defect with contracture of the visual fields and resulting inability to continue at work. Because of its insidious onset, it is often unnoticed until advanced. There is much value in regular eye tests, including tonometry in the over-55s.

*Myopia*

Myopia, or short-sightedness, is characterized by difficulty with distant vision. It can be overcome by the use of spectacles or contact lenses. The large majority of short-sighted people have small degrees of the defect and are not seriously disabled. A minority of myopic people have such a big error that, even with optical correction, useful vision is not possible. Persons in occupations where spectacles or contact lenses cannot be worn are unsuitable for these forms of work. Several new types of treatment are emerging to remodel the cornea, for example radial keratotomy and Excimer laser photorefractive keratectomy.[19]

*Retinal separation (detachment)*

This condition occurs not infrequently, particularly in association with high degrees of myopia such as 12 dioptres or more and after ocular trauma. It should be treated as a surgical emergency and in most cases good vision is restored. The prognosis depends upon the amount of retina which separates and whether or not the macula is detached. Detachment of the macula results in diminution of vision to about 6/60 even if the retina re-attaches. Patients whose retina does not re-attach with surgery lose all vision in that eye. Patients whose retina re-attaches should subsequently avoid the heaviest manual work and some sports, such as boxing or squash.

## Conclusion

To determine fitness for work it is important to assess visual function adequately. Where there is doubt, specialist advice should be sought. There are many occupations which require the highest standards, but defective ocular function does not necessarily prevent people from working in certain other occupations if suitable training and/or equipment are available. Career guidance should ensure that young people do not embark on unsuitable careers, where an uncorrectable or progressive disability will restrict advancement in the future.

### Selected references and further reading

1.  Home Office (1987). Fire Service Circular, No. 8/1987. Home Office, London.
2.  OPCS (Office of Population Censuses and Surveys) (1989). OPCS, London.
3.  Notes for guidance. Record of examination to certify a person as blind or partially sighted, BD8 (1990). HMSO, London.
4.  College of Ophthalmologists (1991). Drivers fields agreed. *College News*, **6.** *Quarterly Bulletin of the College of Ophthalmologists,* London.

5. Munton, C.G.F. (1993). The development of visual standards in the UK. In *Vision in Vehicles,* (ed. A.G. Gale *et al.*), Vol. IV, pp. 17–25. North Holland, Amsterdam.
6. Home Office (1987). Joint Working Party on Appointment Provisions and Visual Standards for the Fire Service. Part III, 3.6, 3.11. Home Office, London.
7. Cross, A.G. (1985). Vision. In *Medical aspects of fitness to drive,* (ed. P.A.B. Raffle), (4th edn). Medical Commission on Accident Prevention. HMSO, London.
8. Commission of the European Communities (1989). Proposals for a Council Directive on the Driving Licence, COM (88) 705 Final.
9. BSI (British Standards Institution) (1983). *Specification for eye protectors for industrial and non-industrial users.* BS 2092. BSI, London.
10. *Paris* v. *Stepney Borough Council* (1951), All ER 42.
11. Cole, B.L. and Vingrys, A.J. (1982) A survey and evaluation of Lantern Tests of Colour Vision. *Amer. J. Optom. Physiol. Opt.,* **59,** 346–74.
12. Fletcher, R. and Voke, J. (1985). *Defective colour vision, fundamentals, diagnosis and management.* Hilger, Bristol and Boston.
13. Norman, L. G. (1960). Medical aspects of road safety. *Lancet,* **i,** 989–94; 1039–45.
14. BSI (British Standards Institution) (1984). *British Standards specification for identification of pipelines and services.* BS 1710.
15. HSE (Health and Safety Executive) (1983). *Visual display units.* HMSO, London.
16. Commission of the European Communities (1990). Council Directive on the minimum safety and health requirement for work with Display Screen Equipment. 90/270 EEC Article 9.
17. Editorials (1989). *'Smokerings'. Model Engineer,* August and November.
18. BSI (British Standards Institution) (1983). Radiation safety of laser products and systems. BS 4803. BSI, London.
19. Marshall, J., Trokel, S., Rothery, S., and Kruger, R.R. (1988). Longterm healing of the central cornea after photorefractive keratectomy using an Excimer laser. *Opthalmol.,* **95**(10), 1411–21.

# 6

# Dermatology

*N.F. Davies and R.J.G. Rycroft*

## Introduction

Less is known about the relationship between skin conditions (dermatoses) and employment than some dermatologists and occupational physicians care to admit. In the everyday practice of dermatology and occupational medicine there are many individual exceptions to most of the current dermatological wisdom. For example, Rystedt in Sweden found that, even in known high-risk jobs, about a quarter of those who had moderate or severe atopic eczema in childhood did not develop dermatitis.[1]

This means that there is often doubt as to whether a particular individual with a dermatosis will be able to tolerate a particular job. It is frequently a sound decision to give the individual the benefit of that doubt, in the interests both of the employee and his prospective employer. The recommendations that follow should not, therefore, be treated as inflexible. A flexible approach allows individual circumstances to be considered properly and fosters good industrial relations.

### Classification of skin conditions

Dermatoses can usefully be divided into two categories:

*Non-occupational*: not primarily caused by skin contact at work, although some (such as atopic eczema) may be aggravated by it.

*Occupational*: primarily caused by skin contact at work, though some (such as allergic contact dermatitis from chromate in cement) may continue even if this contact ceases.

The distinction between occupational and non-occupational dermatoses is often difficult, largely because the majority of occupational dermatoses and a sizeable proportion of non-occupational dermatoses have a similar clinical appearance. This clinical and histopathological entity is termed eczema or dermatitis; the two words are used synonymously by most dermatologists in this country. Until the distinction between occupational and non-occupational dermatoses has been made as accurately as possible, all decisions about fitness for work are severely limited.

The interaction between individual constitution and the occupational environment remains largely ill-defined and unpredictable. That is to say, exogenous (contact) factors and endogenous (constitutional) factors appear to interact differently in different individuals. For example, of two individuals with the same occupational skin contacts, one might notice no adverse effects on a pre-existing psoriasis, while another might find that psoriasis developed on their palms for the first time (see p. 106).

## Skin conditions and employment

Dermatoses and employment may be considered from two aspects:

(1)  the effect of the common *non-occupational dermatoses* on fitness for work; and

(2)  the effect of the common *occupational dermatoses* on fitness for work.

Skin conditions, especially those involving the hands and face, are obvious to prospective employers and fellow-employees. They easily provoke aversion and prejudice from fear of contagion or simply from appearing unpleasant and unhygienic. Thus, Cunliffe has demonstrated that unemployment levels are significantly greater among acne patients of both sexes than controls.[2]

Employers may need to be reassured that, contrary to popular belief, the great majority of dermatoses are not infectious or contagious and that skin conditions need only rarely be a bar to employment. The emphasis should be shifted instead towards the accurate identification of the few dermatoses that can present real problems in specific occupations.

Similarly, fellow-employees may need to be reassured, particularly about the sharing of washing and eating facilities. While the occupational physician or general practitioner may accept the fitness for work of a prospective employee, the personnel manager, supervisor, and fellow-employees still have to be convinced. For some of them it may be their first proper introduction to the true facts about skin disease. The level of accurate information about skin disease in the community is still low in relation to its visibility and prevalence.

# Prevalence

## General

Skin disease is common. Probably the nearest that there has ever been to an accurate survey of the prevalence of skin disease in the general population was that carried out on behalf of the National Center for Health Statistics in the United States.[3] Nearly one-third of a 20 000 general population sample examined were found to have 'some skin pathology that should be evaluated by a physician at least once'. The most common of the skin conditions found were acne vulgaris, tinea ('athletes foot' or ringworm), benign and malignant tumours, seborrhoeic eczema, atopic eczema, contact dermatitis, and psoriasis.

The combined prevalence of seborrhoeic eczema, atopic eczema, and contact dermatitis in the above survey was 6 per cent. The prevalence of psoriasis in the United Kingdom and other Western European countries is around 2 per cent. Skin conditions prompted 22.5 per cent of all attendances at general practitioner surgeries in an inner-city borough in London, and between 20 and 30 per cent of these consultations were for eczema.[4] However, general practitioners' knowledge of dermatology is not always as good as their knowledge of other areas of medicine, which sometimes results in inappropriate medical advice and unnecessarily prolonged absences from work.

### Contact dermatitis

On direct examination of a sample of over 3000 adults from a mixture of urban and rural communities in the Netherlands,[5] 6.2 per cent had eczema on the hands and/or arms, nearly two-thirds of whom were women. Contact irritants were considered to be a factor in more than half, but no patch testing was carried out. Reports on the prevalence of contact dermatitis following patch testing of dermatological outpatients vary widely according to the views of individual dermatologists.

### Occupational dermatoses

The prevalence of occupational dermatoses is not as well known as the prevalence of the common non-occupational dermatoses. This is due to the greater difficulty in diagnosing occupational dermatoses and to the lack of accurate reporting systems, but, as might be expected, more males than females have occupational dermatoses.

In the first six months of 1989, the Health and Safety Executive commissioned a survey based on 73 general practitioners from all parts of the United Kingdom, who recorded the number of cases of occupational dermatitis that they saw in the survey period. The estimate of the number of cases nationally, based on this survey, was 60 000.[6] Five to 15 per cent prevalence rates of occupational contact dermatitis have repeatedly been reported in high-risk groups such as construction workers,[7] although similar rates may occur by chance in non-occupational dermatoses.

The number of premature retirements due to skin disease is not known. Frequently, an alternative occupation can be found. However, some highly trained people, such as toolmakers, laboratory technicians, and nurses with occupational contact dermatitis, may be forced to give up their work. Some atopic eczema sufferers may eventually have to give up working with irritants that are unavoidable, such as shampoos in hairdressing.

# Clinical aspects affecting work capacity

All the comments that follow apply mainly to prospective employees with a past history *and* clinical signs of the skin disease in question. If their conditions have cleared and remained clear without therapy for an extended length of time, a year for example, their dermatosis need not necessarily be considered a significant influence on fitness for work. When a history of skin disease *alone* is relevant and needs to be taken into consideration this will be specifically indicated. Extreme climatic conditions may be contraindicated for practically any of the skin conditions listed.

## Effect of the common non-occupational dermatoses on fitness for work[8]

### Eczema

*Atopic eczema* is now considered to render the potential employee more susceptible to contact irritants only if it was severe in childhood and particularly if it involved the hands.[9] This increased susceptibility is not shared by other atopics with asthma or hay fever only, and does not extend to contact allergens as well as contact irritants. Indeed, there is a certain amount of evidence that it is harder to contact sensitize the atopic than the non-atopic.

There are few jobs where only a history of severe atopic eczema in childhood with hand involvement might be held to constitute an absolute contraindication, but hairdressing (shampoo), catering (wet work and detergent), and production engineering (soluble oil) are three highly inadvisable types of work for such persons. In most other jobs the irritant factor is insufficient, even in employees with active atopic eczema, to constitute a bar unless the hands are currently eczematous. Examples of other occupations with irritant potential are domestic cleaning, nursing, construction work, motor vehicle maintenance, horticulture, and agriculture. The eczema of some atopics worsens in response to hot occupational environments, whether dry or humid.

Involvement of the hands in atopic eczema also raises an entirely separate fitness-for-work problem in certain occupations. Lesions of eczema are very frequently colonized or infected by *Staphylococcus aureus* and sometimes by *Streptococcus pyogenes*. In certain eczematous lesions, carrier rates for *S. aureus* approach 100 per cent and densities may exceed $10^6/cm^2$ and lead to clinically apparent infection. In addition, such patients are colonized on clinically uninvolved skin at rates which may exceed 90 per cent.[10]

Any organism which colonizes skin or contaminates the skin surface is dispersed into the environment on naturally shed skin scales.[11] This has implications in hospitals (patient infection), catering (food poisoning), and the pharmaceutical industry (product contamination). The risk to hospital patients is increased in the immunologically suppressed, although it is not confined to such patients. The hazard presented by active eczema in potential employees in these particular occupations is real and requires individual assessment of risk.

One further consideration may influence the advice given to atopic subjects. Rystedt[9] has pointed out that, even where their work provided no recognizable skin hazard, around half of atopics may develop exacerbations of pre-existing hand eczema, or hand eczema *de novo*. When hand eczema develops in an atopic potentially exposed to any skin hazard at all, it is often difficult for the patient, his trade union representative, or the insurer to accept that the condition is not necessarily occupational. In such cases, industrial injury assessors and expert witnesses giving evidence in claims for compensation may allow the patient the benefit of the doubt. Many essentially endogenous dermatoses are then stated to be aggravated by work exposure, especially if there is known to be a high-risk substance, such as chromate, epoxy resin, or a powerful irritant, in the occupational environment.

*Seborrhoeic eczema* tends, as a clinical impression, to be associated with an increased susceptibility to contact irritants, but to a lesser extent than in atopic eczema. Spread of seborrhoeic eczema from its localized chronic sites can occur in response to hot environments. Discharging otitis externa or profuse scalp scaling may raise problems of bacterial dispersal similar to those in atopic eczema.

*Stasis (varicose) eczema* can be aggravated by prolonged standing. Problematic jobs therefore exist, such as working as a waiter, a shop assistant or a machine operator in engineering. Such postural occupational factors could probably be countered effectively, however, with correct advice about the importance of appropriate exercise and adequately supportive legwear.

*Discoid (nummular) eczema* has little, if any, implications for employment, unless associated with hand eczema, when similar considerations to those in atopic eczema apply.

## Psoriasis

Mild psoriasis not affecting the hands can probably be safely ignored from the point of view of fitness for work, except in extreme circumstances such as those occupations intensely in the public gaze. Aggravation of psoriasis by physical or chemical trauma (Köbner phenomenon) can occur occupationally. It may be elicited on the hands for the first time in psoriasis-prone individuals by occupational factors, although psoriatics vary widely in their liability to hand involvement. If psoriasis already involves the hands, work involving heavy manual labour, such as scaffolding, or contact with irritants, such as in production engineering, may aggravate it.

If psoriasis is or has been at all extensive, physically or emotionally demanding occupations, such as in the armed forces, can be an aggravating factor. When extensive and/or associated with arthropathy, tighter restrictions are applicable.

Colonization of psoriatic lesions with potentially pathogenic bacteria is less of a problem than in atopic eczema and occurs chiefly in those with severe psoriasis who have been inpatients. The density of *Staphylococcus aureus* in such patients has been shown to be three times as heavy on psoriatic plaques as on clinically uninvolved skin, but still to be light in comparison to colonization on eczematous skin.[12]

Psoriasis becomes a potential hazard when lesions involve the hands and forearms or the scalp (common) and face (rare) in those working in hospitals, catering or the pharmaceutical industry, but the lesser degree of staphylococcal colonization in psoriasis compared to atopic eczema, as well as the wider spectrum of suppressive treatments that now exist for psoriasis, allows greater scope for employment of psoriatics even in such high-risk occupations. However, work in special areas, such as operating theatres or caring for immunosuppressed patients, increases the risk.

## Other conditions

*Chronic urticaria* can be made worse by physical or emotional stresses at work. Its control with oral antihistamines, which tend to have the side-effect of drowsiness, may raise the question of fitness for work requiring a constant level of alertness, such as driving or machine operating. Certain newer antihistamines are claimed to be non-sedative and many, although not all, patients can tolerate these safely (Chapter 3, p. 51).

*Photosensitive dermatoses*, and, to a lesser extent *vitiligo*, may be a bar to outdoor work in very sunny environments unless sufficient protection is provided by clothing or by the high efficacy sunscreens which are now available. Dermatological advice can often assist for light-sensitive subjects. Those on drugs such as long-term tetracyclines for acne or amiodarone for arrhythmias may also exhibit photosensitivity.

*Severe nodulocystic acne* may be a contraindication to work involving exposure to hot climatic or microclimatic environments which can severely exacerbate the disorder, e.g., diving in suits heated by hot water. It also probably increases the susceptibility to oil acne, although this should be preventable by other means. Treatment with oral *isotretinoin* (Roaccutane) can now help resolve even the worst cases of acne that were resistant to treatment in the past. There is a strong argument for positively guarding against the unfair discrimination that results in an increase in the prevalence of acne among the unemployed,[2] when recruiting young staff, unless facial appearance is genuinely of crucial importance, as it might be for a hotel receptionist or for other jobs where close customer contact is necessary.

*Multiple viral warts* of the hands can be unacceptable in many occupations involving food-handling, patient care or overt contact with the public. A specific group at risk are wholesale butchers, among whom viral warts can spread to become endemic. It would be unwise to allow anyone with viral warts on the hands to start working in a large butchery without prior treatment. Viral warts on the feet (verrucae) may be contraindicated in occupations involving shared showering or bathing facilities. Dermatological referral should eventually effect the removal of all but the most stubborn warts, allowing the patient to work in areas previously barred to them.

*Tinea pedis* is endemic in occupations involving shared showering or bathing facilities, such as mining, or wearing occlusive footwear, such as diving. This endemic condition is so common that it is not justified to keep new employees away from work until treated and cleared, but it should at least be recognized and treatment initiated before employment starts.

*Impetigo* and other more serious *primary bacterial infections* of the skin, including tuberculosis, have clear implications for employability. Adequate treatment of primary bacterial infections is needed before any bar is removed. Common skin infections, such as impetigo, can probably be regarded as non-infectious after two days of antibiotic treatment, while two weeks might be required as a safer interval for the rarer infections.

*Zoonoses.* It is important to be clear that zoonoses, such as cattle ringworm, can be transferred between animal and man, but *not* from man to man. A zoonosis is not therefore the risk to fellow employees that its appearance might suggest.

*Hyperhidrosis of the hands* may make the individual a 'ruster' in engineering, unacceptable in catering, or disadvantaged in work such as sales or public relations, where frequent hand shaking is required. Dermatological treatment, and even surgery in the form of sympathectomy, can help but often to a limited extent, and may fail to solve the occupational problem. As with acne, however, unfair discrimination at job interviews should be guarded against.

### Race and complexion

Experimental work has detected differences in the susceptibility of skin of different racial origin and complexion to contact irritants. These relatively small differences in practice, however, are not reliable enough to support any rational judgement as to fitness for work.

### Pre-employment skin testing

#### Patch testing

Patch testing prior to employment can detect only previously acquired sensitization and cannot predict future sensitization. A general recommendation for patch testing is therefore often based on a misunderstanding of these fundamental principles, as well as a lack of recognition of the training and experience required to become proficient in carrying out such testing. It is strongly recommended that anyone who carries out any patch testing at all should be properly trained and continue to practise it as part of their regular professional routine. Patch testing may be indicated in individual cases prior to employment if a past or present dermatitis has not been adequately investigated[13]

*Prick testing*

Prick testing prior to employment is not generally of any value from the dermatological point of view. It may help to detect an atopic constitution, but it is the history or presence of atopic eczema which indicates an increased susceptibility to contact irritants, and not an atopic constitution alone (p. 105). Prick testing should never be carried out without full resuscitation equipment being readily available.

*Other skin testing*

Although interesting research applying various standard irritants to the skin has been conducted, there is not yet any simple practical skin test that can be used to predict susceptibility either to irritants or to allergens.

**Effect of the common occupational dermatoses on fitness for work**

Since most of us naturally prefer to continue in our own occupations, an accurate assessment and determination of the causal factors of the dermatosis is the first essential. Once guided by a precise diagnosis, changes in working methods and other preventive measures such as substitution, enclosure, mechanical handling, ventilation, rotation, and personal protective equipment can be helpful. The Control of Substances Hazardous to Health Regulations (COSHH) now provide legislative support to such an assessment, as well as insisting that every employee should have adequate information, instruction, and training on the substances they handle at work. For those at special risk, regular health surveillance may be required to protect individuals and to identify any indication of disease or adverse skin changes at an early stage.

In the majority of cases of occupational dermatoses, continuation in the same employment should be the objective and be achievable, possibly with minor adjustments to work practices. This is particularly important in the many occupational dermatoses where prognosis is known to be little altered by change of job, such as allergic contact dermatitis caused by chromate in cement among construction workers. Carefully considered preventive skin care programmes make both the primary and the secondary prevention of occupational dermatoses more effective.

In a minority of cases a change of occupation may be in the best interests of the individual. It must be stressed again that *this should always be preceded by accurate diagnosis*. There are certain groups in which a change of job is likely to be indicated. Those who have most of their working life still in front of them, such as first-year apprentices, may be well advised to give up a job that is already causing them persistent contact dermatitis. When the prognosis of avoiding further contact with a highly specialized allergen is almost certainly known to be good, as it is in epoxy, acrylic or isocyanate resin dermatitis, a rapid change of job may be indicated once the allergy has been demonstrated by patch testing. Equally, when the prognosis of continuing in contact with irritants is almost certainly bad, as in those with active or previously severe atopic eczema, the best advice may be to give up the unsuitable job as soon as possible. A change of occupation may also be forced on those who have an airborne contact dermatitis, from the Compositae (Asteraceae) group of plants such as chrysanthemums, because of the inherent difficulty in preventing such exposure.

When a change of occupation is decided on, it is vitally important that the new occupation should genuinely be more suitable[14] Clearly, the major requirement should be avoidance of the original contact factor(s). This may need expert guidance, particularly when the contact factor is widely distributed, e.g., allergens, such as formaldehyde, or irritants, such as detergents. A patient with atopic eczema may otherwise change occupation with little if any benefit, as for example a hairdresser becoming a chef.

Up-to-date tables of occupations with a high risk of contact dermatitis and of the irritants and allergens in various occupations are to be found in the textbook reference.[7]

Spurious contraindications to employment on the grounds of common allergies are sometimes met. For example, there is a misconception that nickel allergy, which is currently acquired by about 10 per cent of north-western European women, implies a generally increased risk of dermatitis in the engineering industry. This is probably not so, because of the very low percentages of biologically available nickel in the great majority of metals used in engineering. Only prolonged contact with nickel-plated objects or nickel plating itself is likely to constitute a risk. Few of those working in supermarket checkouts or banks seem to develop hand dermatitis from continual money handling, even though nickel is a constituent of most coinage.

## Special work problems, restrictions or needs

Certain types of work may be considered unsuitable from the point of view of the employer, the insurer, or the safety engineer, although safety itself is never likely to be impaired by any skin condition *per se*. Public health considerations concerning hospitals, catering, and the pharmaceutical industry, as detailed above, may preclude or delay the employment of certain applicants, e.g., those with untreated hand eczema, otitis externa or scalp psoriasis. Persons working with ionizing radiation may not be considered suitable for work in contaminated areas if they have widespread skin lesions which may provide a portal of entry not countered by protective clothing or which could present difficulties if decontamination is necessary.

## Rehabilitation

Rehabilitation of persons with occupational dermatoses rarely requires special facilities. Patients need not necessarily achieve complete clearance of their dermatitis before returning to work, especially if they can temporarily be offered alternative work away from the irritant or allergen which precipitated the condition. Too often employees are advised to stay off work until all trace of abnormality is gone, causing unnecessary emotional and financial strain and endangering the patients' eventual chance of returning to their original job. This action, although taken for what is thought to be the best of reasons, can hinder rather than help the overall prognosis.

The aim of rehabilitation in occupational dermatology is to keep the patient in the same job if at all possible and this can be irretrievably jeopardized by prolonged sickness absence. The foundations of successful rehabilitation are close working relationships between general practitioners, dermatologists, occupational physicians, occupational hygienists, and employers; maintenance of contact between the patient and the place of work during any periods of sickness absence; and monitoring the progress of the employees while their work continues or resumes.

## Conclusions and recommendations

Skin conditions require thorough dermatological investigation in order to diagnose them sufficiently accurately to give reliable medical advice about employment.

Even after full dermatological investigation, there can remain sufficient doubt about the aetiology and prognosis to make medical advice on employment subject to error.

Because of this, it will frequently be sound medical advice to give an individual the benefit of any doubt on fitness for work. Medicolegal considerations may prompt an over-cautious approach that is not truly in the best interests of either the potential employee or the employer. If possible, such prompting should be resisted in a rational manner which can be legally defended.

Dermatological treatment of many common dermatoses, including both acne and psoriasis, has advanced considerably in the last few years. A patient's fitness for work may in certain cases be transformed by dermatological referral and treatment prior to final placement.

From time to time, however, it will remain necessary for prospective employees to be turned down for certain jobs on dermatological grounds; a patient with atopic hand eczema, for example, applying to be a production engineering machine operator working with soluble oil; or a patient with extensive psoriasis applying to be a marine commando. On these occasions it is sometimes invaluable for the physician to be able to quote from previously published material. The emphasis should always be on the accurate identification of the few dermatoses that do have genuine implications for employment, rather than on a general bar on people with skin disease.

Any kind of medical report on a patient, however informal, that is requested for the purposes of pre-employment assessment, should be supplied only with the patient's consent, after due consideration, and with great care not to mislead unwittingly. Uncertainty, which is always likely to exist to some extent, should not be disguised with general statements that cannot be supported either by published evidence or experience.

## Selected references and further reading

1. Rystedt, I. (1985). Work-related hand eczema in atopics. *Cont. Dermat.*, **12**, 164–71.
2. Cunliffe, W.J. (1986). Acne and unemployment. *Brit. J. Dermatol.* **115**, 386.
3. Johnson, M.L.T. (1977). *Skin conditions and related needs for medical care among persons 1–74 years, United States, 1971–1974.* DHEW publications No. (PHS)79–1660 (series 11, No 212). US Department of Health, Education and Welfare, Washington, DC.
4. Champion, R.H., Burton, J.L., and Ebling, F.J.G. (ed.) (1992). *Textbook of dermatology*, (5th edn). Blackwell, Oxford.
5. Coenraads, P.J., Nater, J.P., and van der Lende, R. (1983). Prevalence of eczema and other dermatoses of the hands and arms in the Netherlands. Association with age and occupation. *Clin. Exp. Dermatol.* **8**, 495–503.
6. HSE (Health and Safety Executive) (1991). Health and safety statistics 1989–90. *Employment Gazette*, Occasional Supplement No. 2, September, 60.
7. Rycroft, R.J.G. (1992), Occupational contact dermatitis. In *Textbook of contact dermatitis*, (ed. R.J.G. Rycroft, T. Menné, P.J. Frosch, and C. Benezra), Springer, Berlin. pp. 338–97.
8. Cotterill, J.A. (1985). Constitutional skin disease in industry. In *Essentials of industrial dermatology*, (ed. W.A.D. Griffiths and D.S. Wilkinson) Blackwell, Oxford, pp. 38–46.
9. Rystedt, I. (1985). Factors influencing the occurrence of hand eczema in adults with a history of atopic dermatitis in childhood. *Cont. Dermat.*, **12**, 185–91.
10. Noble, W.C. (1981). *Microbiology of human skin*, p. 325. Lloyd Luke, London.
11. Noble, W.C. (1975). Dispersal of skin microorganisms. *Brit. J. Dermatol.*, **93**, 477–85.
12. Noble, W.C. and Savin, J.A. (1968). Carriage of *Staphylococcus aureus* in psoriasis. *Brit. Med. J.*, **1**, 417–19.
13. Rycroft, R.J.G. (1990). Is patch testing necessary? In *Recent advances in dermatology* (ed. R.H. Champion and R.J. Pye), Vol. 8, pp. 101–11. Churchill Livingstone, Edinburgh.
14. Well, L.M. and Gebauer, K.A. (1991). A follow-up study of occupational skin disease in Western Australia. Cont. Dermat., **24**, 241–3.

# 7

# Neurological disorders

## *J.M. Harrington and F.B. Gibberd*

## Introduction

### Scope of the chapter

Neurological disorders cover a wide range of disease processes and an even larger range of functional disabilities. A review of the congenital and acquired disorders that can affect the central or peripheral nervous system reveals how important an intact system is to the requirements of everyday life let alone the ability to earn a living. An effective system of neurotransmission is essential to psychological and locomotor function as well as to the control that such mechanisms bring to autonomic activities.

Disorders of neurophysiology can be divided into those leading to negative symptoms or to positive symptoms.[1] Negative symptoms arise from a failure of neuronal activity. Such failures may be caused by physical or chemical agents which irreversibly destroy (as opposed to damage) nerve cells or axons. Neural cells are irreplaceable and the limited regeneration which might occur when peripheral nerves are destroyed rarely leads to full recovery of function.

Positive symptoms arise from excessive neuronal or axonal stimulation by an irritative stimulus which is usually biochemical. Such positive symptoms result from malfunction of the inhibitory influences on the system. The importance of an intact synaptic transmission system cannot be overemphasized.

Another way of viewing neurological dysfunction is in terms of the clinical evaluation of the patient. As regards capacity for work the precise diagnosis is less important than the functional consequences. Feldman and Pransky[2] divide functional effects into disturbance of awareness; disturbances of posture, balance, and gait; extremity pain, numbness, and weakness; neurobehavioural impairment; and ophthalmological conditions. These will be dealt with both from the functional and anatomical points of view in subsequent sections of the chapter.

## Prevalence

### The size of the problem

Neurological disorders are an important cause of disability in modern Western society. Estimates from the British General Household Survey, using self-

**Table 7.1** Crude annual mortality and morbidity rates for some neurological disorders per 100 000 population (adapted from Kurtzke 1985[3])

| Disorder | Mortality | Morbidity |
|---|---|---|
| Brain neoplasms | 4–5 | 6–16 |
| Multiple sclerosis | 0–3 | 30–300 |
| Parkinson's disease | 0.5–3.8 | 40–190 |
| Motor neurone disease | 0.4–1.2 | 0.4–1.9 |
| Myopathies | 0.1–0.5 | 2–10 |
| Myasthenia | 1 | 0.5–10 |

reporting procedures, suggest that 6 per cent of the population have a long-standing neurological illness. It is difficult to make valid comparisons with other major disease groupings. This is partly because most neurological diseases are age (and sometimes sex) related. Mortality and morbidity also vary by condition. Diseases that are most common below 65 years and which have prolonged morbidity have greater relevance to work ability than either highly fatal diseases or those whose main clinical impact occurs after the normal age of retirement.

Table 7.1 compares mortality and morbidity rates for some of the more important neurological diseases. The rates cited are crude and adjustment-for-age would produce major variations in the numbers.[3] With the exception of brain tumours and motor neurone disease, the morbidity rates are an order of magnitude larger than mortality rates. Indeed the neurological diseases cited in Table 7.1 pall in comparison to the health impact of cerebrovascular disorders. Here, the comparable mortality rates are in the order of 60–600 per 100 000 per year (12 per cent of all deaths), but only about 10 per cent of these deaths occur below the age of 65. Of the 100 000 'first strokes' each year in the UK, a quarter occur in people below the age of 65. The resultant disability is a major drain on health service resources (5.5 per cent of the total). Overall, nervous system diseases take up 9 per cent of all NHS expenditure—only exceeded by circulatory disorders (13 per cent) and mental illness (20 per cent).[4]

## Non-occupational versus occupational causes of neurological disease

For the occupational physician, the non-work-related causes of neurological disease far outweigh those from occupation. The proven occupational causes are mainly peripheral neurotoxins and the neurobehavioural effects of organic solvents.[5] From the practical point of view, the occupational physician is more likely to be involved with the job adaptation and rehabilitation of patients with neurological disabilities than with eliminating the small number of known occupational neurotoxins from the workplace. Of course, the occupational physician needs to be aware of the possible work related circumstances which could exacerbate a pre-existing non occupationally related neurological disease. The use of organic solvents, therefore, needs to be carefully considered and particularly in patients who already have disturbances of awareness or posture or a neurobehavioural disorder.

## Clinical assessment

If a differential diagnosis is not clear after taking a history, then the clinical examination may be equally inconclusive. Certainly the history of the illness is of crucial importance but by the time the occupational physician sees the patient, the diagnosis is likely to have been established. In these circumstances, the clinical assessment takes on an additional function—that of assessing the individual's ability to perform the job on offer or to return to the job held before the illness began.

In normal subjects, perception and recognition of all forms of sensory stimuli are intact; their balance, posture, and gait can be maintained; they have good control of delicate motor movement; and have no evidence of loss of control of vasomotor, gastrointestinal or genitourinary functions.[2] To this negative symptom review must be added an absence of any positive symptoms or signs such as involuntary movements, abnormal sensations or hallucinations.

Disturbances of awareness include alterations in the ability to stay awake. Whilst classical narcolepsy is rare, sleep apnoea is a common cause of excessive day-time somnolence. Establishing the existence of such a condition can be difficult as the patient is frequently unaware of night-time problems. They may contend that night-time sleep is normal—the problem, in their view, is day-time sleepiness! Such individuals are particularly intolerant of rotating shift work.

Disturbances of posture, balance or gait are usually easy to establish. The patient complains of dizziness, unsteadiness or spatial disequilibrium and their powers of co-ordination may be impaired. Parkinson's disease is a classic variety of this group of disorders. Adjustment of treatment regimes may minimize the work problems but jobs which involve the use of extraocular musculature, such as scanning production lines, or the need for rapid hand co-ordination, may be difficult for these patients. Similarly, the limb spasticity associated with demyelinating disorders may prevent fine manual work or even the ability of the patient to stand for long periods.

Many manual jobs require good muscle power and good peripheral sensation. Lifting or moving objects—particularly if repeated frequently can be a problem for individuals with peripheral neuropathic disorders. This is especially so if the cause is a radiculopathy as the repetitive movements may involve vertebral column movement which could exacerbate the original cause of the patient's disability.

Neurobehavioural disorders following head injury, stroke or encephalitis may range from mild and transient to severe and permanent. Aphasias and apraxias can preclude employment which requires regular communication with other workers. Disturbance of spatial relationships could prevent the patient from driving, whilst memory disturbances will be important for those with intellectually demanding jobs.

**Work assessment**

Establishing an accurate prognosis is particularly important in neurological conditions. The clinical course may be episodic, transient, progressive or static. Such prognostic criteria are important for the patient's job prospects. Although some diseases such as epilepsy (see Chapter 8) have medicolegal implications, most disorders must be dealt with on an *ad hoc* basis. For example, multiple sclerosis is a very difficult disease to evaluate—especially at the first consultation following diagnosis. The disease may never cause more than a transient episode of blurred vision or may progress rapidly and inexorably to quadriparesis. Similarly, cerebrovascular disorders may range from a catastrophic intracerebral bleed to transient ischaemic episodes. Many stroke patients however, recover, at least partially, so it is important, wherever possible, to preserve their original job albeit in a modified form. Such modifications may be temporary or permanent but clearly will require regular re-evaluation.

The consequences of neurological dysfunction will be different for manual and non-manual workers. Sensory impairment or motor dysfunction (with or without a flaccid or spastic component) will make tasks involving power and/or co-ordination extremely difficult. By contrast, a degree of impairment in intellectual function might not be so serious for the manual worker.

The reverse is frequently true of non-manual occupations. A stroke patient with a hemiparesis might still be able to undertake a desk-bound job particularly if he is helped to the desk and stays there. Commuting to work rather than physically getting to the desk from the front entrance of the office may be the biggest problem. However, a stroke patient left with even a moderate degree of dysarthria or dysphasia may have difficulty with communication, memory recall or accuracy of terminology where these are important aspects of the work.

**Rehabilitation**

Much can be done to improve the lot of even the most disabled patient by appropriate rehabilitation which, regrettably, is undervalued and underfunded.[6] Neurological disorders such as demyelinating diseases, extrapyramidal disorders, and cerebrovascular accidents can be greatly ameliorated by rehabilitation procedures. Where the National Health Services fail may be the opportunity—even the necessity—for industry to intervene. Training employees to a task is expensive and it is much cheaper to rehabilitate a partially disabled trained worker than it is to recruit a new one. Add to this the moral responsibility to help a loyal employee and the argument for initiating active rehabilitation is overwhelming. Every neurologically impaired employee should be offered rehabilitation at work. The occupational physician should be actively involved by directly intervening in matching the job to the disabled worker.

**Lay influences on employability**

The commitment of the occupational physician 'to do something' for the employee who has developed a neurological disorder can be undermined, curtailed or even prevented by uninformed lay opinion in the guise of 'management decisions'. Whilst the manager concerned cannot be expected to understand the intricacies of medical problems, it is important that he realizes that occupational health professionals are there to help. He or she should refer all such patients to the occupational health adviser. In a well organized company the latter will be aware of them through the post-sickness absence review procedure. A role of the occupational physician is to ensure that managers have no serious misconceptions about disease processes when they become aware of a diagnosis. Many people, for example, believe that multiple sclerosis will inevitably lead to an incontinent wheelchair-bound existence. Likewise, they often fail to appreciate the improvement in functional ability that can follow a stroke either from the natural recovery process itself or from the effect of an energetic rehabilitation programme.[7,8]

People may also find it difficult to understand the problems of nominal dysphasia or the variable nature of the disability of Parkinson's disease within a patient in a single day. It is the physician's role to explain, to make the relevant clinical assessment and to advise on the necessary job modifications.

**In summary, neurological disease can create a wide variety of disabilities. The clinical assessment of the symptoms and signs and the review of the patient's work capacity are much more important than the diagnostic label. Indeed, the label itself may be an impediment to future gainful employment through misconceptions about the neurological disability as much as failure to provide energetic and intelligent rehabilitation. In all these matters the occupational physician plays a pivotal role.**

## How neurological illnesses influence work

The disability that a patient suffers is dependent on the symptoms and signs that the disease produces and not the disease itself. Injuries, and particularly head injuries, can lead to loss of function anywhere in the nervous system and the occupational physician must be familiar with the patient and his work as well as the nature of his disease before he can determine his work capability.

**Symptoms related to cranial nerves**

Problems relating to the nerves of the eye and ear are considered in Chapters 4 and 5.

*Smell.* Neurological problems with sense of smell most commonly occur after head injuries. Few jobs require a good sense of smell but when it is lost there is usually a loss of taste apart from the four primary tastes of sweet, acid (sour), bitter, and salt. Cooks and professional tasters would therefore have a disability.

*Trigeminal nerve lesions* rarely influence work except for the possibility of trauma to the eye when corneal sensation is lost. Employees working in dusty atmospheres are at risk if there is sensory loss in the ophthalmic division of the trigeminal nerve. In contrast, the pain of trigeminal neuralgia can be so great that concentration at work becomes impossible. The condition needs to be distinguished from psychogenic facial pain.

*Bell's palsy or facial palsy* is common and by itself is not a handicap for most work. It is not painful and usually improves with time. However, it is disfiguring and if the work involves meeting the public it can be embarrassing. The only danger is to the eye. In the early stages the eyelids cannot be closed and the cornea is at risk of becoming dry and ulcerated. When the eyelid cannot be closed it is important to protect the eye. Wearing large glasses helps to protect it from wind which can dry the cornea and dust which can irritate. If necessary a tarsorrhaphy will protect the eye and may even improve the appearance. Fortunately, eyelid closure always recovers even if the rest of the facial paralysis does not. Bell's palsy and other facial palsies should rarely be a cause of a long-term inability to work.

*Swallowing and articulation.* Apart from those who earn their living by talking, such as broadcasters or politicians, these problems are associated with social and home disabilities as much as with difficulty at work so that they rarely affect employment. Difficulty with breathing and paralysis of the respiratory muscles are also matters rarely requiring special consideration at work as the patients so afflicted are usually unable to work.

## Symptoms related to the trunk and limbs

Patients with problems related to their trunk and limbs often find it difficult to describe their symptoms. Therefore it is difficult to categorize their symptoms into the usual neurological groups, appearance (e.g., wasting), power, tone, co-ordination, and the various sensations. Often the word 'weakness' is used to express inco-ordination and sensory symptoms and phrases like 'my hand feels wrong' are used to express weakness when there is no sensory change. The history is particularly important because it helps the patient to express his problem. Having allowed the patient to give his history in his own way other questions often help to disclose any disability. For example 'Is there anything you cannot do now which you could previously do?' 'Is there anything which you would like to do but cannot?'. In making an assessment for work the doctor can often be helped by a physiotherapist or occupational therapist. The doctor should explain clearly which problem he would like assessed by the therapist. He will then be able to establish the patient's disabilities and his opinion will be more firmly based.

*Weakness* can be due to many causes, an upper motor neurone lesion, a lower motor neurone lesion, a neuromuscular junction lesion, a muscle disease (myopathy) or a psychological cause. These causes can usually be distinguished from one another. A hard judgement to make is that between a lower motor neurone lesion and a muscle disease if there is no sensory loss. The management of the different causes is different and the effects on work capability are different.

In an *upper motor neurone lesion* spasticity will often be a major problem and the patient's difficulties can often be helped by physiotherapy and rehabilitation. Retraining of movement patterns and posture and control of the trunk allow the central nervous system to adjust to the lesion and function can be improved. Attempting to make the muscles stronger by using muscle strengthening exercises is usually contraindicated. Physiotherapy at the place of work is of benefit if the doctor and physiotherapist work closely together. Small changes in posture at work and external aids can make a big difference. The type of rehabilitation needs to be carefully formulated but it is often rewarding. The employee should not expect or be expected to have made maximum or full recovery before work is resumed. The rehabilitation process will be helped if the patient can return to the job part-time. The process of going to work and performing a job is a part of the rehabilitation and will allow problems to be identified early. If the patient's intellectual level is preserved employers will often be surprised how much improvement can occur after an acute illness and how the patient's ability to work may be only slightly impaired.

With *lower motor neurone* diseases the situation is different. Unless there is very severe weakness the decreased tone is not a problem and the main difficulty is loss of power. Physiotherapy should be designed to strengthen the appropriate muscles. If there is complete paralysis of a muscle other muscles may be strengthened and trick movements learnt. This will often help the patient to get back to work quickly. The long-term prognosis depends on the pathology but if it is a peripheral acute condition such as Guillain–Barré syndrome full recovery is often possible. In progressive diseases, like motor neurone disease, treatment cannot halt the decline. A physiotherapist and an occupational therapist can be helpful in rehabilitation. If there are localized sites of weakness a splint may help and aids may allow an employee to work. In more severe cases, an environmental control system may allow a severely handicapped person to use office equipment and continue at work.

*Neuromuscular junction disease* is rare and the only one likely to be encountered is myasthenia gravis. Patients with this disease find that exercise makes the weakness worse so muscle strengthening exercises should not be suggested. The disease is difficult to diagnose in the early stages, when it may be misdiagnosed as hysteria if only the limbs are involved. The employee complains first of weakness when asked to do more physical work than usual. Weakness of the eye muscles after repeated movements makes the diagnosis easier but eye symptoms are not always present. If myasthenia is suspected an examination can be carried out before and after exercise but even then the diagnosis may be difficult unless the *edrophonium* test is used and acetylcholine receptor antibodies are tested for. (*Edrophonium* is a short-acting drug which, when given intravenously, transiently reverses myasthenic weakness.) Nevertheless, the occupational physician may be in a better position to make the diagnosis than the general practitioner.

*Muscle disease* is less common than neurological disease. Muscular dystrophies, which are genetic disorders, will rarely become a problem in occupational medicine. The commonest, Duchenne's dystrophy, is usually so severe early in life that the patient never works. However, rarer dystrophies can progress very slowly producing increasing disability. The problem at work is usually confined to weakness and therefore with appropriate aids, for travelling to and moving about the workplace the patient can do sedentary work. With environmental control systems, such as the Possum, it is often possible to set up a work station which will allow the employee to use a word processor, a telephone, and even do simple mechanical tasks, such as opening doors and turning on lights, without moving from his workstation. With adequate access even the weakest person could use an electric wheelchair.

*Weakness due to psychological factors* is usually additional to a physical condition, so that the employee is unable to use his remaining potential for activity. If full recovery is to be achieved rehabilitation programmes for such patients should involve a psychological assessment, although not necessarily by a clinical psychologist or psychiatrist. The problem may be only one of confidence which could be restored by a skilled physiotherapist or occupational therapist. In these situations a therapist at the place of work is helpful. Specialist help from a psychiatrist or clinical psychologist may be needed. It is sometimes difficult to decide when to ask a psychiatrist because the outcome of rehabilitation cannot be easily assessed in its early stages. However, once it is clear that recovery, using ordinary rehabilitation processes, is not going to be satisfactory for psychological reasons there should be no delay in calling in a psychiatrist or clinical psychologist.

Abnormalities of *tone* rarely occur by themselves. Nevertheless, in patients with long-standing upper motor neurone lesions the increase in tone can be out of proportion to the relatively mild weakness. In these cases the hypertonia leads to clumsiness of movement which often affects the fine movements of the hand or the gait. Patients with these symptoms should not be given muscle strengthening exercises as these would increase their disability. Instead, the patients need help with posture and patterns of movement. It is sometimes felt by employers that giving the patient a lighter or sedentary job might help but as power is not the problem a lighter job is not always easier. The patient needs a job which requires less skilful movements. For example, putting in small screws would be more difficult than a heavier, but less precise activity. In *Parkinson's disease* the increased tone and rigidity is associated with bradykinesia. It is the slowness of movements especially when they are not repetitive which is usually the greatest disability. For example, a patient may walk easily for long distances in the open but with great difficulty in a crowded workshop when frequent changes of direction have to be made. The motor skills of patients with Parkinson's disease are considerably impaired. Unfortunately, they are not easily helped by physiotherapy because their ability to retain and relearn motor skills is also impaired. Drug treatment is usually more rewarding. If an employee has Parkinson's disease and is unable to do his work in spite of help from the general practitioner and the occupational physician it is important to seek the help of a neurologist.

*Sensory loss* in the limbs can be a major handicap to employees. The effects can be more disabling than motor lesions. Most normal people rarely use full power and have considerable reserves if they wish to use more force. However, sensation is often used to the full. It is often difficult to compensate for even a mild sensory loss in the fingers and no amount of physiotherapy and training will restore the sensory function. The symptoms and signs, and to an extent the disability, can only become better if the disease improves. Therefore physiotherapy has only a minor role. If the sensory loss involves touch and position sense the therapist can teach the patient about the disability and explain ways of diminishing it by careful use of other sensory organs, for example, using vision when walking rather than relying on the diminished position sense in the legs. A problem that employees are likely to encounter is difficulty with skilled movements of the hands. Using a different type of pen or better lighting or a word processor may help to compensate for the disability.

*Loss of pain and temperature sensation* produces different problems. If touch and position sense are preserved the patient's skilled use of the hands and walking are unaffected. However, the employee with loss of pain sensation is at risk because the normal protective response of withdrawing from dangerous stimuli is lost. The employee may be at particular risk when there are hot surfaces or liquids at the place of work, as he may suffer a burn without realizing that there has been contact with a source of extreme heat. With loss of pain and temperature sensation the patient may remain exposed to a moderate heat source for a long time and so suffer severe injury. Similarly, ill-fitting footwear may not be appreciated and skin damage result. These difficulties occur most frequently in diabetic patients. In more severely disabled employees with a paraplegia the loss of sensation in the buttocks and legs produces a considerable risk of pressure sores. Proper seating to prevent trauma both in the wheelchair and at the workstation is important.

*Ataxia* and uncoordination can produce results similar to peripheral sensory loss, but the disability is likely to be worse because other sensory input, for example vision, cannot be used in compensation. Unless the cause of the ataxia can be corrected no amount of re-training will help. In these circumstances the environment must be changed if the ataxia is a cause of danger to the employee or if it limits his work. Aids are available for typewriters, word processors, and other equipment which make it easier for such employees to carry out their work.

*Poor sphincter control* is a symptom of many neurological diseases. It is a problem at home and at work and the management in both places is the same. By controlling fluid intake and having easy access to toilets it is usually possible for an employee to cope at work. If it is not it is usually because their other disabilities limit work effectiveness. During the acute stage of an illness which causes urinary retention or incontinence a catheter may be necessary, but usually the patient learns how to stimulate bladder reflex activity by abdominal pressure or other stimulus and thereby regain control of micturition. This is more likely to be successful with a spinal cord lesion above the conus, but is less successful when there is a peripheral nerve lesion. If control cannot be achieved the use of a catheter with a bag on the leg or intermittent self-catheterization can allow employees to continue at work without the embarrassment of urinary incontinence. Faecal incontinence is usually unacceptable. If faecal incontinence is a risk a careful bowel regime is essential. Laxatives may help the patient to overcome constipation but make incontinence more likely. One method is for the patient to have no laxatives but to have an enema once or twice a week in the knowledge that he will be continent the rest of the time. This might possibly entail missing half a day a week at work but this can be foreseen and planned.

## Higher (cerebral) functions

*Mental functions* are affected by many neurological diseases, but their influence on work depends very much on the job. A labourer can continue work with a moderate or sometimes even a severe intellectual impairment but an executive cannot. There are no guidelines which can be used generally. *Memory loss* and *dementia* cannot be improved by treatment but can be iatrogenic when treatment for the underlying disease is excessive. For example, anticonvulsants may impair memory. If the epilepsy is only nocturnal or partial, the epilepsy is a lesser handicap than drug-induced drowsiness. Presenile dementia, Alzheimer's disease, is untreatable. With some neurological diseases *changes in mood* can be so severe as to be a handicap. Depression associated with frustration, imposed by the illness, is common and will often be helped by antidepressants, best given at night when unwanted effects on mental function will be least. Occasionally, and especially in multiple sclerosis, euphoria may limit an employee's motivation to overcome his disability and strive to maintain his work potential.

*Speech disorders*, whether dysphasia or dysarthria, can be helped by speech therapy but it is rare for such a major improvement to occur that it becomes the only therapy needed to enable the employee to return to work. It is often more effective to reduce the importance of speech in the job and to provide aids such as a word processor. Speech aids can be used if the voice is very weak as can occur in Parkinson's disease but even then the problem is often the speed of speech as much as the volume. Dysphasia is often associated with dysgraphia, and dysarthria with swallowing problems and therefore the handicap as a whole needs to be considered when planning therapy.

## Drug management

Patients with neurological disease are often given excessive drug treatment which can be a major factor in limiting their ability to work. Therefore, if a patient is unable to work it is important to assess all therapy and if possible stop all treatment that makes work more difficult. The purpose of treatment should be to make work easier. Although the long-term prognosis is important there are times when this might take second place to the immediate symptoms. For example, if a patient who is still at work is found to have a cerebral tumour it might be better to maintain him at work leading a relatively normal life rather than submit him to biopsy and intensive therapy, which would curtail his work, in the slight hope of prolonging his life. There are no clear rules or guidelines for assessing the relative importance of present disabilities against future ones, but the work activity of the patient is an important factor that must be considered.

The use of analgesics to control pain requires as much care as any other medication. Obviously, the underlying cause of the pain must be treated, but great care is required in selecting the correct analgesic. Clear advice must be given on how often the drugs should be taken. Some patients want to take them too often, others inadequately. Only by discussing the situation with the patient can a correct drug regime be agreed. Any pain which is a disability and prevents efficient working must be controlled with sufficient prophylactic medication. If the employee while working takes no analgesia till the pain is bad enough to impede his work then he has waited too long. If the pain is continuous or regular in its occurrence then the therapy needs to be regular and not taken intermittently. Clearly, the type of analgesia will depend on the cause of the pain. Particular causes such as neuralgias may respond to particular therapy, such as *carbamazepine*.

It is rare for pain alone to prevent an employee working but it is common for the pain to reduce the employee's work effectiveness because insufficient regard has been given to relieving it.

*Headache* is probably the most common pain which limits work. Often it is mild and due to tension, and when treatment with weak analgesics is taken sufficiently early in the symptom these will usually be adequate. If the headaches become frequent the home and work environment must be considered for avoidable factors. The prevention of eye strain is considered on p. 95, 127. Smoke, unpleasant smells, and inadequate ventilation make headaches more likely. Migraine is considered on p. 130. Post-traumatic headaches usually decrease over the months following the head injury but may be prolonged if inadequate measures are taken to control them in the early months or if litigation adds to the stress.[9]

## How workplace factors influence neurological function

### Introduction

In considering neurological fitness to work, the most important clinical aspects are to review disability in the light of the work demands. This is how the patient presents and, indeed, how the patient sees it. Nevertheless, we consider it useful to review specific workplace exposures that can cause or exacerbate neurological diseases and we conclude with a section on the main neurological diseases and how they can influence work function. Workplace exposures can be arbitrarily classified as physical, psychological and chemical. The exposures will be dealt with in turn, distinguishing where necessary between factors which exacerbate pre-existent diseases from those which are specific causes of neurological deficit.

### Physical agents

*Noise*

Noise is almost synonymous with mechanized industry. Many people are exposed to noise at work. In the United States it is estimated that 8 million civilian workers are exposed to potentially damaging noise levels and this number is increased by those who work in or live near military or aviation establishments, as well as those who choose to be bombarded with further noise during their leisure time.

Noise is dealt with in Chapter 4 but it is worth noting a few points here to emphasize the neurological features and effects. Although noise-induced hearing loss is the effect of most moment, other effects, such as headaches, diminished ability to communicate, and even perceived difficulties with balance, can be important, particularly in a patient with imperfect neurological function.

The deafness caused by noise is due to damage to the organ of Corti, in the inner ear, but patients with pre-existent deafness (whether conductive or perceptive) should be vigorously protected from further damage. Furthermore, whilst some forms of deafness are ameliorated by the use of hearing aids, noise-induced hearing loss with its specific effects mainly at 3–6 kHz is not.

The problems with communication are twofold: first, there is the difficulty of communicating at all at high ambient noise levels and communication is not improved by ear muffs or plugs unless such devices are sophisticated enough to incorporate radio links. Radio links themselves may, however, add to the noise load. The second feature is that some patients may already have a neurological dysfunction which limits communication. This could be a speech defect or a defective ability to interpret speech. Such patients should, in particular, avoid noisy work situations which will add to their difficulties and which are thus potentially dangerous to them and to their fellow workers.

*Vibration*

Vibration is widespread in industry and, indeed, often accompanies noise. Thus it is no surprise that similar numbers of workers are exposed to vibration at work. The health hazards generally occur at frequencies between 1 and 1000 Hz. The vibration may be whole body, as occurs in truck drivers where the vibration is generally at the lower end of the range (1–10 Hz). Hand-transmitted vibration occurs when the worker holds a vibrating tool—such as a chain saw or pneumatic drill, or holds the workpiece to a vibrating machine—such as in some metal-finishing processes. Such vibrations range from 10 to 1000 Hz. Although little is known about the chronic effects of whole body vibration (apart from specific influences on body organ resonance and perhaps an association with

**Table 7.2**

The two-tier Stockholm classification[10] for hand–arm vibration syndrome and cold-induced Raynaud's phenomenon staging

| Stage* | Grade | Description |
|---|---|---|
| 0 | | No attacks |
| 1 | Mild | Occasional attacks affecting only the tips of one or more fingers |
| 2 | Moderate | Occasional attacks affect distal and middle (rarely also proximal) phalanges of one or more fingers |
| 3 | Severe | Frequent attacks affecting all phalanges of most fingers |
| 4 | Very severe | As in Stage 3, with trophic skin changes of most fingers |

* The staging is made separately for each hand. In the evaluation of the subject, the grade of the disorder is indicated by the stages of both hands and the number of affected fingers on each hand, e.g., 2L(2)/1R(1), --/3R(4), etc.

Sensorineural staging

| Stage* | Symptoms |
|---|---|
| 0SN | Exposed to vibration but no symptoms |
| 1SN | Intermittent numbness, with or without tingling |
| 2SN | Intermittent or persistent numbness, reduced sensory perception |
| 3SN | Intermittent or persistent numbness, reduced tactile discrimination and/or manipulative dexterity |

* The sensorineural stage is to be established for each hand.

osteoarticular disorders), the effects of hand–arm vibration are well known and can be disabling.[10]

In addition to the vascular component leading to *Raynauds phenomenon*, increasing attention has focused in recent years on the neurological effects. Sensorineural staging of the disease process has now been agreed internationally (the Stockholm Classification, see Table 7.2) ranging from intermittent numbness with or without tingling to persistent numbness with reduced tactile discrimination and/or manual dexterity. The pathogenesis of the neural damage is not clear but there is, in addition, an association with *carpal tunnel syndrome*. This may be due to direct median nerve effects or, more likely, to the posture in holding the vibrating tool or workpiece resulting in a type of repetitive strain disorder. Such postures can cause or exacerbate ulnar nerve damage at the elbow.

Whatever the cause, the effects can be severe and disabling. The patient may be unable to undertake fine finger movements and as the vascular component is certainly exacerbated by cold, work is more difficult in the colder months of the year and certain outdoor hobbies may have to be curtailed. Again, a patient who already has a peripheral sensory deficit should be advised to avoid work with exposure to vibration.

### Work-related upper limb disorders

This rather clumsy title has replaced terms such as *repetitive strain injury* or *occupational overuse syndrome*. Nevertheless, there is still much controversy over the pathogenesis of this group of conditions—the most clear-cut links being with tendinitis and tenosynovitis associated with repetitive movements or constrained postures. From the neurological point of view, the main interest lies with *carpal tunnel syndrome*. Whilst the median nerve damage may be caused by similar workplace exposures as the tendon effects, the influence of vibration may be an added feature. Either way, it is important to distinguish this cause of median nerve damage from others—particularly in middle aged female patients who seem to be the group most commonly affected by *carpal tunnel syndrome* (see also Chapter 10, p. 192).

### Temperature

Extremes of temperature may cause a variety of effects but particular interest lies in the influence of temperature on patients with pre-existing neurological disease. Two cases will be cited briefly. At high temperatures the symptoms of *multiple sclerosis* worsen but improve again when the temperature falls. Such patients should, wherever possible, avoid workplaces where high ambient temperatures are common. However, high temperature does not induce exacerbations of the disease or worsen the prognosis. At the other end of the scale, low temperatures, apart from producing a lowered ability for anyone to perform skilled activity, are a particular problem for patients with myotonic disorders especially *myotonia congenita*.

## Light

Poor lighting at work is a particular problem for the visually impaired (Chapter 5). Both poorly lit and dazzlingly bright workplaces may cause headaches in those who have to work there. It is thus vital that the worker has the correct glasses. One particular lighting problem is where flashing lights or even a poorly adjusted visual display screen, induce a fit in those few epilepsy patients who are photosensitive (Chapter 8, p. 149). Flashing lights can also precipitate migraine.

## Pressure

Most of the adverse effects of raised atmospheric pressure in working environments result from the effects of decompression. Neurological damage is associated with the anoxic effect of gas bubbles blocking small blood vessels during the process of decompression following exposure to high pressure. Initial acute symptoms and signs depend on the areas affected but can include sensory and motor dysfunction, dizziness and headaches with convulsions, and coma in the worst affected cases. The chronic effects of repeated damage may be extremely difficult to distinguish from other neurological disorders and can, for example, mimic *multiple sclerosis, Parkinsonism,* or *pre-senile dementia.* The most common source of such exposures is diving either professionally or for pleasure and the effects can be disabling and permanent (see also Appendix 4).

In general, someone with established neurological disease should avoid exposure to raised pressure (diving and compressed air work) or reduced pressure (flying in non-pressurized aircraft). However, the neurological problems associated with changes in pressure are due to inappropriately rapid decompression and so recreational pursuits, if carefully managed, would not be barred automatically.

## Psychological effects

Although psychiatric disorders are dealt with in Chapter 20, it is worth noting here that a number of adverse psychological effects from work could influence patients with neurological disorders. Apart from stress and boredom—perhaps two ends of the same spectrum!—there are effects from shiftwork which could either mimic or exacerbate neurological disorders. The main adverse effect of rotating shiftwork is fatigue. Many workers complain of it and it can result in tiredness or even sleep at work. In practice, these symptoms may be more noticeable in the short-term, than the gastrointestinal or cardiovascular, effects found in large-scale longitudinal surveys of shiftworkers. The circadian rhythm disruption caused by rotating shiftwork, whilst measurable, is rarely translated into overt symptoms other than fatigue. For the patient with pre-existing neurological disease this could worsen their work performance whatever the original deficit might be (motor, sensory or cerebral function). Obviously, a patient with myasthenia or narcolepsy would be particularly affected. It is, therefore, important when evaluating increased fatigue to consider the influence of shiftwork. The financial pressures to continue such a work regime may be considerable and it must be remembered that some shift patterns (particularly the 10- or 12-hour shift) do provide opportunities for a second job on the days off from shiftwork.

**Chemicals**

Neurological damage associated with work is most clearly demonstrated when considering chemical hazards in the workplace. Many may mimic non-occupational neurological disorders and the length of this section emphasizes the importance of workplace factors in the differential diagnosis and management of neurological fitness for work. Similarly, a patient with a non-occupational neurological deficit could have their problems exacerbated by such subsequent exposures. This is particularly pertinent in view of the ubiquitous use of organic solvents in manufacturing industry and their diffuse effects on those who are exposed.

Of all the specific workplace factors which can cause neurological problems, the neurotoxic chemicals are the most important. A detailed list of the agents is beyond the scope of this book but this is adequately covered elsewhere.[5] One of the problems here is the fact that employees are rarely exposed to a single chemical and thus a number of the effects may be due to a mixture of chemicals. Furthermore, it may be impossible to be precise about which chemical is causing which effects. Depending on dose and mixture, it may be possible to discern a dose-response spectrum of disorders ranging from mild slowing of nerve conduction velocity through to frank encephalopathy. Some neurotoxins only produce peripheral nerve dysfunction, others central effects, whilst others can cause both. Although some peripheral neurotoxins such as lead have been known for years, attention has shifted of late to the disorders associated with organic solvent exposure.

*Neurobehavioural disorders and organic solvents*

Organic solvents are an ill-defined group of chemicals but the main ones are toluene, white spirit, xylene, and a variety of alcohols and ketones. Most are used in paint manufacture and it is mainly workers in this industry who have been investigated for neurobehavioural disorders.

The effects of organic solvents range from mild fatigue to frank psychosis. In view of the vague nature of many of the manifestations, psychometric testing has proved useful for both chemical and epidemiological studies. Nevertheless, there is still considerable controversy over the severity of effects that can arise from workplace exposures. Psychosis, dementia, and compensatable disability appear to be frequent in Scandinavian studies but less severe effects have been described in other Western countries. This may be due, for example, to the differences in exposures for house painters in winter-time work between Denmark and the southern states of Europe or North America. Alternatively, some earlier studies tended to record a more severe effect, which may be a reflection of earlier, higher exposure levels. Certainly, in the more recent studies the measurable effects tend to be milder and to include slowed reaction time and diminished ability to concentrate.

Emotional lability and irritability are also consistently reported but are less easy to measure. Indeed, the earliest account of neurobehavioural disorders by Delpeche in 1856 recounts horrific tales of insomnia, nightmares, violent rages, and sexual problems in workers exposed to carbon disulphide in small, poorly ventilated Parisian workshops. Most chlorinated hydrocarbons can produce a 'high' following acute exposures although it is unclear whether the synergism between many of these solvents and ethyl alcohol increases social drinking.

In the clinical context, such a wide range of neuropsychological effects require careful evaluation which involves not only workplace exposures, but also the patient's social habits and previous psychiatric state. The widespread use of anxiolytic and hypnotic drugs in the general population only serves to complicate the clinician's evaluation (see also Chapter 3).

*Neuropathic chemicals*

By contrast, the clear cut peripheral neuropathy induced by chemicals such as inorganic lead compounds, n-*hexane*, and *methyl* n-*butyl ketone*, are relatively easy to evaluate. In these cases, the underlying pathology is either axonal degeneration and/or segmental demyelination. The neuropathy is normally mixed sensorimotor but inorganic lead is unusual in causing a pure motor neuropathy.

*Other neurological effects*

Parkinsonism can be a feature of poisoning by *carbon disulphide*, *manganese* and, possibly, *carbon monoxide*, whereas *epilepsy* is a feature of toxicity associated with organochlorine pesticides and the organic compounds of tin, mercury, and lead.

As usual, common things are the most common, and in the industrial setting, the largest group of workers exposed to neurotoxins are those employed in the industries using organic solvents; in particular the dry-cleaning, degreasing, and paints industry. For these categories, there are an estimated 7–10 million workers in the United States. Thus, it is the neurobehavioural abnormalities which are numerically of great importance and which, perversely, are also the most difficult neurological group to evaluate.

## Conclusions

A number of workplace exposures can cause neurological disease. Whilst physical and psychological factors can produce effects which are usually relatively easily linked to occupation, the chemical neurotoxic agents are more numerous and have the potential to affect a much larger population of people. The neuro-behavioural disorders associated with organic solvents are the most common of these producing a spectrum of illness ranging from mild fatigue and irritability to frank neuropathy or encephalopathy. The range and complexity of the clinical manifestations combined with the complex exposure characteristics of the work-force make clinical evaluation difficult. Such clinical effects are not uncommon in the unexposed general population and pre-existing symptoms of this kind will be enhanced by workplace exposure.

## Specific neurological conditions

### Introduction

On p. 117 *et seq.* of this chapter signs and symptoms of disease and their rela-tionship to work were considered independent of their cause or underlying di-agnosis. The signs and symptoms which will occur in such conditions as head injury or cerebral infarction depend on the site of the lesion. Although the signs and symptoms of disease give a better assessment of work capability than the diagnosis, the diagnosis is important in assessing the prognosis and future work capability. The diagnosis needs to be known when deciding whether a person should be employed, given a long period of time off work or recommended for retirement on the grounds of ill health. Very often it is not possible with brain disease to decide how much of the employee's disability is physical and how much psychological, and it can even be a disadvantage to attempt to be precise in separating them.[6,7]

The diseases in this section are listed in a rough order of frequency.

### Migraine

Page 123 referred to headaches and the use of analgesia, but the management of migraine is more than the treatment of an acute headache. Migraine is frequently familial and usually starts in childhood, sometimes as bilious attacks with ab-dominal pain and vomiting. The onset of headaches for the first time in an em-ployee is unlikely to be migraine unless associated with some other factor, such as commencement of use of a contraceptive drug. Migraine usually presents with a focal neurological symptom and then progresses to a unilateral headache. It is not uncommon for some of the attacks to occur without the aura or for the aura to occur without the headache. The manifestation of the migraine can change with time so an alteration in the character does not mean a new pathol-ogy. If the attacks occur sometimes on one side, sometimes on the other, even if the attacks on one of the sides are rare, it is most unlikely that the migraine is symptomatic of any underlying pathology. However, if all the attacks are on one side then a structural underlying pathology is more likely.

If an employee has headaches due to migraine, management should aim at pro-phylaxis rather than investigation. Many factors, some of which occur at work, can precipitate migraine. It is helpful for the employee to keep an account of ac-tivities in the 24 hours leading up to an attack. It may then be easier to identify any precipitating factor. Precipitation of an attack by specific foods is well recog-nized but less obvious factors may emerge. Missing meals, alcohol the previous night, sleeping in late, as well as environmental factors, such as temperature and humidity, may be implicated. Occupational health professionals can help to eluci-date the factors and possibly remove them. When an attack occurs early treatment with simple analgesics is usually sufficient but for those with more severe symp-toms specific treatment with *ergotamine* or *sumatriptan* may be necessary. The many methods of giving ergotamine is an indication of the variation in response. For those with infrequent but predictable migraine, for example premenstrually, a 2 mg ergotamine suppository, often only a half of one, may prevent the attacks. For those that need rapid relief *Lingraine* which can be sucked and absorbed through the buccal mucosa, or an ergotamine inhaler, may work. Ergotamine can have serious side-effects, especially if used frequently, and therefore the pre-scriptions should be carefully monitored. Recently sumatriptan, which is a 5-hydroxytryptamine agonist, has become available as an injection and even more recently as a tablet for use in the acute attack. It is still too early to assess its long-term value but it appears to be relatively safe.

More important than the medication itself is the way in which the migraine is handled in the workplace. A relatively relaxed attitude by the employer allowing the employee to lie down or rest for a while when the attack starts and a sympa-thetic understanding will mean that the employee spends less time off work. Employees will have greater confidence to go to work if they know that an attack at work will be more acceptable than missing work and staying at home. Psychological factors are less important in migraine than in stress and tension headaches.

Stress (tension) headaches are more a manifestation of psychological prob-lems than neurological problems although neurological opinions are often sought in an attempt to find a physical cause for a non-organic disability. The proper use of analgesia is very important in the management of tension headaches as otherwise the headaches themselves become an additional cause of anxiety which makes them even worse.

## Cerebrovascular disease

Cerebrovascular disease can be conveniently divided into two categories: haem-orrhages and ischaemia; the latter may lead to infarction. The two may some-times occur together as haemorrhage can occur into an infarct or the haemorrhage may precipitate arterial spasm and hence ischaemia and an infarct.

*Ischaemic* events can be minimal with possibly a transient numbness or loss of vision and are unlikely to be a handicap at work unless the employee is a driver or works with dangerous machinery. Because *transient ischaemic attacks* often precede a serious stroke the patient should be investigated in order to insti-gate prophylactic management. Occasionally, investigations demonstrate a mod-erate stenosis of the internal carotid artery without complete occlusion which may be amenable to surgery. If the patient has no contraindication to anticoagu-lants, e.g., hypertension, recurrent transient ischaemic attacks can usually be treated with anticoagulants.

The severity of a cerebral infarct can vary considerably, sometimes there is complete functional recovery; at other times the disability is profound and per-manent and incompatible with a return to work. No conclusion, therefore, about work capability can be made on the diagnosis alone. When the patient has recov-ered to a certain extent, a functional assessment can be made by a physiothera-pist or occupational therapist and, with the occupational physician, a policy for future management can be made. A visit to the workplace by an occupational therapist is helpful in planning a return to work or adjustment of the work practice.

There is a wide range in the time taken to reach maximum recovery which may be a year or more. However, by the end of about four months it is usually possible to give a reliable prognosis because by then the functions which are re-covering are clear and any function which has not started to recover is unlikely to show a significant improvement even with further therapy. For example, if a person is unable to walk, even with mechanical aids, by the end of four months therapy it is unlikely that unaided walking will ever be achieved; but if the em-ployee can walk, say 70 metres after four months it is possible that a year later he will be able to walk more than a kilometre. However, if the employee has not received optimum physiotherapy and rehabilitation a prognosis should not be given. Long-term therapy should concentrate on improving functions. Persisting disabilities should be overcome with mechanical aids or alterations in work practices. Rehabilitation after a cerebral infarct requires considerable skill and if there is any problem the employee should be referred to a rehabilitation special-ist even if the disability is not gross. The prognosis for further strokes depends on the underlying pathology. Cardiac factors, the blood pressure, and medication can all be important in assessing the prognosis. It would be wrong to prevent a person returning to work just because of the anxiety of the employer that a further episode might occur. Each employee needs to have the prognosis assessed individually.

With a *haemorrhagic intracerebral stroke* the clinical situation is usually much more serious, most patients become unconscious and death is frequent. If the cerebral haemorrhage is small some recovery will occur but because of the cerebral destruction by the blood at arterial pressure there is usually a permanent deficit. The rehabilitation process for those who will be able to return to work is similar to those with cerebral infarction, except that with an intracerebral haem-orrhage there is a longer period of acute illness before functional recovery begins.

Decisions about returning to work should not be taken early, especially while improvement is still occurring, which is a cause for optimism. However, once a plateau is reached in the recovery further improvement is unlikely. The prognosis for a further attack depends, as for an infarct, on the underlying cause of the cerebrovascular disease.

A subarachnoid haemorrhage needs to be considered separately. If it is not severe, bleeding is confined to the subarachnoid space and recovery is complete. In more severe cases there may be cerebral damage, which can be transient or permanent. The rehabilitation process is similar to that of a cerebral infarct. If the subarachnoid haemorrhage is due to an aneurysm which is treated successfully by surgery then the prognosis is very good and a further haemorrhage is unlikely.

## Cerebral tumours

Unlike tumours elsewhere in the body, cerebral tumours do not metastasize outside the central nervous system. The malignancy of a tumour can vary from very benign to rapidly malignant. Most benign tumours can be treated successfully by surgery, some of the malignant ones can be halted by radiotherapy, and a few are amenable to chemotherapy.

Following treatment, an assessment of the employee's function and information about the prognosis usually makes a decision about work easy. If function is good, return to work should be automatic but if it is not then the decision to return will rest on two opposing trends. First, there is the natural improvement that will occur with rehabilitation and recovery from the surgery or other treatment and this is not dissimilar to recovery from a stroke. Secondly, there is the natural history of the tumour which if malignant or liable to recur makes the long-term prognosis worse. In practice, information about this is usually available and the decisions are rarely difficult.

## Head injuries

Many patients with severe head injuries will have other trauma such as fractured limbs and this makes management harder and recovery slower. The prognosis is worse when there is associated impairment of vision, hearing or speech. The prognosis is improved if the previous job remains available and the employer is prepared to make special provisions when work is recommenced.

In more severe cases improvement can continue for up to two years while in some cases the injury is so bad and the brain damage so extensive that there is never any possibility of returning to work. However, there are many patients whose injuries are not obviously very severe yet who have difficulty in returning successfully to their previous work.[9]

With concussion there are multiple minor (or major) injuries in the brain with contusion and disruption of the cerebral connections. However, the physical signs of organic disease can be minimal. The patient may look normal but feel unwell. A plaster for a simple limb fracture will often prevent a patient turning up for work but a conscientious employee who has had concussion may seek to return to work too quickly. The plaster encourages sympathy from the employer, but the employee who looks well but says he has a severe headache and cannot concentrate on his work is less well understood. The decision when to advise a person with a head injury to return to work is a difficult one and it is important that the patient should be given sufficient time to recover. If there are any specific problems the advice and help of an occupational therapist may be needed.

Headaches after brain trauma are common and are more severe and more frequent if the patient is under stress or working hard. The patient may feel well when resting at home but headaches develop when he has to cope with commuting and the physical and mental demands of his job. It is therefore helpful to allow the patient to return to work gradually. Returning to work on a Thursday rather than a Monday will mean that after two days work he has an opportunity to rest. It is unfortunate and medically illogical that most patients are asked to return to work at the start of a week. In more severe cases, a planned return to work with advice from the occupational health service may enable half day working, say from 10.30 a.m. to 3 p.m. to be considered; or three days a week for a few weeks so that the long-term recovery is more successful.

Symptomatic treatment for post concussional headaches and other symptoms is important. A small regular dose of an analgesic for a few weeks may be better than waiting for the headache to become severe and then finding that the analgesia does not work. Again this needs to be discussed with the employee at the same time as giving the correct advice on when to take it. Most patients want to return to work and with good management this can be achieved successfully.

Unfortunately, there are significant numbers of patients after head injuries who, without having any demonstrable physical signs, have problems with rehabilitation. This may be because they were encouraged to get back to work too quickly, developed increasing or further symptoms, and lost faith in their ability to recover. Psychological problems are common for many reasons and can be the direct consequence of the injury causing physical changes in the brain, but manifest clinically as psychological problems; or the problem may be less physical and due more to secondary psychological problems. For example, an employee who has been assaulted may suffer from mental trauma as well as the physical trauma and counselling may be necessary. Sometimes the sympathetic encouragement of an employer can help the patient to return gradually to work and so develop a return of confidence, instead of further anxiety. Insomnia in this group is common. Occasionally night sedation is helpful, but should never be allowed to become a habit. More often a tricyclic antidepressant taken only at night will help. The initial dose should be low in order to avoid unwanted effects and then gradually increased as appropriate.

Neurotic patients are not common but do cause considerable difficulties in rehabilitation and take up a disproportionate amount of time and effort of the occupational health and personnel departments. The neurosis may be fostered by a legal claim for compensation. If the head injury occurred at work the complications become even greater and pose particular problems for the occupational physician who has his duty to the patient as an employee, as well as being asked to give advice to the employer. These patients often require specialist help to reach a correct assessment of the problem and for treatment.

Intellectual impairment without other physical signs is not common after head injury, but if it is suspected, especially if work capability might be affected, it needs to be assessed specifically. Psychometric testing will usually resolve the extent of any organic impairment and when this is used in association with an occupational therapist's assessment and the knowledge of the patient's work requirements, appropriate plans for a return to work can be made. As with other organic lesions of the brain, functional improvement does occur but takes time and, depending on the severity of the injury, may not be complete. For an employee in an executive type of job it can be counterproductive to return to work too soon or too suddenly and a gradual return to work is advisable initially; taking on only some of his responsibilities at first and then adding to them. All sedatives and medication which might impair intellectual function or reduce concentration should be stopped unless there is a very strong indication for them. Tranquillizers to reduce anxiety will only make thought processes slower and can be counterproductive. Occasionally there is a good indication for medication, e.g., if there is epilepsy or if depression is reducing intellectual function.

Employees should be advised to do everything they can do for themselves to help recovery. This means eating regularly, going to bed at reasonable hours, and adjusting their lifestyle to improve performance. Alcohol should be prohibited until the employee is working to his own satisfaction and his work is acceptable to his employers. Until his work is acceptable the employee is at risk of losing his job or being downgraded or passed over for promotion. Alcohol-related problems are not uncommon in patients who have had head injuries. A 'catch-22' situation can arise because the employee who has no difficulty in adhering to the ban is the one who probably does not need to; while the employee who does not comply, especially if he disputes it or deceives his medical advisers, is the one who probably needs to keep to it.

*Driving*

Doctors have a duty to advise patients concerning their fitness to drive a motor vehicle. Decisions on this can be difficult for patients with head injuries or neurological diseases. The Driving Licence Regulations and the role of the Driving and Vehicle Licensing Agency (DVLA) are discussed in Appendix 1, and the particular problems arising in relation to epilepsy are discussed in Chapter 8. With neurological disease or trauma to the nervous system, the problem is whether the deficit in neurological function is a bar to driving. The doctor should assess the ability of the patient to operate car controls and to respond quickly, accurately, and intelligently to driving conditions. If a disability lasts less than three months the patient does not have to inform the DVLA and the doctor's advice about driving during these three months is sufficient. This means that only with short-lasting disabilities does the doctor have the duty and responsibility to give a definite opinion on the patient's fitness to drive.

When the disability lasts more than three months and the patient either feels unsafe driving or has symptoms or signs which, in the opinion of the doctor, may impair driving the DVLA should be informed by the patient. The doctor cannot have the final decision on whether or not a patient should drive; this lies with the DVLA and ultimately with the courts if a patient wishes to challenge the DVLA. The doctor's duty is to advise the patient and when appropriate inform the patient of his or her duty to inform the DVLA of the disability. If there is any doubt, the patient should inform the DVLA. The DVLA will seek information from the doctor. The patient may be able to adapt the car, e.g., by installing hand controls so that the feet are not needed, to make driving safer and easier. Adaptations will be considered when deciding whether a licence can be issued or continued. The DVLA may ask doctors with special experience of these cases to test the patient. If the patient is judged unfit to drive he may later re-apply to the DVLA when improvement in the medical condition has occurred.

Employers have a responsibility to ensure that their drivers are medically fit. Generally, if the employee's driving ability is acceptable to the DVLA when they have all the information, the employee should not be prevented from driving. It is important that the insurance covers disabled drivers. On the whole, it is likely that disabled drivers (with valid licences issued by the DVLA when the DVLA is aware of the disability) have no more accidents than drivers without physical disabilities. The regulations for LGVs (large goods vehicles) and PCVs (passenger carrying vehicles) are stricter and are discussed in Appendix 1.

### Birth injuries and congenital cerebral palsies

Cerebral palsy is not a contraindication to work and the patient may have no intellectual impairment even though the physical disability can be considerable. The likely success in employment is usually decided long before the patient seeks to be an employee. Good training and education allowing the child to develop his or her abilities will result in qualifications for an appropriate job. Minor physical disabilities are rarely a problem except when skilled motor activities are needed. Today, with automation and technology there is more need to develop intellectual skills. Many machines can be adapted and driving is usually possible although this may require special adaptations.

For the employer it is easier to assess the long term potential of the employee because birth injuries and congenital cerebral palsies are not progressive. With age, secondary problems may occur earlier than in the normal population, e.g., arthritis in a hip is more likely if the gait is affected, but these changes do not develop quickly. At the start of employment it is advisable to have a full medical and functional assessment so that work can be adjusted to allow the employee to use his skills more efficiently. Congenital disease of the spinal cord, such as in spina bifida, is managed in the same way.

## Spinal cord

Spinal cord disease secondary to vertebral and disc diseases is discussed in Chapter 9. The most usual cause of acute spinal cord lesions is trauma of which a significant proportion occurs at work. Primary spinal canal tumours are rare and are usually benign, neurofibromas being the most frequent. Secondary malignant metastases, especially from the breast and bronchus are common but are usually associated with advanced disease and management is dictated by the primary neoplasm. The most common neurological spinal disease is multiple sclerosis.

## Multiple sclerosis (MS)

Multiple sclerosis usually starts during working life and is therefore likely to develop after an employee has passed any medical examination at the time of initial employment. Clinically, the diagnosis depends on the demonstration of multiple lesions disseminated in time and space in the central nervous system. Modern techniques such as magnetic resonance imaging (MRI) allow lesions to be demonstrated when they are not causing clinical symptoms and hence the diagnosis can be made when only one clinical episode has occurred. Evoked potentials can be used to assess the speed of conduction of the nerve impulse within the nervous system. The most frequently used is the visual evoked potential. The response to flashing or other visual stimulation can be recorded in the posterior part of the brain. Although the response is not a direct measurement of the speed of the nerve impulse from the eye to the occipital cortex, when there is demyelination in the optic pathways the response is delayed.

Other evoked potentials, produced by a sound in the ear or stimulation of a limb, can be measured. A delay in response is not proof of MS because other diseases can cause delay but it can provide evidence of a symptomless lesion and hence demonstrate that there are lesions at more than one site.

A doctor should be cautious before making a diagnosis of MS. In the early stages, as in many other neurological diseases, the findings may be compatible with a variety of illnesses and it is often only later that the diagnosis becomes more clear. Therefore, in the early stages MS should be a differential diagnosis rather than a definitive conclusion. Multiple sclerosis can have a wide range of outcomes. There may be only one clinical episode, with full recovery, and no other trouble throughout life or it may progress rapidly, or any other gradation in between. The manifestations vary enormously, but they are always due to a lesion of the central nervous system and MS never involves the peripheral nervous system. (The optic nerve is a part of the central nervous system and not a peripheral nerve.)

Common manifestations are a single episode of visual deterioration lasting only a few weeks, an area of sensory disturbance in a limb or on the trunk, or an episode of ataxia or sphincter disturbance.

Some symptoms may influence working ability.[8] Because there is such variation it is impossible to predict the prognosis. After a single episode with full recovery the prognosis should be hopeful and an employee should be encouraged to return to normal work. If the attacks are infrequent and there is full recovery after each the amount of time off work over a period of years could be small. No precipitating factors for exacerbations are known and therefore there is no work environment which will alter the prognosis. However, if a patient has not made a full recovery it is possible that certain environments may make the symptoms greater or more obvious. High temperatures are not well tolerated and some patients like to work in slightly colder environments than is usually desired by other employees as this reduces their symptoms. Poor sleep and irregular hours are other factors which may worsen symptoms.

If an employee has established MS then adjustments in work practices may be needed and these will depend on the clinical manifestations and the nature of the work. For those already in work, the majority remain at work for more than five years. The attacks of the disease can be acute with good recovery in which case a limited period of rehabilitation will speed return to work. In more chronic cases, regular assessments to decide about physiotherapy or other ongoing help will be more appropriate. Urgency of micturition is common and if there is easy access to toilets incontinence is rare. In very severe cases of MS special arrangements for the use of a wheelchair may be necessary.

Occasionally, if there is considerable demyelination of the white matter in the brain, there may be intellectual deterioration but usually intellectual function is preserved and this means that if the employee has a sedentary job MS should not mean retirement on medical grounds. There are psychological problems that occur in chronic illness and these need to be considered by the employee's medical advisers. Depression is not uncommon. Euphoria, best defined in this context as pathological contentment, is often mentioned as a symptom of MS. It is not common but as it is rarer in other central nervous system diseases it may be regarded as characteristic of MS. The patient who is not severely disabled will accept the illness and not appear too distressed by his or her problems. This has advantages for the sufferer as a patient but may not as an employee who must have an increased commitment to work if he or she is going to overcome the problems of the disability and continue as a competent and dependable worker. Often euphoria can remove the wish to 'fight' the disability, the employee is content to give in, stops working, and becomes a patient and no longer an employee.

Motivation to work is a very important factor in deciding whether employment can continue, either in its original or modified form. Most patients with continuing symptoms from MS will have attended hospital and their diagnosis and management policy will have been formulated. If this has not occurred referral to a specialist should be made before the employee's future work situation is decided.

## Peripheral neuropathy

Neuropathy is a common condition. About 85 per cent of all patients with peripheral neuropathy have diabetes mellitus and the control of the diabetes is the most important factor in the management of the neuropathy. It is necessary for the employee to take particular care of his or her feet. The second most common cause of peripheral neuropathy is alcohol abuse. In the early stages, alcoholic neuropathy is reversible if the employee ceases taking alcohol and is given vitamin B. Taking vitamin B without stopping alcohol is insufficient— intelligent employees knowing they are taking too much alcohol may put themselves on vitamin B and continue taking excess alcohol so delaying the onset of the neuropathy but making it less easy to reverse when it does occur. Other medical causes of a peripheral neuropathy are rare, but should be sought if no obvious cause is apparent. Subacute combined degeneration, due to vitamin $B_{12}$ depletion, may come on insidiously but the neuropathy always responds to vitamin $B_{12}$ injections. Hereditary motor and sensory neuropathies, one type of which used to be called Charcot–Marie–Tooth disease, can also be insidious, producing gradually increasing disability. A family history makes the diagnosis easier, but as some are due to recessive genes sporadic cases are not uncommon. Usually, the signs precede the disability and poor muscle bulk in the hands or the legs will alert a doctor to the possibility of this disease.

The diagnosis is not a reason to cease work and as the progress is slow the patient can often continue at work for many years and retire in the normal way. In some severe cases, mechanical aids, such as a toe-raising splint, will often increase function. A peripheral neuropathy is a recognized complication of many toxic chemicals. Therefore, the onset of a peripheral neuropathy should always alert the doctor to the possibility of a toxic chemical exposure at work.

## Muscle diseases

Acute muscle disease, such as myositis, is usually associated with some other disease, upon which its prognosis will depend (see Also p. 120).

## Motor neurone disease (MND)

Motor neurone disease although not common, is an important disease in relation to work. It tends to manifest during middle age, before retirement, and progresses relentlessly causing death in an average of three years. In the early stages, it can be difficult to diagnose as it may present with some relatively minor event. For example, if the condition starts with a weakness in one foot, this may lead to a fall and, perhaps, a sprained ankle, and for some time the slow recovery may be attributed to trauma and loss of motivation to return to work. However, with time the progression of the disease to other sites makes the diagnosis easier.

Unfortunately no amount of physiotherapy or medication will improve the weakness of MND. In fact, excess physiotherapy may exhaust a patient making it harder for him to do his work. Management should be aimed at allowing the patient to lead as normal a life as possible. Speech therapy and communication aids are frequently required as the bulbar muscles are often involved and are usually the major reason for physical deterioration and death. Late in the illness the patient is unable to swallow and will inhale saliva. Unfortunately, there is no curative treatment and therefore tracheostomy is rarely justified. The patient's mental ability is unimpaired and with environmental aid systems the patient may be able to manipulate the environment by using a computer-driven motor to open doors, turn on lights or operate a telephone, as well as being able to use the computer for more ordinary tasks such as writing letters.

## Parkinson's disease

Parkinson's disease often starts in the sixth decade especially if it is idiopathic. Its symptoms and signs are discussed on p. 120. Cerebrovascular Parkinsonism starts later and is usually a part of generalized cerebrovascular disease. There are other rare causes. This means that most Parkinson's disease in the working population is idiopathic. It may occasionally be associated with exposure to toxic compounds and therefore an occupational physician should consider this possibility in order to remove the employee from such a dangerous environment and also to protect other employees. Parkinson's disease develops insidiously and initially can be unilateral. The patient may not develop a tremor although this is often the most striking feature to a lay person. The most disabling feature is the bradykinesia. The patient's tremor decreases on voluntary movement and is rarely a disability unless fine movements are needed. However, the bradykinesia makes the employee slower and if there is no tremor his colleagues do not realize that he has a physical illness.

As Parkinson's disease responds to treatment an early diagnosis is important. An astute colleague will realize that the employee is not being lazy because he will be slow at dressing, eating, and doing all his everyday tasks as well as being slow at his work. However, some employers are mistaken in assuming first, that slowness of movement means slowness of thought and secondly, that Parkinson's disease is a contraindication to work. Most patients with Parkinson's disease can stay at work until normal retirement age. A conscientious employee will often compensate by getting to work early or staying late to refute possible suggestions of laziness. The patient's writing will become smaller and it is often found that their writing was getting smaller long before any other disability was noted. In this respect, Parkinson's disease is different from senile or idiopathic tremor where there is no rigidity and no bradykinesia and the writing does not become smaller although it is spidery and tremulous.

Parkinson's disease responds well to *levodopa* preparations, *Madopar* and *Sinemet* being the two most widely used. Adjusting the dosage to give a good response without unwanted effects may be difficult and much care may be necessary to achieve the optimum dose, which should be kept as small as possible and compatible with good functional improvement. The therapeutic index of *levodopa* decreases the longer it is used, so that unwanted effects become worse and its efficacy shorter in duration. Therefore, the administration of *levodopa* should be delayed if the Parkinsonism is mild and the employee has no disability. More recently, *selegiline* has been introduced and is advocated as an early and initial treatment because it is claimed to delay the progress of the disease although this has not been conclusively demonstrated. Most employees who are able to travel to work and perform their duties satisfactorily will not benefit from physiotherapy but if the condition is severe, advice from a physiotherapist can often help them to remain at work.

Patients with Parkinson's disease have difficulty in performing skilled movements and are particularly bad at developing new skills. However, if the motor skill is a longstanding one, such as playing the piano, it may be retained when other apparently much easier tasks are impossible. Employees should not take early retirement because of Parkinson's disease unless it is making work impossible, as continuing at work can help the patient to remain mobile and active. Most employees with Parkinson's disease have normal intellectual function, although there is a group, especially the older patients, who do develop intellectual impairment.

### Essential (idiopathic or familial) tremor

Benign tremor is common but not associated with bradykinesia or rigidity and is rarely a disability except for writing, which may become scrawly but not small. The tremor can be an embarrassment and may be mistaken for Parkinson's disease and therefore the employee and employer may need reassurance. If it is a problem a beta-blocking drug may be used but should be avoided if possible.

### Alzheimer's disease and dementia

Dementia tends to appear in more elderly patients, but when it does occur in someone still at work it is a major problem. The employee has no physical disability and the dementia can develop very insidiously. If the employee has been at the same job for many years the dementia may be less obvious. He or she can work relatively well in familiar surroundings at routine tasks but new tasks are difficult. Colleagues will often be aware of the deterioration. Unfortunately, there is no treatment and a decision needs to be made about continuing employment. Alcohol is an important factor in exacerbating the dementia whether it is taken acutely or over a long period.

## Encephalitis

Encephalitis is relatively rare and its prognosis and influence on work ability vary. Herpes encephalitis can cause much brain damage and these patients may never get back to intellectually demanding occupations. Other, less severe types of encephalitis usually result in full recovery. AIDS encephalitis is a progressive disease which leads to increasing dementia and has a very bad prognosis.

## Post-viral fatigue syndrome

Postviral fatigue syndrome/myeloencephalitis (ME) are less well-defined entities but *postviral disabilities* are common. Fortunately, they usually clear spontaneously during the convalescent stage of the illness. The more protracted symptoms, in the absence of physical signs, are probably due to several factors, both physical and mental.

Following a severe viral illness a period is required for full recovery. During this convalescent phase, exercise and mental and emotional stress are less well tolerated. Exercise is important and should not be avoided as resting muscles cannot increase their strength and endurance. However, excessive exercise leads to increased symptoms. Initially, the amount of exercise should be small and the rate of increase modified according to the symptoms. Similarly, returning too quickly to a stressful job can lead to poor performance, loss of confidence, and exacerbation of the symptoms. The employee should be allowed to work himself back into a job—if a manual worker, possibly by starting work on a Thursday or a Friday so that a weekend's rest follows or, if working at a desk, by only doing undemanding work for the first week. People vary in the amount of convalescence they need and the doctor needs to give individual advice. However, the symptoms should decrease. A serious problem arises when either the symptoms persist without improvement or there has been no definite viral illness. This syndrome has been labelled ME but without any clear criteria of its severity and without laboratory tests to support it, there is considerable uncertainty as to whether it is, in fact, a single clinical entity. If an employee is possibly suffering from this condition it is important to exclude other illnesses, and to formulate a policy for management which might include the help of occupational and other physicians, occupational therapists, physiotherapists or psychiatrists depending on the exact symptoms.

## Selected references and further reading

1.   Matthews, W.B. (1986). Neurology. In *Oxford textbook of medicine*, (ed. D.J. Weatherall, J.G.G. Ledingham, and D.A. Warrell), (2nd edn). Oxford University Press.

2.  Feldman, R.G. and Pransky, G.S. (1988). Neurological considerations in worker fitness evaluation. In *Occupational medicine: state of the art reviews*, (Eds. Himmelstein, J.S. and Pransky, G.S.), Vol. 3, No. 2, pp. 299–308. Hanley & Belfus, Philadelphia.
3.  Kurtzke, J.F. (1985). Neurological system. In *Oxford textbook of public health*, (ed. W.W. Holland, R. Detels, G. Knox, and E. Breeze), Vol. 4, pp. 203–49. Oxford University Press.
4.  Secretary of State for Health (1991). *The health of the nation*, (Cmnd. 1523). HMSO, London.
5.  Baker, E.L. (1988). Neurological and behavioural disorders. In *Occupational health*, (ed. B.S. Levy and D.H. Wegman), (2nd edn). Little Brown, Boston.
6.  Ward, C.D. (ed). (1992). Hither neurology—meeting the challenge of neurological disability. *J. Neurol. Neurosurg. Psychiat.*, **55** (Suppl.)
7.  Illis, L.S., Sedgwick, E.M., and Glanville, H.J. (1982). *Rehabilitation of the neurological patient*. Blackwell, Oxford.
8.  Mitchell, J.N. (1981). Multiple sclerosis and the prospects of employment. *J. Soc. Occup. Med.*, **31**, 134–8.
9.  Johnson, R. (1987). Return to work after severe head injury. *Int. Disabil. Studies*, **9**, 49–54.
10. Gemne, G., Pyykkö, I., Taylor, W., and Pelmear, P.L. (1987). The Stockholm Workshop scale for the classification of cold-induced Raynaud's phenomenon in the hand–arm vibration syndrome (revision of Taylor–Pelmear Scale). *Scand. Work Environ. Hlth.*, **13**, 275–7.

# 8

# Epilepsy

*I. Brown and S.D. Shorvon*

## Introduction

The World Health Organization's definition of epilepsy is: 'a chronic brain disorder of various aetiologies characterized by recurrent seizures due to excessive discharge of cerebral neurones.'[1] In practice, the diagnosis of epilepsy is applied to a person who has a persisting tendency to recurrent epileptic seizures. Neither single nor occasional epileptic seizures, febrile seizures nor acute symptomatic seizures (those occurring during an acute illness) are usually classified as epilepsy. A single unprovoked seizure is not considered sufficient evidence to justify a diagnosis of epilepsy, unless other evidence of a tendency to recurrence is found (e.g., EEG evidence of epilepsy or a structural lesion on neuroimaging). Epilepsy can cause medical, psychological, and social problems, each of which can have an important impact on everyday life. It is a common condition which affects large numbers of working people. In about one-third, epilepsy is the only handicap, and in the others there are additional neurological, intellectual or psychological problems.

## Classification of epilepsy

Epileptic seizures can take highly variable forms, of which the well-known grand mal (tonic-clonic) convulsion is only one example. Thus, epilepsy is commonly classified according to seizure type.[2] Seizures are divided into two main categories: *generalized seizures,* in which initial epileptic discharges involve widespread areas of both cerebral hemispheres simultaneously; and *partial seizures,* which focus in a small area of the cerebral cortex. *Generalized seizures* are subdivided into tonic-clonic seizures, absence seizures (petit mal), myoclonic seizures, tonic seizures, and atonic seizures, each with differing clinical forms but consciousness is lost in all. The clinical features of partial seizures are highly variable, reflecting the function of that part of the brain involved in the epileptic discharge. *Partial seizures* are subdivided into three main types: (1) simple partial seizures in which there is no alteration of consciousness; (2) complex partial seizures in which consciousness is lost or impaired; and (3) secondarily generalized seizures in which the epileptic discharge starts focally and then spreads triggering a generalized convulsion.

## Prevalence and Incidence

There are practical problems in establishing the prevalence and incidence of epilepsy. First, the condition is episodic. Between attacks the patient may be perfectly normal, with normal investigations. Thus, the diagnosis is essentially clinical, relying heavily on an eye-witness account of the attacks. Secondly, there is a large number of other conditions in which consciousness may be transiently impaired and which may be confused with epilepsy. Thirdly, the condition may be unreported, for several reasons. The patient may be unaware of the nature of his attacks, and so not seek medical help. Patients with mild epilepsy, or partial seizures, in particular, may not consult a doctor, and may be missed in surveys. Finally, the term 'epilepsy' needs to be clearly defined in such studies. The question of whether to include single seizures arises, as does the issue of whether people who have been seizure-free for several years still have epilepsy. Febrile convulsions which affect up to 3 per cent of all healthy children between the ages of 18 months and 5 years, are usually excluded from population statistics.

Even with a restricted definition, epilepsy is a common condition. A British study documenting first seizures recorded in 67 general practices found an annual incidence rate, across all ages, of 63 cases per 100 000 persons per year, and other surveys and studies in other countries have found similar rates.[3,4] Throughout working life, from the ages of 16 to 65 years, first seizures occur at a rate of approximately 40 cases per 100 000 persons per year. The cumulative incidence of epilepsy, i.e., the risk of having a seizure at some point in life, has been estimated to lie between 2 and 5 per cent.[4]

The prevalence of active epilepsy has usually been found to be between 5 to 10 cases per 1000 persons, depending on the definitions and methods of investigation; epilepsy is thus amongst the most common of serious medical conditions.[3,4] Its prevalence is approximately similar at all ages after early childhood, and it affects all races and classes. The majority of patients suffer tonic-clonic (grand mal) seizures, either generalized or secondarily generalized. A recent British-based population prospective study (the National General Practice Study of Epilepsy: NGPSE), has provided definitive data on the characteristics of epilepsy in an unselected population.[5,6] In this investigation, 62 per cent of patients had tonic-clonic seizures (grand mal seizures, either primary or secondarily generalized), 11 per cent complex partial, 12 per cent mixed partial seizure types, while other seizure types were uncommon. A similar breakdown of seizure types has been recorded in other community-based studies. The frequency of seizures in a population is highly variable. About one-third of cases suffer seizures less than once a year, and about 20 per cent more than once a week.

### Causes of epilepsy

Traditional studies have shown that a cause can only be confidently established in only a minority of new cases of epilepsy (20 to 40 per cent). The likelihood of

**Table 8.1**   Common causes of adult onset epileptic seizures

- Genetic propensity
- Developmental anomalies (especially neuronal migrational defects)
- Head trauma (and neurosurgery)
- Structural cerebral lesion (e.g., tumour, haemorrhage, arteriovenous malformation)
- Cerebrovascular diseases (e.g., infarction, hypertensive vascular disease)
- CNS infection (e.g., meningitis, encephalitis, abscess)
- Degenerative disorders (e.g., Alzheimer's disease)
- Systemic diseases (e.g., renal, hepatic, haematological)
- Birth trauma
- Congenital/developmental disorders (e.g., cortical dysplasia)
- Toxic/iatrogenic (e.g., alcohol, psychotropic drugs, drug abuse)
- Metabolic disorders (e.g., hypercalcaemia, inappropriate antidiuretic hormone secretion)
- Drug withdrawal (e.g., psychotropic drugs)

establishing the underlying aetiology in a given patient is clearly dependent to a large degree on the extent of investigation. The wider use of MRI scanning will greatly increase the pick-up rate of previously undetectable underlying structural cerebral disorders, especially of the developmental type. The cause of epilepsy varies with age. Thus, epilepsy developing in young adults is most frequently due to alcohol or cerebral tumour, and, in late adult life, to cerebrovascular disease in those in whom a cause is found. Table 8.1 is a list of the most common causes of epileptic seizures in adults.

Toxic causes of epilepsy are rare. Seizures may occur as a result of lead encephalopathy, almost always in children. Seizures have occurred in employees over-exposed during the manufacture of chlorinated hydrocarbons, and ingestion or gross over-exposure to organochlorine insecticides has resulted in status epilepticus.[7] EEG abnormalities of epileptic type have been recorded in the absence of any clinical abnormality in workers exposed to methylene chloride, methyl bromide, carbon disulphide, benzene, and styrene, although the significance of these observations is uncertain.

### The recurrence of seizures

Usually, a person who has suffered a single seizure is not regarded as having epilepsy, which, by definition has a tendency to recurrence. Estimates of the risk of a second attack after a first have varied from 27 to 80 per cent, the variation reflecting selection bias in the study population. The NGPSE calculated recurrence rates by actuarial analysis in 564 unselected patients with newly presenting non-febrile seizures.[6] Overall, 67 per cent of patients had a recurrence within 12 months of a first attack and 78 per cent had a recurrence within 36 months. Seizures associated with a neurological deficit presumed present at birth had a

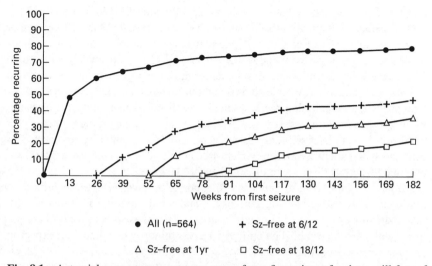

**Fig. 8.1** Actuarial percentage recurrence rates after a first seizure for those still free of recurrence at 6, 12, and 18 months, and for all patients. Three-year recurrence rates for all patients was 78 per cent, which fell to 44 per cent if a second seizure had not occurred within the first 6 months, and to 32 and 17 per cent for those seizure-free for 12 and 18 months, respectively.

100 per cent rate of relapse within the first 12 months, whereas seizures associated with a CNS lesion acquired postnatally carried a risk of relapse of 75 per cent by 12 months, and 85 per cent by 36 months. Seizures occurring with an acute insult to the brain carried a risk of relapse of 40 per cent by 12 months, and 46 per cent by 36 months.

It is well known that the risk of seizure recurrence is much higher in the first weeks or months after an initial attack, and the hazard rates for recurrent seizures in the NGPSE were 0.033 each week for the first 6 month period after the first attack, 0.007 each week for the next 6 month period, and 0.004 each week for the next 12 months. The longer the time period which passes without a second seizure, the less is the overall risk of subsequent recurrence; a fact which is often of great importance in resolving issues concerned with safety at work (see Fig. 8.1)

## Chances of remission of epilepsy

Although there is a high risk of recurrence after a first attack, most people developing epilepsy become seizure-free.[6,8] A simple comparison of prevalence and cumulative incidence rates shows that seizures cease in the great majority of patients who develop epilepsy.[8] Similarly, hospital-based studies of initial therapy in newly diagnosed patients, show that seizures are rapidly controlled in about 60–70 per cent of patients.[9] Population-based studies have also revealed that, 10 years after diagnosis, about 65 per cent of epileptic patients were in remission from seizures (defined as a 5 year period without attacks), and by 15 years from diagnosis, about 75 per cent were in remission. Most patients who enter remission, do so in the first 2 years after diagnosis. As time elapses without seizure control, the prospect of entering subsequent remission decreases markedly. In one British study, the probability of a patient whose epilepsy was still active at five years being in a two year remission 5 years later was only 33 per cent, and 38 per cent 10 years later. This contrasts with patients who were seizure-free at five years, amongst whom 100 per cent and 95 per cent were in remission 5 and 10 years later.

About 20–30 per cent of patients will continue to have seizures, regardless of treatment, and suffer chronic epilepsy. The good outcome in patients with newly diagnosed epilepsy is in sharp contrast to the subsequent prognosis of patients with chronic established epilepsy, only a minority of whom can expect to become seizure-free. Factors indicative of a poor prognosis include: a long duration of uncontrolled epilepsy; a combination of different seizure types; frequent seizures; partial epilepsy; structural cerebral disorder; mental handicap or the presence of associated neurological or psychiatric deficits.

*Benign Rolandic epilepsy* occurs in adolescence and does not usually recur after the initial manifestation. From an employment point of view it is important that these young people are not labelled epileptic.

## Prevention of epilepsy in the workplace

### Primary prevention

The prevention of head injuries is the most important preventive measure and is fundamental to safety at work, in the home, and on the road. Epilepsy does not follow a trivial head injury; however, if the head injury is associated with a depressed fracture (especially if the dura is torn), an intracranial haematoma, or focal neurological signs, then there is a significant risk of later epilepsy.[10]

The wearing of seat belts for all motorists and the introduction of a comfortable and strong safety helmet when appropriate are the obvious first preventive measures. This paradoxically reverses the usual order of safety steps used in occupational health and makes personal protection top of the list. Making the working environment safe should be the first step, but often the unpredictability of events makes this impossible. It should be compulsory that safety helmets are worn at all times in areas specified by the works' safety officer or safety committee. As a second step, the workforce should be made aware of areas above which other employees are operating at heights, so that these can be avoided if possible. A safety helmet will not protect an individual from serious head injury if anything heavy is dropped from a great height. If work has to be performed underneath such a hazard steel netting should be rigged to catch anything that falls.

## Secondary prevention

Patients who have had penetrating head injuries, or a cerebral abscess, have such a significant risk of seizures in the first two years after the acute event, that there are good arguments for choosing work for them, during this period, along the same lines as for someone who has already had a seizure, including a ban on driving. Although it is customary to give prophylactic anticonvulsants after a head injury of the type that is likely to be followed by epilepsy, controlled trials have yet to show any advantage.[11] The other main preventive measure is the avoidance of precipitating factors. Some of these are discussed below.

### Shiftwork

Seizures are common just before and just after waking, especially with primary generalized epilepsy, and so it might be felt that the introduction of a shift system into the work programme of a person with well-controlled epilepsy would predispose him to an increased frequency of seizures. Firm documentary evidence of a change in seizure frequency has not been found. This may be due to people with epilepsy opting out of shiftwork, as indicated by Dasgupta *et al.*[12] Many people with well-controlled epilepsy, however, can work rotating shifts without problems.

Patterns of sleep are disturbed by night-work and to a lesser extent by other types of shiftwork. Night-workers sleep for shorter periods during their working week and sleep longer on rest days, to make up the deficit.[13] Sleep deprivation is an important precipitant of seizures for some individuals, and is best avoided by those with epilepsy.

### Stress

An association between stress and seizure frequency has been the subject of many anecdotal reports. Changes in brain arousal lead to changes in excitability and this may affect neuronal discharges, particularly of those neurones that surround an epileptic focus.[14] Is there any scientific evidence to support this association? Substantial numbers of patients report that the frequency of their seizures increases if they are exposed to stress but stress itself may also be associated with other seizure-provoking factors such as alcohol and sleep deprivation. Conversely, inactivity and drowsiness may also be related to an increase in seizure frequency. The possibility that stress and its associated factors may have an adverse effect should be considered when employees with epilepsy are moved to different areas of responsibility.

### Photosensitivity

Photosensitive epilepsy is rare and usually associated with primary generalized epilepsy. It may need to be considered where a light source flickers. The overall prevalence is 1 in 10 000 but it is twice as common in females. Ninety per cent of patients have suffered their first convulsion due to photosensitivity before the age of 22 years.[15] Photosensitivity may be increased following deprivation of sleep.

The diagnosis of photosensitive epilepsy is supported by performing an EEG recording with photic stimulation and eliciting a photoconvulsive response. This is usually a generalized discharge of spike wave activity elicited by the flickering stimulus, persisting after the stimulus has ceased. Spontaneous seizures may occur in photosensitive subjects. It must be remembered that some individuals have a paroxysmal EEG response to photic stimulation, without any evidence of having had a seizure.[15]

Television is a common precipitant of photosensitive epilepsy. The provocative stimulus is the pattern of interlacing lines formed by the flying spot from the electron gun. Nearness to the set appears to be an important factor, as this enables the viewer to discriminate the line pattern. Background illumination is another factor. Flickering sunlight (e.g., through the leaves of a tree), faulty and flickering artificial lights, and glare are also occasional precipitants. **It would be unwise for a person with photosensitive epilepsy to work in a situation where television or video screens are in common use.** Swimming in bright sunlight may constitute some risk because of glare and flicker patterns on the water surface. Helicopter rotor blades and aeroplane propellers may also provoke episodes.

The use of a visual display unit (VDU) in employment constitutes a much smaller risk than that incurred while viewing television. The majority of VDUs have relatively slow phosphors in the tubes to reduce apparent flicker, and, in addition, they usually do not use an interlaced line pattern. **The probability of a first fit being induced by a VDU is exceedingly small and, even in the established photosensitive subject, unlikely to occur.**

The Civil Aviation Authority (CAA) has recognized the special risks that may be associated with flying, especially to the slow flicker that is visible through helicopter blades. The CAA performs an EEG investigation as part of its routine medical screen on all helicopter pilots applying for commercial licences. This is not presently required for professional fixed-wing aircraft pilots, but once harmonization of aviation medical standards is achieved throughout the European Union, possibly in 1996, it will almost certainly become mandatory for all professional pilots.

*Other types of reflex epilepsy*

Although reflex epilepsy may occasionally be induced by reading, concentrating, sudden startle or hearing music or bells, this is rare.

*Alcohol and drugs*

Alcohol consumed as beer appears to be a potent precipitant of seizures, especially if large volumes are consumed. This may be due to the moderate overhydration that occurs and a similar mechanism is possibly at work just before menstruation (although hormonal factors also contribute here).

A number of drugs have been incriminated as epileptogenic agents. By far the most common are the tricyclic antidepressants. Others include *isoniazid*, bronchodilators such as *theophylline* and *terbutaline*, and antipsychotic drugs such as *haloperidol* and *chlorpromazine*.

Fluctuating levels of anticonvulsant drugs, due to failure of compliance, interaction with other drugs *or sudden withdrawal* may also result in a seizure.

## What to do if a seizure occurs

If a seizure is likely to occur at work, supervisors and workplace colleagues should be warned and instructed in appropriate first-aid measures. Convulsive seizures are almost always short-lived and do not require immediate medical treatment. The person should be made as comfortable as possible preferably lying down (eased to the floor if seated); the head should be cushioned and any tight clothing or neckwear loosened. During the attack, the patient should not be moved, unless they are in a dangerous place, in a road, by a fire or hot radiator, at the top of stairs or by the edge of water, for instance. No attempt should be made to open the mouth or force anything between the teeth. After the seizure has subsided, the person should be rolled on to his or her side making sure that the airway is cleared of any obstruction, such as dentures or vomit and that there are no injuries which may require medical attention. When the patient recovers consciousness, there is often a short period of confusion and distress. The person should be comforted and reassured and allowed to rest. **An ambulance or hospital treatment is not required unless there is a serious injury, or the seizure lasts more than 10 minutes, or the person has a series of seizures without recovering consciousness between them.**

## The responsibility of the physician at the workplace

The first task is to establish without doubt that a seizure has occurred. The employee should attend the occupational health department as soon as possible and remain off work in the interim period. A detailed history of the event should be obtained and information sought from the patient and any reliable witness to try and establish the nature of the attack. Interviewing work colleagues and relatives who witnessed the event can be extremely useful, as the subject usually remembers very little beyond the first few seconds. It is very unwise to rely solely on written reports and second-hand information. Relevant points about family history and consumption of drugs or alcohol, should also be obtained. The patient should be fully examined, as a seizure may occasionally be the first symptom of a serious systemic illness such as meningitis, or of a local cerebral condition; detailed medical assessment is always necessary.

Permission to contact both family doctor and hospital consultant (if referral has taken place) should be obtained from the patient. It is often useful to contact these physicians informally and discuss the situation that has arisen. This should be followed by a formal letter giving a concise account of events, the examination findings, and requesting any further relevant information.

Not all episodes of unconsciousness are epileptic seizures: other possible diagnoses include syncope, drug overdose, paroxysmal cardiac arrhythmia, transient cerebral ischaemia (TIA), and simulated attacks.

Prolonged cerebral anoxia due to syncope may produce some twitching and even incontinence, although a generalized seizure is unusual. The focal ischaemia of a TIA does not usually involve loss of consciousness and is often a neurologically negative event, causing loss of function such as aphasia, and only rarely producing a convulsion. The possibility of a simulated attack may need to be considered.

Once it has been established as far as possible that a single, unprovoked, convulsion has taken place at work, the following procedure should be adopted:

1. The medical notes must state clearly the course of events and that a single seizure has taken place.

2. Management should be contacted and given clear and concise recommendations, in writing, regarding placement of the employee, without any breach of confidentiality. Such written recommendations should be constructed with the agreement of the employee. Some employees prefer to inform their immediate supervisor that they suffer from epilepsy and that this is well controlled with medication; it is worth discussing the possibility of such disclosure, which is usually agreed to by the patient.

3. The occupational physician and occupational health nurse must become familiar with any anticonvulsant prescribed and have a sound knowledge of both unwanted and toxic effects.

## Consideration of potential new employees

The most significant factor in recruiting a new employee is how well qualified is that individual for the job. It would be unrealistic to state that all jobs are suitable for a candidate with epilepsy but it is reasonable to state that the majority of jobs are suitable. Individuals should be considered on their merits and the reader is strongly recommended to a training manual prepared by the International Bureau for Epilepsy.[18] This gives some excellent practical advice, provides an assessment questionnaire and illustrates some typical cases with vocational scenarios.

## Sensible restrictions on the work of people with epilepsy

Restrictions must be discussed fully with the employee and with management. Clear written instructions should be given regarding placement, responsibilities, and review. Confidentiality must not be breached (see above). Restrictions should be no more than is necessary on common sense grounds, as would apply equally to any individual subject to sudden and unexpected lapses in consciousness or concentration, however infrequent.

In the United States it is illegal to deny employment to an otherwise qualified applicant because of disability, provided the disability does not impair health and safety standards at the workplace. However, this begs the question 'for what type of work is someone with epilepsy qualified?' The Epilepsy Foundation of America (EFA) has developed a comprehensive interview guide summarized by Masland.[16] The guide helps to define the important characteristics of a person's epilepsy, and draws attention to both advantageous and disadvantageous features. A consistent warning of attacks is certainly an advantageous feature, but is unusual. Conversely, sudden loss of consciousness without warning must be considered disadvantageous. The frequency of attacks is another important consideration and the success rate in placing people with epilepsy is far greater if they have fewer than six seizures per year.

In general, minor attacks are less disruptive than major ones, but periods of automatism (performance of acts without conscious will) may upset colleagues. Other particularly disadvantageous characteristics are prolonged periods of postictal confusion, and sudden akinetic attacks where the possibility of serious injury is increased.

It is impossible to be dogmatic for all occasions, as individuals and industries are infinitely variable. Sensible restrictions, however, include the following: climbing and working unprotected at heights, driving or operating motorized vehicles, working around unguarded machinery, working near fire or water, and working for long periods in an isolated situation. Hand-held power tools may be a hazard if they can be fixed in the 'on' position.

There are certain jobs with special hazards where the risk of even one seizure may give rise to catastrophic consequences. These jobs fall into two groups. The first of these is mainly in transport, and includes vocational drivers, train drivers, drivers of large container-terminal vehicles, crane operators, aircraft pilots, seamen, and commercial divers. The second group are jobs that include work at unprotected heights, e.g., scaffolders, steeplejacks, and firemen; work on mainline railways; with high-voltage electricity, hot metal, or dangerous unguarded machinery, e.g., chain saws; or near open tanks of chemical fluids, see Table 8.2.

The working environment and any equipment to be used by the employee with epilepsy should be inspected by the occupational physician. The safety officer and the employee's immediate supervisor should be involved in any decisions.

**Table 8.2**    Examples of jobs with special hazards (from Espir and Floyd 1986[17])

- Vocational drivers, i.e., of large goods and public service vehicles, and taxis
- Drivers of trains, cranes, straddle carriers
- Aircraft pilots, seamen, coastguards
- Work at unprotected heights, e.g., scaffolders, steeplejacks, and firemen
- Work with high-voltage electricity
- Work with dangerous unguarded machinery, e.g., chain saws
- Work with valuable fragile objects and equipment
- Work near tanks of water or chemical fluids

It is important to remind the employee that contravention of agreed restrictions may not only put his own life in danger, but also those of his colleagues and friends. The employee should also be reminded that it may be impossible to make any insurance claim for financial compensation for personal injuries should an accident occur as a result of evasion of agreed restrictions.

A policy should be established for terminating any restrictions on work practices. This policy should be made known to the affected employee and not altered unless circumstances are exceptional. There is little place for partial lifting of restrictions: the employee is either considered safe or not. If a work restriction is removed after a period of freedom from seizures, the employee should be instructed to report any further attack to the occupational health staff or to a personnel officer or manager. If anticonvulsant medication is stopped or changed, consideration should be given to close monitoring at work for a period, or to the temporary re-introduction of a suitable work restriction.

It may be found that following the introduction of medication, control is still poor with an unacceptable rate of seizure recurrence. It is important that every effort is made to improve control before the individual is rejected for employment or promotion. Perhaps there are certain precipitating factors that can easily be avoided, e.g., alcohol. Has an appropriate anticonvulsant been chosen, and an adequate serum level been achieved? (see pp. 51–2, 155).

Perhaps the employee is forgetful or actively non-compliant? Is there a correctable structural cause? All these possibilities should be explored and the occupational physician or occupational health nurse should co-ordinate their efforts with the family doctor and hospital consultant.

There should be a specific timescale for the removal of restrictions. A de-restriction review date should be offered, as this will ensure that the employee's future is being seriously considered and confirm that he or she is still a valuable member of the workforce. In this respect it seems reasonable to follow, for employment, those guidelines used by the Department of Transport for ordinary driving licences (see Appendix 1). If an employee is safe to drive a machine as dangerous as a car, he should be safe to undertake virtually all industrial duties. Jobs with special hazards are listed in Table 8.2. After an initial seizure, the Department of

Transport advises that a subject may not drive a motor car for one year, and it would seem reasonable to follow the same practice for restrictions in industry.

## The effect of anti-epileptic drugs on work performance

A clear distinction must be made between chronic side-effects and acute toxicity. The latter occur when doses are too high, they are rapidly reversible, and can be prevented easily by medical intervention. The chronic side-effects of anti-epileptic drugs are, unfortunately, less easy to control, and may be an unavoidable penalty of effective long-term drug therapy. These effects, however, should be slight, and not prove a major handicap in the working environment; indeed, the drug should seldom be prescribed if serious toxic effects are experienced. Minor effects on concentration, speed of reaction, and other cognitive measures may be recorded in people on drug therapy, but these should not be allowed to impair performance significantly. Some anti-epileptic drugs have a sedative effect or can cause depression or irritability, but again this should not be of a degree which interferes with daily activity. In most patients with epilepsy, monotherapy in conventional dosage ensures seizure control, and in this situation no side-effects should be expected. In patients with uncontrolled epilepsy, however, drug treatment often needs to be more complex, and minor side-effects are acceptable. The balance between efficacy and toxicity depends upon individual factors and it is difficult to generalize. An appropriate level of toxicity for one person may be unacceptable to another. In patients with mental impairment and cerebral damage causing epilepsy, side-effects are more common and more severe; most such individuals will be in a sheltered working environment, where some degree of drug-related impairment of work performance should be expected. Drug level monitoring provides a guide to appropriate dosing and a check on compliance.

## The disabled person's register

Should a person with epilepsy register as disabled? This very much depends upon the degree of disability as the register is intended for individuals who have a substantial health problem which significantly affects employment prospects. Being on the register will help in getting and keeping a job and provide 'travel to work grants' if public transport cannot be used. There may also be an opportunity to receive a Disability Working Allowance if the qualifying criteria are met. Further information on the above is provided in Chapter 2, p. 38, and can also be obtained from the local job centre.

## Opportunities for sheltered work

The majority of people with epilepsy are capable of normal employment without need for supervision or major restrictions. There exists a minority group with additional handicap who may only be able to work in a more sheltered environment. Such additional handicap often includes poorly controlled seizures, physical disability, low intelligence, and poor social adaptive skills. The following specialised facilities are available in the United Kingdom for people with epilepsy:

## MEDICAL SERVICES

The National Health Service (NHS) provides medical services for people with epilepsy through its general practitioner and hospital services. Most patients will be seen in neurological, paediatric or mental handicap clinics, and the great majority of people with epilepsy are satisfactorily managed in this way. Residential care, where needed, is usually provided by the Social Services Departments, as part of their community care responsibilities. In addition, there are, however, epilepsy charities, residential centres and special assessment centres which cater for the particular needs of patients with epilepsy; these are outlined below.

## EPILEPSY CHARITIES

### National Society for Epilepsy

National Society for Epilepsy (NSE): was founded in 1892, and is the oldest epilepsy charity of its type in the world, and the largest epilepsy charity in the United Kingdom. Its aims are:

1. To provide services for people with epilepsy nationally, and this includes NHS outpatient and inpatient assessment services (in association with the National Hospital for Neurology and Neurosurgery), residential care, medium-term inpatient rehabilitation, community nurse services, and a network of community support groups.

2. To provide education services for the general public, employers, the media, and the medical and paramedical professions. This is provided via a telephone help-line, study days, lectures, and written and visual material.

3. To carry out medical research, in conjunction with the Institute of Neurology, and the Postgraduate Neurological School of London University.

### British Epilepsy Association (BEA)

This is an epilepsy charity which provides a telephone help-line to the general public and a system of lay self-help groups. Its activities are particularly aimed at modifying regressive attitudes to epilepsy, and to social support. It also provides written and visual material.

## RESIDENTIAL CENTRES AND SCHOOLS FOR EPILEPSY

In the United Kingdom, there are a number of special schools and centres for epilepsy, the largest of which are the Chalfont Centre (National Society for Epilepsy, Chalfont St

Peter), the David Lewis Centre, and St Piers Lingfield. These provide residential care for people with epilepsy, usually associated with other handicaps, with a condition so severe that independent life in the community is not possible. Some include provision for sheltered employment or daily activities, in which residents perform useful and satisfying jobs. The financial support for the residents is usually through local authority grants, health service grants or private or charitable funds.

### SPECIAL MEDICAL ASSESSMENT CENTRES

There are three NHS special Assessment Centres in the United Kingdom. These provide short-term medical and social inpatient assessment for people with severe or complicated epilepsy, funded through the NHS. The largest is at the Chalfont Centre for Epilepsy, run jointly by the NSE and the National Hospital for Neurology and Neurosurgery (a Special Health Authority). The paediatric special centre is run from the Park Hospital in Oxford, administered by the Oxfordshire Regional Health Authority. The other centre is at Bootham Park Hospital in York. Referral to any of the centres is through the normal medical channels, usually from general practitioners, paediatricians or neurologists. The centres admit patients from anywhere in the United Kingdom. (For full addresses, see Appendix 9.)

## Special work problems

### Disclosure of epilepsy to employers

In an ideal world, an individual with epilepsy would start work armed with an account of how his seizures affect him, how often and when they occur, details of his medication (and possible side-effects), and an estimate of likely prognosis. The occupational physician could then, from his own knowledge of the work processes at the factory or office, advise employment in a sector which maximized the employee's production and opportunities for promotion, and minimized any risk to him or to his colleagues.

Only about a third of the working population have even a nominal contact with an occupational physician, however, and in reality the situation is often quite different. The person with epilepsy is aware that in open competition his opportunities are impaired, and that his choice of vocation is limited. His opportunities of mobility and promotion within a company may also be limited. He may have suspicions that he will not be allowed to join the pension fund. Finally, he has to face the possible condescension of his fellow workers who, he feels, may have been told to watch out for his fits.

From this perspective, therefore, it is not surprising if epilepsy is often concealed from an employer or a potential employer. A survey of people in London with epilepsy[19] showed that over half of those who had had two or more full-time jobs after the onset of epilepsy had *never* disclosed their epilepsy to their employer, and only 1 in 10 had *always* revealed it. If seizures were infrequent, or usually nocturnal, so that the applicant considered that he had a good chance of getting away with concealment, then the employer was virtually never informed. Two variables in this survey correlated with failure to gain employment: frequent seizures, and lack of any special skill.

This state of affairs will be improved only slowly by educational programmes. Another possible way forward includes a clearer definition of jobs that can safely be done by people with epilepsy. Such a definition has been considered and published by the International Bureau for Epilepsy[20] and they considered that the vast majority of jobs are suitable for people with epilepsy, especially where the person possesses the right qualifications and experience. Blanket prohibitions should be avoided and the organization of work practice should be examined to reduce potential risk to an acceptable level.

### Accident and absence records of those with epilepsy

It is widely held that people with epilepsy are more accident-prone and have worse attendance records than other workers. However, this view is not substantiated from the little literature available. Many studies must be inherently biased, as the person already known to have epilepsy has declared his or her condition, either voluntarily or involuntarily by having a seizure at work, and therefore eliminated himself or herself from many potentially hazardous jobs which in themselves lead to increased accidents and sickness absence. The most significant study of work performance which attempted to eliminate this bias was conducted by the US Department of Labor 45 years ago. A statistical comparison was made of 10 groups with different disabilities, including people with epilepsy, with matched unimpaired controls. Within the epilepsy group, no differences were found in absenteeism, but their incidence of work injuries was slightly higher. The differences noted in accident rates were not, however, statistically significant. The general conclusion of this study was that people with epilepsy perform as well as matched unimpaired workers in manufacturing industries.

In 1960 Udell hypothesized that people with epilepsy were capable of normal work performance. Although his sample was small, this work demonstrated that discriminatory practices against the recruitment of people with epilepsy are unwarranted, if based on the notion that as a group they have high accident rates, poor absence records, and low production efficiency. Udell also made the point that any applicant with epilepsy must be appraised individually with regard to the degree of seizure control, and any other associated handicap. He also added that employers should have a receptive policy for recruitment and job security. This may encourage employees to admit the problem, and allow industry an opportunity to appraise their abilities and place them most appropriately.

The more recent study of epilepsy in British Steel (BS)[12] generally supports these previous findings. There was no significant difference between epilepsy and control groups with regard to overall sickness absence and accident records. This report also analysed job performance, and showed that there was no major overall difference between epilepsy and control groups using five job performance factors. Work performance, however, was significantly reduced when people with epilepsy and an associated personality disorder were compared with the remainder of the epilepsy group. The BS study emphasized that, although some degree of selection has to be applied when employing people with epilepsy, the overall performance of those with epilepsy compared with that of their colleagues was satisfactory.

The major problem is not to prove that performance at work is satisfactory, but to challenge and change the firmly held and deeply entrenched prejudices of employers.

## Current employment practices

An informal survey of current attitudes and practices with respect to epilepsy within the previously nationalized industries, armed forces, teaching profession, National Health Service, and Civil Service, revealed an interesting dual approach adopted by most occupational health departments. There was often a carefully worded and apparently inflexible regulation, yet many occupational physicians used a more sympathetic approach. This was usually only obvious, however, if the physician was contacted personally. Such manoeuvres were only undertaken by doctors in industries and services that could allow the flexibility of relocation to different jobs.

Not unreasonably, the armed forces were found to be the least flexible. In the case of new entrants, proven cases of epilepsy are not accepted for service and those who had suffered a single seizure less than four years before entry, are also not acceptable. For serving personnel, a single seizure after entry necessitates full examination of the individual, restricted activities, and observation for a period of 18 months. Full re-instatement is awarded only after assessment by a senior consultant. Aircrew, who have suffered a single seizure after entry, are grounded permanently and servicemen who suffer more than one seizure will be considered for discharge on grounds of disability.

Epilepsy is also a contraindication for employment in the police force. The police expect all their officers to be fit for all duties. Officers developing epilepsy in service are usually discharged, but only after careful individual assessment (personal communication to I.B.).

Many of the large and often previously nationalized industries follow similar codes of practice and are able to pursue a more sympathetic and accommodating approach. Epilepsy declared at the pre-employment stage may be a contraindication to employment, but is not an absolute bar. The discretion of the examining physician allows some compromise to be achieved if the applicant has a special skill or quality to offer, and if the job is suitable. Epilepsy developing in service can often be accommodated if the employee is willing to be relocated, but this may involve some loss of earnings and status. If unacceptable, retirement on grounds of ill health is usually offered. A good example of such practices is demonstrated by the current policy of British Coal's medical service.

The Department of Education and Science has a flexible policy for the employment of schoolteachers with epilepsy and allows its locally appointed part-time medical officers to use reasonable discretion. Difficult cases are referred to the Department's medical advisers, and each is judged on its own merits.

The National Health Service (NHS) has made considerable progress since the first edition of this book in 1988 but still has no national guidelines. This is by virtue of the numerous separate employers which, as a whole, form the entity of the NHS.

Virtually all Trusts and Health Authorities have an Occupational Health Service and many have the benefit of a consultant adviser in the specialty. Guidelines on occupational health issues, as they may affect NHS employees, have been constructed by the Association of National Health Occupational Physicians (ANHOPS) and they discuss, in general, many of the common conditions that can affect fitness for work, including epilepsy. In essence, the guidelines state that all individuals are assessed on their merits. They emphasize that the epilepsy should be well controlled and the care of the patient must not be compromised.

The Civil Service has an open and documented policy on the recruitment and employment of people with epilepsy. The health standard for appointment in the Civil Service requires that a candidate's health is such as to qualify that person for the position sought and that the person is likely to give regular and efficient service for at least five years or for the period of any shorter appointment. The Civil Service Occupational Health Service stress that epilepsy *per se* is not a bar to holding any established appointment, apart from those posts with special hazards.

### Getting employers to understand about epilepsy

Many of those with epilepsy are unemployed. Even if employed, many workers with epilepsy are frequently denied promotion because of their disability or because of misconceptions about it. In a survey of employers in the United States it was found that few would employ persons known by them to have had a generalized seizure within the previous year. In this study, Hicks and Hicks recorded a consistent reason given for the failure to offer people with epilepsy employment, that 'they create safety problems for themselves and other workers'. Such reasoning has not varied for more than two decades. These authors point out that this assumption is misconceived, and not supported by published data. An encouraging feature of this study was evidence of a positive change in attitude. Although the cause remains uncertain, changes in the law in the United States and the continued efforts of public and private agencies may well be responsible.

Regular informal health education seminars could take place at work. A well thought out programme that involves the personnel department, occupational health team, and interested union representatives may prevent some problems occurring. Topics such as epilepsy, stress, or alcohol abuse could be discussed openly, with the benefit of expert advice being immediately available. The occupational physician or occupational health nurse can play a major role in informal health education and in changing attitudes. Health education is concerned not only with the prevention of disease, but in the understanding of disease in others. Problems, such as epilepsy, are often shrouded in mystery, or considered as too unsavoury to discuss in detail. For such a common complaint, with a prevalence of about 5–10 per 1000 of the population, the ignorance demonstrated is astonishing. Many employees, both on the shop-floor and in management, consider that someone with epilepsy also has some degree of mental handicap combined with a lesser or greater physical infirmity. Certainly such problems may coexist, but they are the exception rather than the rule. It is of paramount importance that health professionals should dispel myths and bring a sense of proportion to problems.

The hard work of agencies such as the British Epilepsy Association, the National Society for Epilepsy, and the Employment Medical Advisory Service has done much to inform employers. Misconceptions about epilepsy are slowly disappearing and attitudes changing.

### Relationship between the occupational physician, consultant neurologist, and GP

Recommendations received from the neurologist may differ from those acceptable to the occupational physician, who must consider the best interests of the patient in his particular working environment. The family doctor, who may have cogent views and is likely to have closer knowledge of the patient can liaise with both these two specialists. It is advantageous if all the physicians involved work together to avoid conflicting advice.

In companies with an occupational health service, an employee with epilepsy should be encouraged to contact the nurse and discuss problems as they arise. The nursing service at work is often readily accessible to the employee and has a special role in counselling and health education. Confidential notes should be kept and the case discussed with the occupational physician at the earliest opportunity. Employees with epilepsy should be reviewed regularly by the occupational health service.

## Existing legislation and guidelines for employment

For a more detailed discussion of legal aspects, see Chapter 2, and also Carter.[21]

The Health and Safety at Work, etc., Act 1974 makes no specific references to the disabled, and applies to all employees regardless of their health. The dual responsibility of employer and employee is entirely reasonable, but may create problems. Many people with epilepsy do not disclose it to their employer for fear of losing their job, or to a prospective employer for fear of not being offered the job.[19] Under these circumstances the employee with epilepsy may contravene Section 7 of the Health and Safety at Work Act, if he knowingly accepts a job that is unsuitable for a person with epilepsy. An employer, however, may legally refuse to employ an applicant for a job on any grounds except those of sex and race (see Chapter 2) without necessarily giving reasons for his decision. The law relating to discrimination does not at present protect disabled applicants whose only recourse is in relation to voluntary moral obligations assumed by some employers under Equal Opportunities Policies.

What are the legal implications if a worker develops epilepsy while in service? All employees are covered by the Employment Protection (Consolidation) Act 1978. This Act protects against unfair dismissal, but such protection is only operable after two years continuous employment. Is dismissal on medical grounds unfair? The employer may be obliged to justify his decision to an Industrial Tribunal by at least one of five fair reasons for dismissal. Two of these are pertinent to this situation:

1.   Is the employee capable of performing his duties safely and efficiently?

2.   Has it become impossible for the employee to continue to work without contravening a statutory duty or restriction?

Incapability and illegality are both fair grounds for dismissal. The Industrial Tribunal makes the final decision, subject to an appeal to the Employment Appeal Tribunal, but will be concerned that the employer has discussed with the worker his state of health if possible, and made absolutely sure that the employee is incapable of doing the job in question, and that an alternative job is not available.

Some employers are under the misconception that an applicant with a history of epilepsy will not be accepted into the pension fund. The view of the Occupational Pensions Board, however, succinctly states the situation: 'Fit for employment—fit for the pension scheme' (see also Chapter 1, p. 7).

No special insurance arrangements are necessary for a worker with epilepsy. The Employer's Liability Insurance covers everyone in the workplace, provided that the employer has taken the disability into account when allocating the individual to a particular job. Failure to disclose epilepsy will, of course, render the employer's insurance invalid and should an accident occur as a direct result of the condition, it is unlikely that a claim for compensation will be met.

To summarize the legal position, the employee with epilepsy is protected by the same legislation and should enjoy the same pension rights as any other employee. He can be dismissed from employment if the disability seriously interferes with his capability to perform his duties satisfactorily. Dismissal can also take place if the employee's medical condition contravenes statutory regulations governing the job.[21] It is unfortunate that employers can discriminate against a suitably qualified applicant with epilepsy purely on the grounds of potential disability. A satisfactory solution to the employment of someone whose epilepsy is well controlled is unlikely to be achieved by legislation alone. Changing the legal position on discrimination would help, particularly if the employer had to justify his decision to reject an applicant, if it appeared that such a decision was made purely on medical grounds unrelated to the job in question.*

## The Driving Licence Regulations and their effects (see Appendix 1)

The broad intention is to allow driving licences to be granted, in suitable cases, to people with epilepsy who have been free of any attacks for two years with or without treatment, or who have a history of at least three years of attacks but only during sleep. It is also important to note that an individual should also refrain from driving for a period if a change in therapeutic regime occurs. This is especially so if the dose of anticonvulsant has been reduced. The current recommendation from the Driving and Vehicle Licensing Agency, Swansea (DVLA) is that if undergoing planned withdrawal of anticonvulsant medication the patient should be advised to cease driving during the withdrawal period and for six months after cessation. If further epileptic attacks occur the epilepsy regulations will need to apply.

Van, crane, and minibus drivers will need to be found alternative employment within the company, as will those whose job also involves driving. The safety of fork-lift truck drivers will depend on individual circumstances.

A single unprovoked seizure, as defined on p. 146 is not epilepsy, but the subject is still obliged by law to inform the DVLA of the event as it clearly is, in view of the high recurrence rate, a 'disability which is or may become likely to affect your fitness as a driver'.[23] The DVLA will invariably advise at least one year of ineligibility to hold a licence. Initial seizures are often followed by others (p. 146).

For advice on driving with other neurological disorders and after head injuries see Chapter 7, p. 135.

## Conclusions and recommendations

Many people do not disclose a past or present medical history of epileptic seizures when applying for a job, or during a routine examination at the work-place.[19] This may well cause major problems for the individual and the em-

---

*A recent report by Dickey and Morrow indicated that a group of patients with epilepsy had a poor appreciation of their legal responsibilities and frequently failed to comply with them.[22]— *Editor*.

ployer and, on occasions, inadvertently contravene the Health and Safety at Work Act or invalidate insurance cover. The unenlightened attitudes of some employers have led understandably to such secrecy or even denial by the employee or applicant. The possibility of dangerous situations arising at work, or dismissal without recourse to appeal may be the outcome. A competent occupational health service, trusted by both shop-floor and management, can be invaluable in sorting out conflicts and giving advice.

Responsibility for the employment and placement of a person with epilepsy rests with the employer and he should have appropriate medical advice. Each case must be judged on its merits in the light of all available information. Any attempt to advise management without a sound and complete understanding of the requirements of the job is unfair to both employee and employer. Each employee with epilepsy must be regularly reviewed. The development of good rapport and mutual trust will encourage the employee to report any changes in his condition or medication and discuss anxieties that have developed.

A sensible approach by management, with access to medical advice, should help the individual to come to terms with his condition, appreciate the reasons for any restrictions, and understand that decisions taken on the basis of such medical advice are in his best interests. The employer should drop old prejudices in favour of current concepts about epilepsy. This will only occur when all those concerned with epilepsy undertake the responsibility of educating employers, the general public, and perhaps some members of the medical profession.

## Acknowledgments

We would like to thank Dr J.W.A.S. Sander for his help in preparing this chapter as well as Mr C.G.D. Bradley LL B, Solicitor, and Dr R.J.M. Irvine, Medical Advisory Branch, DVLA, for their advice.

## Selected references and further reading

1.  Hopkins, A. (1987). Definitions and epidemiology of epilepsy. In *Epilepsy*, (ed. A. Hopkins), pp. 1–18. Chapman & Hall, London.
2.  Dreifuss, F.E. (1987). The different types of epileptic seizures, and the international classification of epileptic seizures and of the epilepsies. In *Epilepsy*, (ed. A. Hopkins), pp. 83–113. Chapman & Hall, London.
3.  Shorvon, S.D. (1988). Medical services. In *A textbook of epilepsy,* (ed. J. Laidlaw, A. Richens, and J. Oxley), pp. 611–30. Churchill Livingstone, Edinburgh.
4.  Sander, J.W.A.S. and Shorvon, S.D. (1987). Incidence and prevalence studies in epilepsy and their methodological problems: a review. *J. Neurol. Neurosurg. Psychiat.*, **50**, 829–39.
5.  Sander J.W.A.S., Hart, Y.M., Johnson, A.L, and Shorvon, S.D. (for the NGPSE) (1990). National general practice study of epilepsy: Newly diagnosed epileptic seizures in a general population. *Lancet*, **336**, 1267–71.

6. Hart, Y.M., Sander, J.W.A.S., Johnson, A.L., and Shorvon, S.D. (for the NGPSE) (1990). National general practice study of epilepsy: Recurrence after a first seizure. *Lancet*, **336**, 1271–74.

7. Davies, J.E., *et al.* (1983) Lindane poisonings. *Arch. Dermatol.*, **119**, 142–4.

8. Shorvon, S.D. (1984). The temporal aspects of prognosis in epilepsy. *J. Neurol. Neurosurg. Psychiat.*, **47**, 1157–65.

9. Goodridge, D.M.G. and Shorvon, S.D. (1983). Epilepsy in a population of 6000. *Brit. Med. J.*, **287**, 641–7.

10. Jennett, W.B. (1975). *Epilepsy after non-missile head injuries*, (2nd edn.). Heinemann, London.

11. Jennett, W.B. (1987). Epilepsy after head injury and intracranial surgery. In *Epilepsy*, (ed. A. Hopkins), pp. 399–409. Chapman & Hall, London.

12. Dasgupta, A.K., Saunders, M., and Dick, D.J. (1982). Epilepsy in the British Steel Corporation: an evaluation of sickness, accident, and work records. *Brit. J. Indust. Med.*, **39**, 146–8.

13. Wilkinson, R.T. (1971). Hours of work and the 24 hour cycle of rest and activity. In *Psychology at work*, (ed. P.B. Warr), pp. 31–54. Penguin, Harmondsworth.

14. Betts, T. (1992). Epilepsy and stress. *Brit. Med. J.,* **305**, 378–9.

15. Jeavons, P.M. and Harding, G.F.A. (1975). *Photosensitive epilepsy: a review of the literature and a study of 460 patients*. Clinics in developmental medicine. Spastics International Publications, No. 56. Heinemann, London.

16. Masland, R.L. (1983). Employability. Part VIII. Social aspects. In *Research progress in epilepsy*, (ed. C. Rose), pp. 527–32. Pitman, London.

17. Espir, M. and Floyd, M. (1986). Epilepsy and recruitment. In *Epilepsy and employment*, (ed. F. Edwards, M. Espir, and J. Oxley), pp. 39–46. Royal Society of Medicine, London.

18. Troxell, J. and Thorbecke, R. (April 1992). *Vocational scenarios: A training manual on epilepsy and employment*. Second Employment Commission of the International Bureau for Epilepsy. International Bureau for Epilepsy, P.O. Box 21, 2100 AA Heemstede, The Netherlands.

19. Scambler, G. and Hopkins, A.P. (1980). Social class, epileptic activity and disadvantage at work. *J. Epidemiol Commun. Hlth.*, **34**, 129–33.

20. *Epilepsia*, **30**(4), 411–12. Employing people with epilepsy. Principles for good practice, Employment commission of the International Bureau for epilepsy (1989).

21 Carter, T. (1986). Health and safety at work: implications of current legislation. In *Epilepsy and employment*, (ed. F. Edwards, M. Espir, and J. Oxley,) pp. 9–17. Royal Society of Medicine, London.

22. Dickey, W. and Morrow, T.I. (1993). Epilepsy and driving: attitudes and practices among patients attending a seizure clinic. *J. Roy. Soc. Med.*, **86**, 506–38.

23. DOT (Department of Transport) (1982). Conditions of United Kingdom Driving Licence. DOT, London.

# 9

# Spinal disorders

## *E.B. Macdonald and J.A. Mathews*

### Introduction

Back pain is the largest single cause of time lost from work, and low back pain will affect about 70 per cent of the working population at some time during their working life. There are few tests which are of use in predicting who is going to get pain in any particular working environment, and pre-employment screening is therefore of limited value.

While back pain can occur spontaneously it is more common in occupations which involve heavy manual work. Most individuals with short-term pain in the back can be successfully rehabilitated to their normal work but the outlook is much worse for chronic pain. The emphasis should therefore be placed on prevention by a combination of improving workplace design, setting up good work practices, and providing adequate training for the worker.

The vertebral column is the jointed bony core of the spine. It allows movement in addition to providing strength and rigidity. The jointed bony structures are supported by muscles which provide strength with flexibility. Extra strength is provided at the thoracic and lumbar levels by the muscles of the chest and abdomen. The constant demands made on the spine in nearly all activities lead to recognizable changes. The changes, which result from normal wear and repair are often termed 'spondylosis' and can be seen on an X-ray. This is generally asymptomatic but when use is excessive or injudicious, symptoms may result.

The symptoms have several cardinal characteristics. The most common is pain. This is generally intermittent, related to movement, and clearly emanates from the spine. The pain usually arises from the joints themselves when it is often axial; it may derive from the dural covering of the nerve roots and be proximally referred, or it may arise from true nerve root irritation or damage when it is often distal and shows classical neurological features. Similarly, the abnormal signs may be related to the joints—asymmetrical production of pain or restriction of movement; dura pain on nerve root stretching, or nerve root pain with reflex weakness, or sensory changes.

By contrast, a minority of spinal disorders are congenital, inflammatory or neoplastic. Inflammatory disorders may be idiopathic (e.g., ankylosing spondylitis) or infective, and neoplastic disorders generally arise from secondary deposits. In these patients pain will be constant and progressive, and restriction of movement symmetrical, increasing to complete rigidity.

Disorders of the spine are very common and their occupational significance is frequently an issue for individuals, their medical advisers, and employers. Despite the reduction in employment in heavy industry, some problems, such as low back and neck pain, appear to be an increasing cause of absence from work. Low back pain is the major cause of retirement through ill health in many industries ranging from mining to health care and has a huge individual and social cost. Conversely, the employment opportunities of those with inflammatory back disorders such as ankylosing spondylitis are now much wider with the growth in the service and retail sectors and the introduction of information technology.

## Prevalence and morbidity

Between 70 and 80 per cent of the population will experience low back pain causing absence from work during their lives but most of these episodes will be self-limiting and of short duration albeit with a tendency to recur. Low back pain of acute onset tends to improve spontaneously and the recovery rate in a cohort of back pain sufferers has a half life of about 20 days (i.e., half the sufferers will be better in 20 days), whatever the treatments delivered and the skills of the therapists.

The certified incapacity due to back pain is summarized in Fig. 9.1.[1] The National Back Pain Association estimated that in 1987–8, about 46.5 million working days were lost due to back pain at a cost to society of £2000 million. The UK sickness and invalidity benefit for back pain has escalated since 1975. Diagnosis of spondylosis and allied disorders and intervertebral disc disorders account for 50 per cent of the total. There is little difference in the prevalence of back pain in different occupational groups and it is likely that an equivalent amount of disability occurs in the non-insured population. Low back pain occurs maximally in the 5th decade. The accuracy and relevance of precise diagnosis is questionable, but within this total, about 50 per cent of low back pain is attributed to prolapsed intervertebral disc.[2]

About 4–6 per cent of the patients of general practitioners will seek advice about spinal problems each year, about 10–20 per cent of these will be referred to hospital and of these about 30 per cent are admitted at some time. Fifty per cent of the average hospital physiotherapy treatments are for spinal conditions. About one-third of those referred to hospital with a disc problem will have operative treatment.

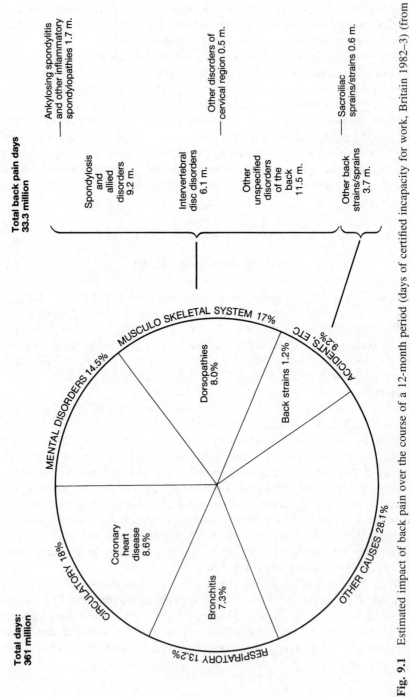

**Total back pain days
33.3 million**

Ankylosing spondylitis
and other inflammatory
spondylopathies 1.7 m.

Other disorders of
cervical region 0.5 m.

Spondylosis
and
allied
disorders
9.2 m.

Intervertebral
disc disorders
6.1 m.

Other
unspecified
disorders
of the
back
11.5 m.

Other back
strains/sprains
3.7 m.

Sacroiliac
sprains/strains 0.6 m.

MUSCULO SKELETAL SYSTEM 17%

MENTAL DISORDERS 14.5%

ACCIDENTS, ETC 9.2%

Dorsopathies
8.0%

Back strains 1.2%

CIRCULATORY 18%

Coronary
heart
disease
8.6%

Bronchitis
7.3%

OTHER CAUSES 28.1%

RESPIRATORY 13.2%

**Total days:
361 million**

**Fig. 9.1** Estimated impact of back pain over the course of a 12-month period (days of certified incapacity for work, Britain 1982–3) (from Wells[1]).

# Clinical aspects affecting work capacity

## Neck pain

It has been shown in a population survey that 28 per cent of males and 34 per cent of females give a history of neck–shoulder–brachial pain.[3]

The majority of the population over the age of 40 will have some spinal radiographic changes. These include narrowing of one or more intervertebral disc spaces in the middle or lower cervical regions often with osteophytic outgrowths. The apophyseal and neurocentral joints are also affected. However, there is a poor correlation with symptoms and many people remain symptomfree. Radiology is of value in assessment and important in the investigation of injury, possible infection or malignancy. Its value as a guide to prognosis, treatment or fitness for work is debatable. **There is no place for the use of spinal X-rays as a pre-employment screening test to exclude potential back problems.**

### Symptoms

Pain is the most common feature but deformity (torticollis) or neurological factors may dominate. The intermittent nature and provocation by posture are important and reassuring features. In many patients a history of an unaccustomed activity or an injury e.g., 'whiplash', may be elicited. If sustained at work the problem is often more persistent. Most pathology is in the low cervical spine, C5-6, C6-7, but the symptoms of pain are often referred away from the actual level. The pain may be entirely local, or referred to the occiput, towards the shoulders, or to the interscapular region. Restriction of movement is usually asymmetrical. The delineation between articular and dural pain is often unclear, but true nerve root pain is usually more distal by nature of the sclerotomes supplied from the lower cervical levels usually involved.

### Signs

Physical examination should start with observation of posture and any deformities and swellings. The range of neck movement should be examined in the three standard planes: flexion–extension, lateral flexions, and rotations. Next, shoulder movements are examined partly to check for shoulder pathology but also to look for dural tension signs, and this should be followed by a neurological examination of the arms. In addition, a history of bladder or bowel symptoms should be sought, and the long tracts and plantar responses examined.

### Treatment

The basic treatment for a physical condition due to injury or wear and tear is rest. This rarely needs to be total (i.e., bed rest) but frequently a restricting collar is very helpful. Collars need to be carefully fitted so as to achieve at least a 70 per cent reduction in neck movement as opposed to merely providing warmth and draught-proofing (comforting though this may be). Non-steroidal anti-inflammatory drugs may help the minor inflammatory component of the disorder, and do have a modest analgesic action. 'Muscle relaxants' are often used. There is a great deal of evidence that manipulation or traction by physiotherapists or osteopaths can hasten recovery from individual episodes, and prophylactic advice is important in preventing a recurrence.

*Occupational factors*

The symptoms and degree of disability vary considerably. The provoking occupational factors are not well understood, but disability is more frequent in jobs where there is restricted headroom, work in awkward and confined places, work requiring the head and neck to be held in a constant position, and strenuous work using the arms. All of these may aggravate neck stiffness, pain in the neck and arms, and paraesthesiae.

After an exacerbation it is wise initially to avoid tasks which involve heavy carrying (e.g., over 20 kg, or less depending on the individual and the frequency of the task), lifting, shovelling, manual loading and unloading, the use of heavy vibratory tools, and working with the arms elevated and the neck extended. Attention should be paid to the ergonomics of display screen equipment workstations, seating and the organization of clerical work. Clerical workers can be helped by having raised and tilted work surfaces, so that flexion of the neck for long periods is avoided. Document holders should be supplied for workers who require to refer to documents while working with display screen equipment.

Those with persisting neck stiffness may not be fit for their jobs if these require a good and free range of neck movement, as in driving a motor vehicle, crane, or forklift truck. However, symptoms usually improve in the majority and therefore occupational restrictions should be reviewed and reduced whenever possible.

## Ankylosing spondylitis

Ankylosing spondylitis is an important cause of chronic pain and disability in young adults. It affects males and females in the ratio of 4:1 and women are less severely affected. The overall prevalence is about 1 per cent, many will remain undiagnosed and 6 per cent of cases will have a family history. The age of presentation is usually between 18 and 30 years. It may occur atypically as an accompaniment to Reiter's syndrome, psoriasis, and chronic inflammatory bowel disorders. There is a close relationship to the B27 tissue antigen.

In many cases the disease will remain mild and will have little impact on functional ability and will not cause absence from work.

*Symptoms*

The disease classically starts as inflammation of the sacro-iliac joints with back or posterior thigh pain, and often immobility stiffness. It may be unilateral, bilateral or alternate from side to side. In the more severely affected there will be widespread inflammatory change spreading up the spinal joints, causing in the most severe patients virtually total spinal fusion. In some patients a severe kyphosis and general ill health may occur, and the disease is occasionally complicated by amyloid deposition. The two main pillars of treatment are non-steroidal anti-inflammatory drugs and physiotherapy.

*Occupational prognosis*

Work is beneficial for people with ankylosing spondylitis as increased activity reduces discomfort and the risk of permanent deformation. Eighty per cent can work full-time and heavy manual work is not contraindicated, although ultimately only about 10 per cent will remain in such work, and most will be employed in sedentary, professional or light manual work.

In one series, after 30 years of ankylosing spondylitis, 31 per cent were still working at their original jobs and 22 per cent had changed to lighter work. However, even in the armed forces, 70 per cent were able to follow a full service career.[4] The majority will cope with work for at least 20 years and minimal work adjustments are required. The prognosis is less good in those with severe hip involvement, or fixed and extreme flexion of the thoracic spine, or in the few who develop a severe peripheral polyarthritis.

The specific limitations at work are usually related to joint stiffness and thus individuals without free neck movements and all round vision may be unsuitable for some tasks such as drivers of cranes, heavy goods vehicles, public service vehicles or fork-lift trucks. Work requiring agility or working in confined spaces may be contraindicated, but any restrictions should be recommended only on an individual basis. Patients do well if they are kept under regular review, symptoms are adequately treated, they participate in regular physiotherapy classes, and are encouraged to remain physically active. The National Ankylosing Spondylitis Society has local branches and self-help groups and provides information and support. Some regional centres are still able to arrange short courses of inpatient treatment for groups of patients, with considerable benefit. Where workplace physiotherapy is available this should be used on a routine basis to maintain maximal function.

## Low back pain

Low back pain is defined as pain in the region of the lumbosacral spine. It is generally intermittent. In most patients it arises from a mechanical disorder of the lower lumbar joints most often at the L4-5 and/or L5-S1 levels. Occasionally it may be referred from an intra-abdominal or retroperitoneal lesion—neoplastic or vascular. Other lumbar pathology, such as inflammation or neoplasm, will produce more relentless features. Cauda equina claudication may result from narrowing of the lumbar canal and gives rise to leg pain or weakness on exercise.

*Symptoms*

Pain is the dominant feature. It is generally centred on the low lumbar spine, especially when arising from the intervertebral joints themselves. It will classically be intermittent and related to movement. Irritation of nearby dural coverings or nerve root sheaths may produce chronic referred pain. This is felt in the buttocks or thighs but sometimes radiates up the spine. True nerve root symptoms are generally more severe, and more distal as the L5 or S1 roots are usually involved, and are more closely related to changing cerebrospinal fluid (CSF) pressure—as in coughing or straining. In these patients there may be bladder and bowel symptoms.

*Signs*

Initially one should look for deformity. Paraspinal muscle prominence due to spasm is common, as is loss of the expected lordosis. Local tenderness is a frequent feature. Movements are examined in the two main planes; flexion–extension and lateral flexions. In these mechanical disorders restriction of movement is classically asymmetrical. Dural tension signs are elicited by checking the straight-leg-raise and the femoral nerve stretch tests which relate to L5/S1 and L3/L4 nerve roots respectively. Restriction of movement or production of pain are sought. Finally, a standard neurological examination should be conducted from L1-S4 with particular attention to checking the L5 dermatome (which has no reflex) and the saddle area for anaesthesia.

Computed tomography (CT) scanning and magnetic resonance imaging (MRI) define the dimensions of the spinal canal and usually confirm the nature of the lesion.

Low back pain is a symptom rather than a diagnosis, is remarkably common, often poorly understood in individual cases, and causes much morbidity. Twenty three per cent of the total number of patients consulting their general practitioners during a year will be seeking advice on rheumatic complaints and of these back troubles account for 27 per cent. However, this does not reflect the true size of the problem as half of the patients attending osteopaths will do so for back pain, and of these, one-third will not have attended their own doctors.

In the workplace, absenteeism due to back pain is common in all occupations. In mining it accounts for 12–18 per cent of all certificated absence, in nursing about 50 per cent will experience some back discomfort in a year, and there are high rates of back pain in manual workers, drivers, helicopter pilots, and many other groups. Office workers experience almost as much back pain as manual workers although their associated sickness absence will be far less.

In considering the fitness for work of back pain sufferers a number of aspects must be considered including the physiological cause of the back pain, the occupational and individual risk factors, and an appreciation of the ergonomics of the workplace and the task requirements.

*Treatment*

As a mainly mechanical disorder the basic conventional treatment is rest. This may be complete as with bed rest, or partial with a fitted lumbosacral spinal support. In patients with severe back pain a few days of enforced bed rest may be mandatory, but most patients cannot achieve this at home, and so need to compromise with a corset which can, in any case, be used for longer periods. Longer spells of bed rest are often counter-productive. Analgesics and non-steroidal anti-inflammatory drugs may be useful for symptomatic relief.

Many accessory treatments are available for particular painful aspects of the syndrome.[5] Manipulation has been shown to hasten the relief of pain when the patient has marked asymmetry of spinal restriction, and particularly if there is a dural tension abnormality, e.g., restricted straight-leg-raise. Traction is probably helpful when root pain is a prominent feature. When root features are severe and a root lesion is detectable, then epidural anaesthetic-steroid injections can hasten relief.

Frequently, patients go directly to osteopaths or chiropractors. These people are often skilled and highly trained in the art of manipulation and may hasten relief when the underlying pathology is not too severe. Acupuncturists and faith healers also have success in similar situations.

There is rarely need for surgery. This should be considered on the occasions when a grossly unstable joint can be shown to be causing pain. A fusion is then indicated. More often sciatica can be shown to be due to nerve root pressure due to disc prolapse. The offending disc protrusion can then be removed by surgery or by chemonucleolysis.

# Special work problems

*Accidents*

Low back pain is frequently attributed to the effect of injury in an accident at work and studies in various occupational groups have shown with surprising consistency that while accident rates vary, about 20–25 per cent of 'accidents' affect the back, and of these manual handling, (e.g., lifting, loading or carrying) is a factor in about 50–60 per cent. However, detailed analysis of 236 back injuries showed that in 48 per cent the back pain arose spontaneously and was 'non-accidental'. The precipitating causes in the remainder were slipping and stumbling on rough or unstable surfaces and loss of balance in 75 per cent, a sudden unexpected load in 12 per cent and blows to the back in 7 per cent.[6]

*Manual handling*

Tasks involving much heavy lifting are associated with increased back pain. The risk of injury is not linear as those who lift infrequently are at greater risk than those who perform a moderate amount of lifting regularly, probably because of a training effect. Thus back pain occurs frequently in the sedentary worker during weekend gardening or other unaccustomed physical activity.

The size and shape of the load is important—a 10 kg block of lead being much safer to handle than a 10 kg box of feathers. The presence or absence of handles is clearly significant.

*Body space*

Work, particularly involving manual handling, in restricted headroom or confined environments greatly reduces a worker's safe lifting capacity, and a 3 per cent reduction in headroom has been shown to reduce the maximum lifting capacity of the individual by 50 per cent. Other physical constraints can prevent the use of safe handling techniques.

*Driving*

Professional drivers, lorry drivers and salesmen driving over 24 000 miles (38 000 km) a year have an increased risk of low back pain, possibly because of a combination of vibration, prolonged sitting, and the task of loading and un-loading. Vibration in other environments is an established risk factor.

**Personal risk factors**

A number of personal risk factors have been defined which have relevance in the occupational setting.[7] Men are more likely to experience disc protrusion than women, but during pregnancy women are particularly at risk of back pain because of their lax ligaments.

Height and weight are important. One study of a large group of military re-cruits who were followed up over 20 years showed that those with both height above 182 cm and a weight over 82 kg were more likely to experience back problems. Effects of age has already been discussed above, with disc lesions being maximal between 35 and 55 years, but absence from work due to back problems increases with age. Fitness is inversely related to risk of back injury as is muscle strength. The amount of space available in the spinal canal for the nerves is a factor and thus measurement of spinal canal diameter measurement can be useful, although it is difficult to obtain. Smoking is definitely a risk factor although whether this is because of an association with other adverse lifestyle behaviour e.g., smokers are generally less fit and active, or whether it is due to smoking alone is still debatable.

**Prevention of low back pain**

Much effort has been invested both by industry and medical research in the pursuit of effective strategies to prevent low back pain at work. On the basis of the morbidity statistics it would not be unreasonable to conclude that these have failed. However, there have been some examples of a reduction of back pain problems in industry, but usually only with a multifaceted approach including good ergonomic design of workplaces, appropriate attention to selection and training, and effective treatment and rehabilitation.[8]

# Existing legislation and guidelines for employment

## Lifting limits

Recognition of the potential impact of heavy manual work has led to much legislation, although usually of a general rather than a specific nature. Thus, the Factories Act 1961, states that 'a person shall not be employed to lift, carry or move, any load so heavy as to be likely to cause injury to him'. Specific regulations apply to some industries including the woollen and worsted textiles, jute, pottery, agriculture, and construction industries. Some of these have proposed specific weight limits and in 1967 the International Labour Conference adopted the International Labour Organization (ILO) Convention 127 recommending a maximum permissible weight to be lifted by one person (male) of 55 kg, with smaller limits for women and young people. This recommendation was not ratified by the United Kingdom and many other countries.

In recent years the legislation has been more general than specific. The Health and Safety at Work, etc., Act 1974, requires all employers to provide and maintain a system of work that is safe and without risks to the health of all their employees, so far as is reasonably practicable.

Further directives on health and safety have emanated from the European Union including one on manual handling. This has led to the Manual Handling of Loads Operations Regulations 1992 (see Appendix 7), which requires employers to minimize manual lifting, establish a process to assess the risks in any manual handling task, control or minimize those risks, provide information and training to employees, and regularly review the arrangements.

This approach is preferable to the imposition of arbitrary limits, although some organizations establish their own. Thus one information technology company has established a limit for a one person lift of 55 lb (25 kg) and a major pharmaceutical company has a limit of 30 kg, while a cement manufacturer may expect employees to handle 50 kg bags all day. Clearly, arbitrary limits would be quite impracticable in mining, nursing, and construction work and, given the significant risk which can be present in certain tasks with very much smaller loads, the general approach of assessing and controlling the risk associated with each task, is to be preferred.

However, useful recommendations have resulted from medical research. The guidelines to the *Manual handling regulations*[9] include a chart showing the weights which may be lifted at different heights and distances from the body (see Fig. 9.2).

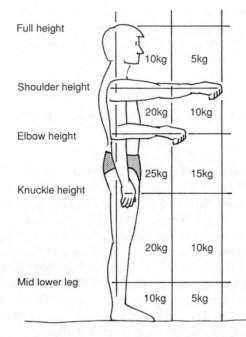

**Fig 9.2**   Lifting and lowering heights and distances from the body.[9]

In *Force limits in manual work,* Davis and Stubbs[10] took the same approach publishing sets of diagrams indicating acceptable loads at different distances from the erect trunk. These were based on studies of intra-abdominal pressure while the lifting tasks were being performed and on earlier work which showed that lifts which caused intra-abdominal pressures to rise above 90 mmHg were associated with increased rates of back injury.

These guidelines are, however, based on laboratory studies of healthy volunteers, and can only be extrapolated to workplaces with caution. Because of their inadequacies the risk assessment approach, which is the basis of most current legislation, is preferred.

### Risk assessment

To assess the risks of any particular activity the individuals must be considered in the context of the task and the working environment. In some occupations, such as dock work or community nursing, certain aspects of the working environment in ships or patients' homes, for example, may be outside the control of the employers. In all working situations the potential hazards can normally be identified and control measures established. The factors to be considered in performing an assessment are given in Table 9.1.

**Table 9.1**  Task assessment

*The tasks—do they involve*:
Holding loads away from the trunk?
Twisting or stooping?
Reaching upwards?
Large vertical movement?
Long carrying distances?
Strenuous pulling or pushing?
Unpredictable movement of loads?
Repetitive handling?
Insufficient rest or recovery?
A work rate imposed by a process?
Lifting patients?

*The loads—are they:*
Heavy, bulky, unwieldy?
Difficult to grasp?
Unstable/unpredictable?
Intrinsically harmful e.g., sharp/hot?

*The working environment—are there:*
Constraints on posture?
Poor floors?
Variations in levels?
Hot/cold/humid conditions?
Strong air movements?
Poor lighting conditions?

*Individual capability—does the job*
Require unusual capability?
Endanger those with a health problem?
Endanger those who are pregnant?
Call for special information/training?
Require special clothing?

*Instruction and training—does it include:*
Use of mechanical aids?
Principles of good task design?
Good handling methods?

## Reducing risks at work

The priority in the prevention of back pain at work must always be to remove or minimize the hazard, by changing work practices, providing lifting aids, or simple modifications to the workplace layout. Most risks can be reduced by simple and inexpensive changes. If this is not possible, the use of mechanical aids, such as levers, barrows, and trolleys, will reduce the demands of the job. Fork-lift trucks may be required. Simple rollers and conveyors can assist loading and unloading. Consideration should be given to reducing the size of the load and any load which is either large, e.g., a large cardboard box, and/or heavy, e.g., over 20 kg, should preferably have handles.

Loads should not be stored above shoulder height as the biomechanical stresses of lifting to this height are considerable and reduce by about 75 per cent what would be a 'safe' load at lower levels. Whenever possible heavy loads requiring manual handling should not be stored on the floor, and not lower than knee height.

Loads held at arms length exert a fivefold increase in back strain, compared to being held against the body and frequent lifting reduces the 'safe' load to about 25 per cent of the acceptable maximum lift for any individual.

Reasonable space in which to move and work are essential and many accidents occur in situations where the worker has restricted room to stand or move.

A particular hazard to the spine is the bending twisting lift which can provoke annulus rupture with the lightest loads, such as when the housewife reaches down to pick up the bottle of milk, or the seated employee reaches down and to the side to lift without moving from the chair. Other common hazardous tasks include lifting loads into or out of the boot of a car, or out of high-sided boxes, bins or stillages.

### Seating

It is likely that tasks involving minimal manual handling may adversely affect the back if they involve poor seating postures, or standing and leaning over a work surface for long periods. Elevating the work surface, or the object being worked on (the ideal height for a work surface when standing is 8 cm below the elbows), providing a stool or appropriate seating, and encouraging frequent changes in posture, are all beneficial. The Display Screen Regulations 1992,

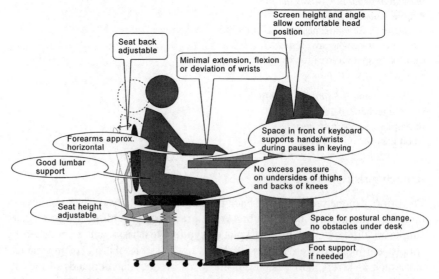

**Fig. 9.3**   Correct sitting position at a display screen workstation.

address the importance of correct seating at workstations (see Fig. 9.3) and detailed guidance is available[11]. (see also Appendix 7.)

Badly designed chairs can aggravate pre-existing back pain, and contribute to its onset. Seats for prolonged sedentary work should be adjustable for height and back support. The seat should allow the worker to rest the feet on the floor, and if not, as with workers of short stature, a foot rest should be provided. The seating should be firm and the back support appropriately curved and supporting the lumbar spine.

The seat should be horizontal and a forward tilting ability is preferable to a rearward inclination. Back pain sufferers are frequently helped by tilting the seat forward so that the front edge is about 10–15 degrees below the horizontal. The extreme version of this is the Scandinavian 'kneeling chair' which can provide relief to some back sufferers by increasing the pelvic-femoral angle. However, a simple back support fitted to a chair can often improve comfort and the doctor should resist making firm recommendations about alternative seating for a back sufferer, as no one chair is suitable for all, and simple remedies should be tried first. Seats with arm rests are preferable.

The classical luxurious soft 'directors chair' is often the least ergonomically appropriate. Many unsatisfactory chairs can be improved by the provision of a simple ergonomically designed back support such as the 'Backfriend' available from Medesign Ltd (see Appendix 9 for the full address).

Sedentary workers should be encouraged to move around, stretch, and do simple exercises, and the Japanese tradition of periodic group exercises in the workplace may have some physiological merit.

## Driving

As mentioned earlier, driving is a risk factor for back pain, and particularly affects those travelling long distances, who are often driving company cars.

The choice of company car, and choice is often possible, is normally influenced more by issues of image and self-esteem than by practical considerations. Thus, the older or very tall employee, or the back pain sufferer may choose a car completely unsuitable for their condition. Ample headroom, easy access, and good adjustable seating should be of primary importance in the choice of car. Power steering can help some people with cervicobrachial pain, and automatic transmission may also be beneficial for low back pain and sciatica sufferers.

## Training

Implicit in all the above is the need to educate the worker in safe working practices, safe manual handling techniques, and self-preservation. However, training cannot compensate for poor workplace and task design and these should be addressed first. All too often the provision of training is seen as an easy option by some employers who think that the purchase of some off-the-shelf package, or video, and the provision of a short training session is sufficient to discharge their obligations. As a result, training is often completely ineffective.

Successful training requires to take into account:

- The specific task to be performed
- The established work practices
- The perception that new methods are difficult or time-consuming
- The poorly understood mechanisms of injury
- The weight, shape, and general handling properties of the material/articles
- How any improved job methods might be constrained by poor workplace layout and job design.

Training on the job with a more experienced colleague is rarely adequate and encourages the acquisition of bad habits which may have evolved. There is much evidence to show that the training which has been delivered in the past is not effective in reducing the incidence of back injuries.[8]

The number of preferred training methods is almost as large as the number of trainers and there is little objective evidence that any of the specific lifting techniques are better than others. The traditional technique with a straight back, feet apart, and flexed knees imposes less stress on the lumbar spine than lifting with a bent back and is confirmed by studies of intradiscal pressure. Avoidance of the turning twisting lift by turning with the feet rather than twisting with the trunk has also a good anatomical and pathological basis. Large entities, such as oil drums and people, require entirely different techniques of lifting and training needs to be tailored to the task. Therefore, the following steps need to be taken to provide effective training:

- Analyse the job
- Identify the risks/unsatisfactory postures
- Correct the existing methods and identify training objectives
- Provide training, encourage practice of new methods
- Ensure acquisition of necessary skills
- Ensure there is support from supervisors
- Refresh training regularly and audit the process

New employees require more time for training and should not be expected to perform at high work rates initially but allowed to build up work speed gradually, especially if the task is repetitive.

Frequent review of techniques and re-training when necessary should be an established part of a prevention programme. The single session of training in manual handling techniques is as ineffective as would be one golf lesson to impart the perfect swing.

## Fitness for work

### Pre-employment screening

Self selection usually ensures that persons with unfit backs do not take up heavy manual work. Additional measures such as pre-employment screening, whether by questionnaire or examination, are of very limited value and should only be considered in special circumstances such as work in some types of heavy industry, the fire and rescue services or as required by law, such as in coal mining.

Although many large organizations have an occupational health nurse or doctor, most industries do not have regular access to professional medical advice. In these circumstances the recruiting officer, manager, or foreman may depend on the opinions and advice of the local general practitioners. However, it is usually possible to establish contact with a local group occupational health service or local occupational health nurse or doctor and these and the Employment Medical Advisory Service can provide authoritative advice.

Generally, however, everyone tends to err on the side of caution, which is a mistake, and there are many heavy manual workers who have been told at some time in the distant past, that they would never be fit for the task they are now happily performing!

In assessing fitness for work the minimum information required is as follows:

- *A detailed medical history.* Has the recruit had any major illness, injury, or occupation likely to reduce his ability to undertake manual work?
- *The occupational history.* What previous manual work has the applicant performed successfully. Has there been a back injury or prolonged or recurrent absence from work due to back pain or other medical condition?
- Does the individual appear fit to do the job on offer?

In general, if the recruit has a normal range of movement of the spine and limbs, an absence of significant musculoskeletal deformity and has no other abnormalities, he is acceptable for manual work.

Guidance note MS20 from the Health and Safety Executive deals with preemployment screening and indicates that refusal of employment on health grounds should only be on the basis of defined job specific criteria.[12]

### Specific screening tests

There are a number of biological variables that may affect lifting capacity and which may be useful in certain circumstances.

Strength is obviously significant and strength testing may be valuable sometimes. Chaffin *et al.*[13] showed that isometric testing can be useful in predicting subsequent back injuries as these were less common in those who had a wide margin between their individual maximum strength and the largest force they had to exert at work. More recently, dynamic strength tests have been developed as these are thought to replicate the work task more accurately. However, strength testing is prone to inaccuracy and sophisticated equipment is necessary to perform testing adequately.

Height and weight are also important and have some weak predictive power but recent studies have confirmed that there is no justification for excluding tall men from heavy manual tasks.[14]

Studies of the relationship between spinal canal diameter and back pain have shown that those with the narrowest spinal canals are more prone to back pain and have longer associated absence. However, measurement of canal diameter is difficult and prone to inaccuracy and because of this, is not a strong enough predictor to be of value in the occupational setting.

Many years ago, radiology of the spine was widely used in the belief that screening out those with radiographic abnormalities was worthwhile, but numerous studies have confirmed that radiographs are of no value in predicting who will get back pain at work, and the radiation hazard is unacceptable.[15] Personality tests have been used to investigate chronic back pain sufferers, but are notoriously unreliable, and have no place in pre-employment testing in relation to back pain.

### Screening after sickness absence

Careful management, both medically and generally, is required for the employee returning to work after illness or injury, especially after back or sciatic pain or other illness affecting manual handling ability. Absence may be self- or doctor-certified and with each the significance of any disability is equally liable to miscalculation. At one extreme the absence may be spurious, while at the other, the individual may be trying to return to work too early for financial or other reasons. The general practitioner or hospital doctor is unlikely to have any real idea about the nature of the work task and its physical requirements, and the decision to return to work will often be made on subjective information from the patient.

Many employers contribute to the unnecessary prolongation of absence by adopting an inflexible approach to fitness—the worker is either fully fit or unfit. Medical advisers should try to influence this attitude by communicating with the employer at an early stage when they feel that the patient is capable of lighter work. If it is advised that the functional restriction is temporary, some employers can be persuaded to make some accommodation and provide alternative work.

If the back problem has been caused by work, this should also be communicated so that the workplace can be assessed and preventive action taken. The following signs and symptoms are useful in the prediction of recurrence of back pain in those returning to work after an episode.[16]

*From the history*
- Two or more previous attacks
- A fall on the buttocks or back as a cause of injury
- Sickness absence of 5 weeks or more in the current attack
- Residual pain in the leg on return to work

*From the examination*
- Restriction of pain free straight leg raising to 45 degrees or less
- Pain or weakness on resisted hip flexion

- Inability to sit up from lying flat
- Back pain on lumbar extension

If any of these features are present, the patient should be employed initially on lighter work or be considered for further rehabilitation. (For a further review of this subject see Troup and Edwards.[17])

## Treatment

A significant proportion of patients with back pain threaten to develop a chronicity in their symptoms which is not easily explicable on a physical basis. For these patients a longer period of rehabilitation treatment may be useful. Indeed it may be the only alternative to seeking fringe methods of relief that are available, such as osteopathy, chiropractice, and acupuncture. The conventional treatments used involve a blend of psychiatry, physical methods, occupational therapy, and exercises. At one extreme might be the patient whose problem is thought to be due to a mixture of pain leading to weakness and symptoms of mild depression, and at the other, a patient who is clearly clinically depressed. This leads to diminished *vis a tergo*, weakness, and pain. Diminished *vis a tergo* and weakness may be helped by a mainly very physical approach such as isometric exercises, hydrotherapy and an exercise regime, and pain by methods based mainly on psychotherapy and drugs.[18] The role of back schools is controversial but the formation of small groups who are taught the principles of back care, isometric exercises, and avoidance of harmful stress is popular. Back schools offer an holistic approach to coping with back pain, minimizing disability and maximizing functional potential. The principles are both physically and psychologically sound and assessment to establish their value should be encouraged.

## Spinal cord injuries

The incidence of spinal cord injuries in Britain is about 3 per 100 000 of the population. Motor vehicle accidents account for 50 per cent. Spinal cord injury occurs most often in teenagers and young adults at the beginning of their careers.

The functional independence which may be achieved in the end depends on the level and completeness of the lesion and the adequacy of training (see Table 9.2). Excluding those with a high cord lesion, paraplegics should be able to lead an independent life, though this is only achieved by rehabilitation in a special unit where there is rigorous training in self-care and no concessions to dependence or invalidism.

Spinal cord injury is not simply a malady of the spine—physical, psychological, and social adjustment continue indefinitely. Paraplegics are likely to stay in the spinal injury centre for 4–6 months and quadriplegics about eight months.

**Table 9.2** Functional expectations at different levels of spinal injury

| Level of injury | Functional expectation |
| --- | --- |
| Above C5 | Totally dependent: special respiratory equipment is required; speech is restrained; a powered wheelchair may be controlled by head or mouth microswitches. |
| C5 | Some assistance is needed in all activities. |
| C6 | Can propel manual wheelchair with difficulty; a powered wheelchair is needed on slopes; sometimes driving is possible; in males, bladder drainage is to a leg bag after bladder outlet surgery. |
| C7–T1 | May achieve bladder evacuation by reflex bladder contraction; bowel evacuation is by suppository and rectal stimulation; can be completely independent from a wheelchair. |
| T2–T6 | Fully independent with a wheelchair. |
| T7–T12 | By using a wheelchair is completely independent; can 'walk' wearing orthoses to brace the lower trunk and legs, but not far. |
| L1–L3 | Can walk using knee–ankle–foot orthoses and crutches. |
| L4–S1 | Can walk using ankle/foot orthoses and two sticks or crutches; bladder is emptied by straining and applying suprapubic pressure; lower bowel is emptied by straining or manual removal of faeces. |
| S2–S4 | Only urinary control is difficult. |

Quadriplegics are liable to:

(1) orthostatic hypotension;

(2) autonomic hyper-reflexia with increased sympathetic activity usually provoked by over-distension of a viscus causing hypertension, severe headache, flushing, goose-flesh, and sweating;

(3) thromboembolism;

(4) spasticity; and

(5) impaired respiratory function.

All with spinal injuries lose control of the bladder and bowels, have impaired genital function, and are liable to pressure sores and successive emotional reactions of shock, denial, depression, and hostility before gradual acceptance. After spinal injury, capacity for physical work is low at first. Endurance and muscle strength are regained by physical training. Subsequently, medical complications and social isolation are lessened. The goals of rehabilitation may not be reached for several years. Return to work may be delayed by psychological, physical, environmental, and opportunity constraints, and by claims for compensation. Vocational counsellors in the spinal injury centres work closely with the Disability Employment Adviser, previous employer, training services, and institutions for further education. Rehabilitation must include the acquisition of new skills. Open employment may prove difficult for many, especially quadriplegics, who may consider sheltered employment where productivity is geared to capabilities. Rather than severity of disability, the best predictors of successful occupational resettlement in rank order are previous employment status and ability, previous attitudes towards work, maturity, and verbal ability.

If attention is paid to removing the architectural barriers to employment and by maintaining a positive attitude throughout, many should be able to return to useful employment. In one large series of 2012 paraplegics and tetraplegics, 65 per cent were in employment and 20 per cent in some home occupation; only 14.6 per cent were not working.

In assessing paraplegics who depend on wheelchairs, their abilities to propel them, open, go through and close doors, go up and down ramps, transfer from wheelchair to lavatory, chair, or bed must be ascertained. Their independence in dressing and the time taken to prepare for work in the morning should be measured.

## Conclusions and recommendations

The disorders of the spine are many and varied and continue to present an enormous challenge to the individual sufferers, their medical advisers, and employers. The treatment of many of the degenerative conditions is largely symptomatic and the emphasis must be on support to the individual to help improve symptoms and psychological well-being until remission which usually occurs. Rehabilitation is vital and employers should be encouraged to accommodate the disabled worker in the knowledge that the 'rehabilitation of work' may be more effective than occasional visits to physiotherapy departments, and will often speed recovery and return to normal function.

Much back pain can be caused or exacerbated by poor workplace design or organization and employers must continually strive to reduce occupational hazards by assessing and controlling risks and by monitoring the health of employees at work and thereby making improvements: in other words, a 'quality' management approach to the largest single cause of disability in British industry. Investment in this area is almost always cost-effective.

### Selected references and further reading

1. Wells, N. (1985). *Back pain.* Studies of current health problems, No. 78. Office of Health Economics, London.
2. Lawrence, J.S. (1969). Disc degeneration, its frequency and relationship to symptoms. *Ann. Rheum. Dis.*, **28**, 121–38.
3. Mathews, J.A. (1993). In *Neck pain in Rheumatology*, (ed. J.H. Klippel and P.A. Dieppe). Gower, London.
4. Wynn Parry, C.B. (1965). Management of ankylosing spondylitis. *Proc. Roy. Soc. Med.*, **59**, 619.

5. Mathews, J.A. *et al.* (1987). Back pain and sciatica. Controlled trials of manipulation, traction, sclerosant and epidural injections. *Brit. J Rheumatol.*, **26**, 416–23.

6. Manning, D.P., Mitchell, R.G., and Blanchfield, P.L. (1984). Body movements and events contributing to accidental and non accidental back injuries. *Spine*, **9**, 734–9.

7. Porter, R.W. (1986). *Management of back pain.* Churchill Livingstone, Edinburgh.

8. Graveling, R.A. (1991). The prevention of back pain from manual handling. *Ann. Occ. Hyg.*, **4**, 427–32.

9. *Manual handling. Guidance on the manual handling operations regulations.* (1992). HSE Books.

10. Davis, P.R. and Stubbs, D.A. (1980). *Force limits in manual work.* Science and Technology Press, Guildford.

11. HSE (Health and Safety Executive) (1992). *Display screen equipment. Guidance on regulations.* HMSO, London.

12. HSE (Health and Safety Executive) (1982). Pre-employment Health Screening. Guidance note MS20. HMSO, London.

13. Chaffin, D.B., Herrin, G.D., and Keyserling, W.M. (1978). Pre-employment strength testing—an updated position. *J. Occup. Med.*, **20**, 403–8.

14. Walsh, K., Cruddas, M., and Coggon, D. (1991). Interaction of height and mechanical loading of the spine in the development of low back pain. *Scand. J. Work Environ. Hlth.*, **17**, 420–4.

15. Rowe, M.L. (1982). Are routine spine films on workers in industry cost or risk benefit effective? *J. Occup. Med.*, **24**, 41–3.

16. Lloyd, D.C.E.F. and Troup, J.D.G. (1983). Recurrent back pain and its prediction. *J. Soc. Occ. Med.*, **33**, 66–74.

17. Troup, J.D.G. and Edwards, F.C. (1985). *Manual handling and lifting.* (An information and literature review with special reference to the back.) HMSO, London.

18. Franks, A. (1993). Low back pain. *Brit. Med. J.*, **306**, 901–9.

# 10

# Limb disorders

*C.J. English and G.M. Cochrane*

## Introduction

This chapter is about common diseases of the limbs which hamper work, their incidence and prevalence, the courses that they are likely to take, their prevention and management at work, and pre-employment screening where that is appropriate. Emphasis is given to their effects on function of the upper limb to reach, feel, grasp, control, lift, carry, manipulate, place, propel, and balance; and of the lower limb to feel and by moving to control, impel, support the body in standing, maintain equilibrium, walk, climb, kneel, and run. These functions are diminished by pain, altered sensation, stiffness, disordered control of movement or absence of any part of a limb.

Although musculoskeletal diseases account for a substantial proportion of medical consultations and heavy costs in prescribed medicines, sickness benefit, and lost productivity, they are often diagnosed with uncertainty, and treated inadequately with rest and anti-inflammatory analgesic medicines in the hope of spontaneous resolution. Correct diagnosis and early treatment result in reduced morbidity and an early return to work.

Some occupations demand locomotor normality at entry, e.g., mining and tunnelling, the armed forces, the merchant navy, the police, and the fire and ambulance services. When disabled people are not excluded by established criteria or specific occupational hazards any pre-employment screening should be sensitive to their need for modifications of the job or introductory training. Management may need reassurance to employ those with disorders of their limbs and more still those with unsightly defects and deformities, involuntary movements or socially unattractive characteristics. The motivation, commitment, attendance, and safety records of disabled people match in full those of their able-bodied colleagues. The principal barriers are lack of understanding and prejudice. The advising physician has a crucial role in appreciating and explaining to the reluctant employer the functional abilities and potential for work of a disabled person and how the employer and employee can receive advice and financial assistance from the Department of Employment in overcoming architectural barriers, adapting the workplace, and providing necessary tools and equipment. Examples of diseases that may cause difficulties in employment are considered under five headings.

1. Conditions present from birth or childhood which may impede entry to work.

2. Disorders of the upper limb during the years at work.

3. Disorders of the lower limb during the years at work.

4. Arthritis, gout, and connective tissue diseases.

5. Paget's disease of bone (osteitis deformans)

## 1. Conditions present from birth or childhood

Disabled young people need help in their transition from school to work. They have poorer chances of being employed and receiving training and further education than able-bodied school leavers. It is essential to think ahead to prevent the physical and psychological harm that comes with rejection and unemployment. Early in the final year a discussion concerning the school leaver establishes the child's aptitudes, preferences, intellect and educational achievements, manipulative skills, and mobility. If open or sheltered work is not feasible the disabled school leaver becomes eligible for Invalidity Benefit from the age of 16 and may attend a day centre provided by the local authority.

Commitment and discussion should enable the correct career to be chosen with appropriate training and further education. Young disabled people who are trained are much more readily accepted by the labour market.

### Dwarfism

Growth may be severely retarded because of an inherited defect or a disorder which arises during childhood. Achondroplasia which has an incidence of 1 per 20 000 is a single gene defect with autosomal dominant inheritance and a high mutation rate. Most achondroplasics are born to parents of normal stature with no family history. The incidence of fresh mutations increases with paternal age. An adult achondroplasic woman may reach a height of around 123 cm and a man 132 cm. The limbs are disproportionately short, but the trunk is normal in length with increased lumbar lordosis and thoracic kyphosis. The bridge of the nose is depressed and the forehead and vault of the skull enlarged. Life expectancy, intelligence, and personal independence are no different from those of normal stature.

Turner's syndrome is a form of proportionate small stature in girls, due to the complete or partial absence of one of the two X chromosomes. Its incidence is about 1 per 3000 live female births. Features may include webbing of the neck, low hair line at the back of the neck, short fourth metacarpals or metatarsals, hypoplastic nails, multiple naevi, broad chest with widely spaced nipples, failure of sexual development, and cardiac abnormality. Sensory and visuo-motor perception are below average but verbal ability is good. Many choose caring work.

The illnesses in childhood which stunt growth are prevented or their effect diminished by improving social conditions and nutrition and by early recognition and treatment. Among them are endocrine disorders of the anterior pituitary, thyroid and pancreatic islet cells, rickets, coeliac disease, fibrocystic disease or neglect.

For people of restricted growth, as for others, the choice of career should depend upon talent and inclination. The major problem is convincing a potential employer. Insurance may be a barrier where it is considered that heavy machinery or laboratory equipment create a special risk. Ergonomic assessment, adaptations to the workplace and the provision of special handling aids should be considered to achieve employment. The ability to drive by simple pedal extensions and seat adaptations is particularly important when mobility is restricted.

The Restricted Growth Association provides social contact and advice and acts as a pressure group. (For the full address see Appendix 9.)

### Osteogenesis imperfecta: the brittle bone syndrome

The incidence of this inherited disease is 1 per 30 000 births. The synthesis of type 1 collagen, the only collagen of bone, is defective causing bones to be excessively fragile. Other tissues which contain type 1 collagen are also involved: the sclerae, skin, dentine of teeth, heart valves, tendons, and ligaments. Four main types are recognised.[1] The most common and mildest is type I, having family history, blue sclerae, and discoloured teeth with enamel breaking off the defective dentine; deafness is frequent; fractures may be few, occurring late, and stature is often normal.

The majority of those with osteogenesis imperfecta achieve a high rate of employment. The severely affected need to attend a special school. In all cases, further education and training should be encouraged. If the disease is severe, special career advice should be sought. In job placement the risk of developing deafness as part of the disease should be heeded.

### Haemophilia and arthritis

Haemophilias are the commonest disorders of blood clotting, affecting all races with incidence of around 80 per million of the population. (See Chapter 17, p. 335)

In some haemophiliacs the disease is mild, causing little inconvenience, but in others there may be recurrent haemorrhages. The severity of bleeding is related to the residual level of Factor VIII in plasma. Bleeding usually follows injury, which may be trivial. Clots form slowly and break up easily. Bleeding into joints occurs with distressing frequency and intense pain. The knees (70 per cent), ankles, and elbows are most often affected, usually only one joint in each bleeding episode. One haemarthrosis predisposes to another, and repeated exposure of a joint's surfaces to blood accelerates destruction of cartilage and underlying bone, proliferation of synovial membrane, atrophy of muscles, and progressive damage and deformity of the joint. Bleeding occurs also under the periosteum, within bone, and in muscles, causing severe pain, swelling, and neurovascular compression, notably in the forearm, leg, and iliopsoas muscle when the femoral nerve may be involved presenting with pain and swelling in the groin and flexion at the hip.

Treatment to arrest bleeding is intravenous replacement of the coagulant factor as soon as possible after onset. This is also the best analgesic: addiction to narcotics was common in haemophiliacs before an effective haemostatic agent was available. Rest initially is followed by graded exercise to restore function. Chronic pain of haemophilic arthropathy can be relieved by *Ibuprofen* or *Indomethacin*. Aspirin is contraindicated as it compounds the bleeding tendency and can cause gastrointestinal bleeding. **Intramuscular injections are absolutely prohibited in haemophilia.**

Ignorance and misconceptions have kept boys from school and men from work. Since there have been haemophilia centres in all regions in the UK haemophiliacs have relied less on local hospitals. They take reasonable care to avoid trauma, recognize the first sign of bleeding, and know how to achieve immediate control. Self-treatment has radically improved the management of severe haemophilias A and B and most sufferers in Britain can now inject themselves intravenously with factor concentrate whenever they suspect bleeding. This has resulted in increased independence, reduced reliance on hospital treatment, better academic achievements and attendances at school, and improved prospects of employment. For self-treatment only a 15 minute break from work is required. Good haemophilia care has led to a threefold reduction in days lost from work.

Through fear of unemployment there has been a tendency to hide the diagnosis. In one survey[2] the unemployment rate of 502 respondents was 17.5 per cent when the current UK rate of unemployment was 6.9 per cent. Of those unemployed, 76 per cent attributed to haemophilia their failure to be appointed; 1 in 4 of those in work had not told their employer; yet 80 per cent of those who had disclosed the diagnosis found their employers and workmates helpful. Forty-eight per cent were registered disabled but 75 per cent considered that they had received no advice from teachers, career officers, doctors or disablement resettlement officers; 76 per cent had been in the same job for more than three years.

The occupational physician has a vital role in advising the potential employer about the good prospects for the haemophiliac, assessing suitable work, mainly sedentary for the severely affected and avoiding, for all, heavy manual labour and obvious risks of injuries, and ensuring suitable arrangements for self-treatment. Advice is readily available from the local haemophilia centre on particulars of management and from the Haemophilia Society (see Appendix 9, p. 514 for the address) on vocational training, employment, and employer's insurance; and from the local disablement employment adviser on assistance with essential facilities, equipment, and transport.

*Congenital limb deformities*

Deformities may occur as complete absence (amelia) or malformation of any part of the limb. In transverse deficiencies all elements beyond a certain level are absent and the limb resembles an amputation stump. Prosthetic devices are most valuable in lower extremity deficiencies. With effective support most people with congenital amputation lead normal lives.

1. *Upper limb deficiencies* are less frequent than those of the lower limb. Some deformities benefit from surgery to secure the best functional position. Sensation is normal and through using the limb to its limit from infancy, the child acquires adroitness and prostheses are frequently rejected. Ergonomic assessment should be undertaken with measurements of power, manipulative skills, and reach; and advice from a Placement Assessment and Counselling Team (PACT) of the Department of Employment (see Chapter 2, p. 37) should ensure that career choice is not severely restricted.

2. *Congenital deformities* of the lower limb are corrected early in life by splinting, surgery or prosthesis to encourage standing and walking. Persistent congenital dislocation of the hip occurs in 1.5 per 1000 live births, six times more frequently in girls than boys, and the left hip more than the right. With inadequate treatment the disability is severe with instability, short leg, limping, restricted movements, and pain. Work should be sedentary and skilled to give security of tenure.

3. *Arthrogryposis multiplex congenita* occurs in about 3 per 1000 live births but is not genetic. The fibrous ankylosis of many joints arises from defective development of fetal muscle or from atrophy of lower motor neurones. The limbs are in abnormal positions with most joints fixed in flexion with the exception of the knees where hyperextension is usual. Scoliosis and a deformed chest are likely. Limbs are used to their limits and a stick, brush or pencil may be held in the mouth, fingers or toes to operate a keyboard, paint or write. Intelligence is usually normal and special training for a career will be rewarded.

4. *Marfan's syndrome* is an inherited disorder of connective tissue, transmitted as an autosomal dominant disorder, affecting about 1 in 10 000 of the population. Thirty per cent are through mutations and the incidence increases with paternal age. The features are tallness with arm span exceeding height, sparse subcutaneous fat, digits which are disproportionately long and thin, lax ligaments, hypotonia, long thin face and narrow maxilla with high arched palate and crowded teeth, dislocated lenses and tremulous irises, severe myopia, and weakness of the aortic valve and aorta with liability to dissecting aneurysm. Death usually occurs before the age of 50. The intellect is normal and higher education and training are recommended in choosing a career.

### Juvenile rheumatoid arthritis

Rheumatoid arthritis beginning before 16 years of age affects 1 in 1000 children, and girls more than boys. About 20 per cent of cases have systemic onset Still's disease, 40 per cent have polyarticular onset similar to adult rheumatoid arthritis, and 40 per cent have an arthritis limited to a few joints. Some children in the latter group develop iridocyclitis with risk of cataract, adhesions of the iris, secondary glaucoma, visual impairment, and sometimes blindness. Other serious complications of juvenile chronic arthritis are involvement of the large joints, retarded growth, muscle atrophy, joint contractures, underdevelopment of the lower jaw, and fusion of the joints of the cervical spine. The prevalence of this form of severe disability is about 1 in 20 000 of the population. Females are affected twice as often as males and 1 in 10 has defective vision. Education is commonly interrupted and emphasis should be on extending education and realistic work opportunities and career.

## 2.   Disorders of the upper limb

### *Non-articular rheumatism*

The extent of any association between upper limb symptoms and work continues to be debated. The introduction of terms such as 'repetitive strain injury', 'cumulative trauma disorders', and 'overuse syndromes', has misled and confused. They have been seized upon by the popular press, trade unions, employees, and lawyers but the diseases commonly occur unrelated to work, repetition, strain, and injury.[3] The terms should be abandoned, being inaccurate and vague, when by careful examination exact diagnosis is possible.

**To suggest on the balance of probability that the activities at work are responsible, several criteria must be satisfied: the absence of any history of a potentially causative activity not related to work, the duties at work must seem likely to stress the affected part, the onset and occurrence of symptoms should show work association following a change in working practice or return to work after holiday or extended leave, the work rate is rapid, the duties arduous, and the same activity is continued for long periods without breaks.** Before concluding that upper limb symptoms and the patient's work are causally related the occupational physician is advised to examine the workstation and the process as well as the patient.

*Fibromyalgia* describes pain in fibrous connective tissue of muscles, tendons or ligaments induced by physical or mental stress, poor sleep and exposure to damp or cold and in association with occupational or recreational strain. Primary fibromyalgia is more likely to occur in young women who are tense, depressed, anxious, and striving. In older adults the symptoms are associated with vertebral osteoarthrosis. The diagnosis is made on a history of diffuse discomfort with discrete tender points and by exclusion of other disease. The treatment is explanation of its benign nature, reassurance, stretching exercises, and amitriptyline at night to improve sleep.

Defined non-articular rheumatic disorders, which diminish performance, are considered below.

*Shoulder*. Pain at the shoulder may have a local cause in or around the joint or be referred from disease in the chest, upper abdomen or cervical spine. Cervical radiculopathy causes diffuse pain when nerve roots are irritated, usually by facet joint arthritis and spondylosis in which degenerative changes and the formation of bony osteophytes narrow the neural foraminae. Damage to the rotator cuff in the shoulder joint causes a painful arc between 70 and 120 degrees on elevation of the arm when the supraspinatus tendon is involved; and pain on external rotation denotes that the infraspinatus tendon is inflamed. The peak incidence is in middle life and affects women more than men. Plaques of hydroxyapatite may be laid down in the tendon (calcific tendinitis) and may discharge into the subdeltoid bursa with severe pain on movement and at night and exquisite tenderness. Treatment by intrasynovial injection of corticosteroid with lignocaine is usually quickly effective in tendinitis and bursitis.

Bicipital tendinitis is inflammation of the synovial sheath surrounding the tendon of the long head of biceps causing pain on resisted supination of the forearm and on flexion at the elbow.

'Frozen shoulder' means inflammation of the capsule of the glenohumeral joint with its adhesion to the head of the humerus completely limiting glenohumeral movement. Adhesive capsulitis is a better term. This occurs over the age of 35, and is triggered by injury to the shoulder or upper limb or by pain referred from the cervical spine or heart. Exercises should begin as soon as possible to prevent this complication. Local injection of corticosteroid and analgesic may help. Pain diminishes first but full movements may not be regained for over a year.

*The elbow.* Tennis elbow describes pain in the region of the lateral epicondyle, aggravated by grasping and lifting and extension of the wrist. There is point tenderness over the lateral epicondyle where the extensor muscles of the wrist and fingers are attached. The treatment consists of eliminating aggravating factors and intralesional injection of corticosteroid with local anaesthetic. Golfer's elbow is a comparable syndrome involving the attachment of the flexor muscles of the wrist and fingers to the medial epicondyle. Postural and ergonomic adjustments, task modifications or job rotation may be necessary to prevent recurrence. Inflammation of the olecranon bursa may occur after injury and from infection, gout or rheumatoid arthritis.

*The wrist and hand.* Tenosynovitis is inflammation of the tendon sheath and enclosed tendon, causing pain on movement, swelling and friction rub. The usual aggravating factor of inflammation of the extensor tendon is excessive repetitive hand work. The treatment is intrasynovial injection of corticosteroid and local anaesthetic and avoidance of causal and aggravating movements until relief. De Quervain's disease, stenosing tenosynovitis, involving extensor pollicis brevis and abductor pollicis longus, causes disabling pain at the radial side of the wrist. Surgical release may be required. If the employee can establish that traumatic inflammation of the tendon was caused by manual labour Industrial Injury Benefit may be claimed under the Social Security (Industrial Injuries) (Prescribed Diseases) Amendment Regulations 1991.

Where groups of staff complain of similar symptoms an ergonomic survey will be required. Major alterations may be needed to work practices, procedures or workplace design and in extreme situations this may extend to automation of the process.

Tenosynovitis of the finger flexors is less often due to trauma and occurs in rheumatoid arthritis, gout, and neisserial and mycobacterial infections. Trigger finger and trigger thumb are due to nodules on the flexor tendon and sheath causing intermittent locking in flexion. Surgical excision of the sheath may be necessary if injection of steroid into the sheath is not effective. A ganglion (a synovium-lined cyst containing gelatinous fluid) often occurs at the wrist. It can be ignored, unless symptomatic when surgical excision is required.

Cramp of the hand or forearm due to repetitive movements is another prescribed disease (A4) in any occupation involving prolonged periods of handwriting, typing or other repetitive movements of the fingers, hand or arm. Prevention rests on changing working practices, introducing variety of tasks, and rest breaks.

*Working with visual display units.* Keyboard users may complain of discomfort in the neck and upper limbs related to prolonged, constrained static posture, the intensity and duration of work, repetitive movements, psychological stress associated with the demands of the job, lack of autonomy, poor employer/ employee relationship, piece-work payments or fear of redundancy. The Courts place great weight on publications from the Health and Safety Executive (HSE).[4–8] A good preventive strategy has two main components (see also chapter 5, p. 96):

(i)   assessment of the work task, the workstation, and work procedures; and

(ii)  pre-employment screening for similar past conditions, education, instruction, training, supervision, monitoring procedures, and appropriate record-keeping.

## Peripheral nerve injuries

Brachial plexus traction injuries occur mostly in young men involved in motorcycle accidents and are covered in Chapter 11, p. 209.

Winging of a scapula, because of isolated weakness of the serratus anterior muscle, may arise from damage to the long thoracic nerve by wearing a heavy backpack. A more frequent cause is neuralgic amyotrophy, in which pain around the shoulder is followed by weakness and wasting. Recovery proceeds slowly over 12–18 months.

Wrist drop may be due to damage to the radial nerve. The nerve is most vulnerable in the spiral groove of the humerus, in fractures of the humerus, or to external pressure as in 'Saturday night paralysis'.* A wrist splint is needed to allow good use of the hand until conduction in the nerve returns. A severed radial nerve must be explored and repaired. Weakness of extension of the thumb and index finger may be caused by compression of the posterior interosseous nerve

---

*Paralysis of the wrist caused when the arm hangs over the edge of a chair and the owner is inebriated!

at the elbow by the supinator muscle. The nerve should be surgically released. If reconstructive procedures are necessary involving transfer of one or more flexor tendons to act as extensors of the fingers and thumb, good function can be restored. The median nerve may be damaged at the elbow in 'pronator syndrome', or its motor branch, the anterior interosseous nerve may be compressed in the forearm but more commonly the median nerve is injured at the wrist.

The nerve is the most vulnerable structure in the carpal tunnel to compression by tenosynovitis, fluid retention in pregnancy, rheumatoid arthritis, venous engorgement, lymphoedema, local trauma or osteoarthritic deformity. Carpal tunnel syndrome is three times as common in women as in men, may be bilateral, and the features are burning pain or tingling in the hand, mostly at night and relieved by vigorous shaking. There is diminished sensation in the radial three digits and weakness of the muscles of the thenar eminence. Cervical nerve root damage may coexist. Conservative treatment is rest, diuretics, and wearing a splint at night to hold the wrist, hand, and fingers in neutral positions. Definitive treatment is surgical decompression. It is always prudent to confirm the diagnosis by nerve conduction studies.

The ulnar nerve is also vulnerable to damage at the elbow and wrist and the most common site is at the elbow. The features are wasting and weakness of the interossei, the fourth and fifth lumbricals, the muscles of the hypothenar eminence and adductor pollicis. (Note Froment's sign, which is an inability to adduct the thumb strongly to the radial side of the index finger without flexing the terminal phalanx of the thumb.) Sensation is diminished over the little finger and adjacent side of the ring finger and the ulnar side of the hand but not above the wrist crease. If there is proven delay in nerve conduction simple decompression is indicated; if the elbow joint is abnormal and the nerve dislocates anterior transposition is chosen. If the nerve is divided in open injury primary suture is imperative. Damage to the ulnar nerve at the wrist occurs in open injuries as by laceration, through recurrent occupational trauma as in thumping with the heel of the hand, or pressure of a ganglion. If there is a history of occupational trauma, its avoidance is advised. If a ganglion is palpable it should be excised.

If lack of key grip is disabling, the extensor indicis can be transferred into the first dorsal interosseous muscle. (For further discussion of peripheral nerve injuries see Chapter 11, p. 207 *et seq.*)

*Vibration white finger or hand–arm vibration syndrome*

Workers most at risk are users of chain-saws, hand-held rotary grinding, polishing and sanding tools, and percussion tools for metal work, mining, quarrying, and demolition. The disease develops over several years, progressing from intermittent blanching of one finger, with or without tingling and numbness, to frequent episodes of extreme blanching of all fingers in summer and winter. Pre-employment screening should identify those with a history of primary Raynaud's disease who are at increased risk and should be excluded from any exposure to hand/arm vibration. Health surveillance procedures are required.

Employee information leaflets should ensure understanding and encourage early reporting of symptoms. Safety considerations are of importance where a secure grip on tools is required. Total re-training and re-location may prove difficult if there are sensory and functional impairments of the hands. Despite change of occupation the damage to the arterial wall may progress.

### Degenerative joint disease

Osteoarthritis of the glenohumeral joint in middle age is more common in foundry workers, divers and compressed-air workers (from aseptic bone necrosis), and others engaged in heavy manual work and in the dominant limb, with pain, restriction of movements, and crackling as the joint is moved.

Osteoarthritis of the acromioclavicular joint with synovitis may cause a prominent cystic swelling above the shoulder. Degenerative changes in the elbow joint cause deformity, restricted flexion and extension, and sometimes ulnar neuropathy. In the first carpometacarpal joint at the base of the thumb osteoarthritis causes bony enlargement and deformity, pain on gripping, wringing, and grasping large objects. Pain may be relieved by a thumb base splint extending to the proximal phalanx and intra-articular injection of corticosteroid. If these fail the trapezium bone may be excised. In the distal interphalangeal joints of the fingers osteoarthritis is common and gelatinous cysts may form Heberden's nodes over bony spurs at the dorsolateral and medial sides of the joint, with flexion and lateral deviation of the terminal phalanx. They rarely cause functional disability.

### Dupuytren's contracture

Painless thickening and shortening of the fascia in the superficial compartment of the palm leads to progressive flexion deformity of the fingers. One or both of the hands may be affected, the right more often, and usually the ring finger first and the little finger before the middle finger. The skin adheres to the fascia and becomes puckered and extension of the finger becomes impossible. Men are affected more than women in the ratio 5:1, and the incidence increases with age after 40. There is hereditary predisposition and associations with alcohol, epilepsy, diabetes mellitus, and liver disease. The evolution of the disease is unpredictable. The treatment of choice is local fasciectomy before there is severe deformity. Similar lesions may occur in the plantar fascia. If manipulation or grip are affected and are essential for work, changes should be made in the workplace or to manual controls before relocation.

### 3.   Disorders of the lower limb

### Pain and limited movements in the hip

Disease at the hip joint is likely to cause limping because of pain, shortening of the leg, flexion contracture or muscle weakness, notably of the gluteus medius.

Pain commonly radiates in the territory of the obturator nerve down the inner side of the thigh to the knee.

1. *Ankylosing spondylitis* is a cause of pain in the hip and is dealt with in Chapter 9 (see p. 170).

2. *Osteoarthritis* is the most common of all disorders of the hip joint. Pathological changes, usually without symptoms, begin in most people before the age of 40 and are universal by the age of retirement. Causal factors include obesity, trauma, aseptic necrosis of the femoral capital epiphysis in childhood (Perthes' disease), slipped epiphysis, inflammatory arthritis, and prolonged overuse in certain occupations. Agricultural workers are particularly liable to osteoarthritis of the hip.[9] Those with a history of predisposing conditions should be discouraged from heavy manual work.

The load on the hip is reduced by losing any excess weight and holding a walking aid in the contralateral hand. A raise should be added to the heel to compensate for shortening. Selected progressive exercises increase the range of motion at the joint and strengthen the muscles acting on it. Consideration should be given to the nature of the person's occupation and the environment at work, travelling and car parking, reducing the distance that must be walked, avoiding stairs, and providing a high working seat and a rail, and raised lavatory seat.

The indications for total hip replacement are restriction of walking distance to 100 m, reliance on a walking aid, pain-disturbed sleep and analgesics by day, and increasing difficulties with everyday personal care. The success in freedom from pain is 95 per cent and most who are in sedentary work can return in six weeks and in manual work within six months, capable of all but heavy lifting, carrying, climbing, and crouching.

### Pain and instability at the knee

1. *Patellar pain* in young adults, more commonly in women, may be caused by compression arthropathy in the lateral patellofemoral joint, due to relative weakness of vastus medialis allowing lateral displacement of the patella. Usually conservative treatment suffices—strengthening the vastus medialis by selective exercises and increasing knee flexion. Work activities need not be restricted permanently.

2. *Chondromalacia patellae* is a softening degeneration of the articular surface of the patella after direct injury, strenuous athletic activity especially in girls, prolonged immobilization or recurrent dislocation. The knee hurts on standing after sitting and going up and down stairs. Active movement of the knee against resistance produces crepitus and grating, more if the patella is pushed against the femur. Chondromalacia may be followed by osteoarthritis. Exercises to strengthen the vastus medialis selectively will help and many recover spontaneously, although in some people disabling pain persists for years. Until the discomfort abates, activities have to be restrained and work should not demand crouching, kneeling, climbing or heavy carrying.

3. *Osteochondritis dissecans* is the separation through injury of an island of subchondral bone. The knee is the most common site, at the lateral face of the medial femoral condyle. The condition is mostly in males in the second and third decades. Additional trauma may cause the fragment to loosen and discharge into the joint. Before a fragment loosens the symptoms are mild aching and intermittent swelling. The loose body may result in mechanical locking. X-rays and arthroscopy confirm the diagnosis. In adults, replacement or removal of the segment will be necessary. Over the following 30 years 80 per cent will develop degenerative arthritis.

4. *Injuries* to the menisci are common and result from twisting sprains applied to the flexed knee. The medial meniscus is more commonly affected. The cartilage may be torn or its peripheral border ripped from the capsule. The torn or detached portion may jam between the articular surfaces causing locking. Miners, agricultural workers, and labourers who must repeatedly rotate on flexed knees are at risk; however, most tears occur in sport outside work. The diagnosis may be confirmed by arthroscopy or magnetic resonance imaging (MRI). Resection of the torn fragment is usually possible through the arthroscope. With diligent rehabilitation manual workers may return to their full employment two weeks later when they can squat fully without holding. Sedentary workers can return much sooner, and as soon as they can depress the brake and clutch pedals if they are required to drive.

5. *Cruciate ligament injuries* are common, the anterior ligament more frequently and this may be overlooked. Anteroposterior laxity causes instability and predisposes to injury of the medial meniscus. Assistance is needed to change from heavy manual work. Assiduous physiotherapy and orthopaedic advice are required.

6. *Bursitis* may occur through repeated physical injury, acute or chronic infection, gout or inflammatory arthritis. Bursae are sac-like cavities filled with synovial fluid, located where friction occurs. The infrapatellar bursa enlarges in those whose work involves kneeling, for instance carpet-layers, and they should use thick foam knee pads. 'Beat knee' is an acute inflammation of a bursa with haemorrhage which may be complicated by infection with surrounding cellulitis, usually from kneeling in cramped, damp, and cold conditions. It is recognized for compensation under the Industrial Injuries Act although it has become much rarer with mechanization and the decline of the coal industry. Treatment must be prompt and thorough with antibiotics and immobilization followed by exercises to recover muscular strength. It may be imprudent to return to the same work.

7. By the age of 40, almost everybody has some early degenerative changes in the knees although few have symptoms. Frequency increases with age. Heredity, obesity, excessive joint use, and injury contribute to susceptibility. The symptoms are pain, stiffness eased by exercise, diminishing range of

movement, tenderness, and grating. As ligaments become lax the joints become unstable and deformed.

Treatment includes explaining the nature of the problem and selecting suitable work which avoids heavy labouring, carrying, climbing, and walking long distances, particularly over rough ground, relieving excess weight, and strengthening muscles acting on the joint. Severe cases may now benefit from the insertion of a prosthetic joint.

### *Pain in the ankle and foot on standing and walking*

Diagnosis and management depend on determining the site and the structure involved and whether the disorder is the result of injury, systemic disease or abnormality of form or function.

1. *Inversion sprain of the ankle* is a common injury and may damage the anterior talofibular ligament. If the talus can be displaced forwards the ligament has ruptured. A mild inversion sprain is treated by strapping in eversion by a 40 cm long stirrup of one-way stretch elastoplast: no time should be lost from work. Partial rupture of the lateral ligament is treated by immobilization of the ankle in a below-knee walking plaster for three to six weeks with a temporary change to sedentary work. Subsequently, an outside flare may be added to the heel of the shoe to protect against further injury.

2. *Pain under the heel*, especially at the start of the day and on direct pressure over the inner weight-bearing tuberosity of the calcaneus, is caused by inflammation at the periosteal attachment of the plantar fascia. A thick, foam rubber pad in the shoe under the heel and precise injection of corticosteroid with local anaesthetic bring relief. Temporary change of duties should only be necessary where work involves much walking, standing or heavy lifting.

Pain at the back of the heel with a red, tender thickened area, often in young women, is due to inflammation of a bursa over the insertion of the Achilles tendon caused by friction of the shoe. Lifting the heel by a foam rubber pad and stretching the back of the shoe usually suffice.

3. *Mid foot problems* are mainly foot strain and flat feet. Obesity and occupational stress overstretch muscles and ligaments leading to pronation of the foot and valgus position of the heel. Reducing weight, adding a 5 mm inside wedge and Thomas heel to the shoe, and an insole support, which lifts the longitudinal arch, will relieve discomfort: the nature of the work should be reviewed if symptoms persist or recur.

4. *Metatarsalgia*, pain in the ball of the foot, is common in those with deformed, pronated feet, hallux valgus, and the lateral four toes displaced upwards on the metatarsal heads. A valgus and metatarsal insole support helps to restore the position of the foot and by lifting the shafts of the metatarsals relieves pressure on the metatarsal heads.

5. *Osteoarthritis of the first metatarsophalangeal joint* at the base of the big toe is very common causing pain, bony enlargement, and hallux rigidus. A rocker bar built into the sole of the shoe under the metatarsal heads is the first treatment and surgery is the second. Return to work can be expected within two months of surgery, wearing protective footwear.

6. *Hallux valgus* is a deformity at the first metatarsophalangeal joint predominantly in females and is often due to abnormal positioning of the toe in fashionable footwear. Corrective osteotomy is the treatment of choice for persistent pain and the deformity. Return to sedentary work in two months is possible or slightly longer if prolonged standing or walking is required.

*Nerve compression syndromes*

1. *Nerve root disorders.* Pain in the leg may be due to dysfunction of a lumbar or sacral nerve root and is dealt with in Chapter 9 (p. 171 *et seq.*).

2. *Pressure on peripheral nerves.* The common peroneal nerve is superficial behind the head and neck of the fibula and may be compressed against the fibula by external forces, e.g., prolonged squatting or sitting cross-legged for lengthy periods. The consequences are paresis of dorsiflexion and eversion of the foot and occasionally sensory deficit over the web between the hallux and second toe. Recovery will occur if causal factors are rectified.

*Metatarsalgia and interdigital pain.* Repeated pressure on an interdigital nerve between two metatarsal bones, most often the third and fourth, may produce a Morton's neuroma, causing pain in the forefoot radiating to the tips of two toes. The neuroma may be excised if local injection of corticosteroid and a metatarsal insole support do not relieve the pain.

*Peripheral vascular disease*

1. *Atherosclerosis* is silent until narrowing, aneurysm or occlusion of the vessel occurs. The first symptoms are aching and tiredness in the calf or other muscles on walking causing limping, worse on walking quickly or uphill. Occlusive disease may progress so that ischaemic pain occurs in the leg at rest. The pedal pulses are absent or reduced. The foot becomes pallid after one or two minutes elevation, and red when it is dependent. More extensive obliterative disease leads to necrosis and gangrene.

Acute obliteration by embolus or thrombosis causes sudden pain with a cold, white or blue foot, absent pulses and weakness with diminished sensation below the obstruction. Urgent surgery is required to prevent irreversible ischaemic damage to the tissues.

Collateral circulation may be increased by muscle demand and people with intermittent claudication should walk for 60 minutes daily, stop when uncomfortable, and walk again. Tobacco in all forms should be eliminated. Prophylactic foot care is crucial and may require the attentions of a chiropodist.

Stockings should be loose, wool in winter and cotton in summer; shoes should fit well; and extremes of temperature should be avoided. Chosen work should be in a dry, comfortable environment, allow sitting and limit walking to short distances, without stairs or hurrying.

Intermittent claudication which prevents the person from working indicates the need for operative treatment. If arteriography demonstrates widespread arteriopathy surgery is unlikely to succeed. Walking will become increasingly restricted and only sedentary work can be undertaken.

2. *Venous thrombosis* may occur due to injury to the epithelium of the vein, hypercoagulability which may arise with oral contraceptives or stasis—even prolonged immobility with the legs dependent during air flight. Most thrombi begin in the valve cusps of deep calf veins. Deep vein thrombosis may be symptomless or cause pain, oedema, tenderness, and prominent superficial veins. Deep vein thrombosis demands rest in bed with the foot of the bed elevated and immediate anticoagulation with heparin succeeded by warfarin for two to six months. Work can be resumed as soon as anticoagulation control is stabilized.

Superficial thrombophlebitis can be palpated as an indurated cord and requires only compression support and a non-steroidal anti-inflammatory drug. Absence from work should be brief.

3. *Varicose veins* are superficial veins which are dilated and tortuous because venous valves are incompetent, allowing reverse flow. In health, the direction of venous flow is from superficial to deep by perforator veins. Previous deep vein thrombosis and vein recanalization result in incompetent valves.

Varicose veins are a common problem that can cause much concern and sickness absence in factories employing large numbers of women who have to stand for long periods. Prolonged standing without walking aggravates existing varicose veins. Varicose veins may cause aching and fatigue, worse at menstruation, and relieved by elevation which is an important sign, and by compression stockings. The person should avoid standing still, walk much more every day, lose excess weight, and regain movements at the ankle joints and in the feet. The indications for surgical treatment are pain, recurrent phlebitis, eczema, superficial and very painful ulcers. Treatment options include sclerotherapy, local ligation of varicosities with or without ligation of the saphenofemoral junction or complete or partial stripping of the long saphenous vein. Treatment choice will depend on the number, size, and location of varicosities, the competence of the saphenofemoral valve and whether there are predisposing factors to coronary artery disease. Although the internal mammary artery is now preferred for coronary artery bypass grafting, the long saphenous vein may also be required if multiple bypass grafts are undertaken.

Successful sclerosing therapy requires total obliteration of the vein by fibrosis. The vein must be empty of blood during and after the injection of a 1 or 3 per cent solution of sodium tetradecyl sulphate. Rubber pads are applied over the injected veins and compression bandages from the base of the toes to above the highest injection site; they remain on for three weeks. Normal activities and walking activate the muscle pump and promote venous drainage from the limbs. Absence from work may not be necessary. The complications of injection therapy are few.

Multiple ligation of varicosities and ligation of the saphenofemoral junction is most likely to be undertaken as a surgical day case procedure. Support stockings require to be worn for six weeks but a return to work can be foreseen within 24 hours following recovery from anaesthesia.

Stripping of the long saphenous vein may also be undertaken as a day case procedure or possibly may require an overnight stay. Absence from work of less than a week is to be expected except where working conditions could be considered dirty when return should be delayed until removal of sutures on the seventh postoperative day.

### 4.  Arthritis, gout and connective tissue disease

1. *Rheumatoid arthritis* affects 1 per cent of all populations, women two to three times more often than men. Onset may be at any age, most often between 25 and 50. Genetic factors predispose to this auto-immune disorder. Most often the onset is insidious but may be abrupt. Any synovial joints may be affected and are painful, tender, swollen, warm, and stiff. Symmetrical involvement of peripheral joints is usual.

Symptoms vary from day to day and within a day. The first hour or two after waking are particularly punishing. Those engaged in heavy manual work are forced, before others, to seek less demanding work. The use of the arm may be seriously impaired by arthritis of the elbow and shoulder. Arthritis of the wrist joints is especially disabling. Carpal tunnel syndrome may result from synovitis at the wrist. Much can be done to protect and preserve the use of the hands, providing aids for using keys, opening doors and turning taps, and teaching the correct ways of handling and lifting, not using the knuckles when rising from a chair, and supplying splints to support the wrist. Carpal tunnel syndrome may require surgical division of the flexor retinaculum.

In the lower limbs, the knee is among the most frequently affected joints with effusion, stiffness, pain aggravated on bearing weight, instability, and varus or valgus deformity. Arthritis at the mortice joint at the ankle causes pain on flexion and extension of the foot. Subtalar involvement causes pain on inversion and eversion. Synovitis at the metatarsophalangeal joints is particularly common, causing pain, like treading on a marble, under the ball of the foot. Correcting the posture of the foot by supporting orthoses, well-fitting shoes or surgery can make walking tolerable.

The best indication of the value of treatment is the ability to work. It is imperative whenever possible to avoid becoming unemployed, modifying work if necessary or relocating within the firm. Few employers will be willing to take on a person with progressive disease, physical limitations, a chequered work record, and uncertain future. Successful employment depends more on social and environmental factors than on the degree of disability.[10] The best jobs are those indoors which call for skill not strength.

2. *Systemic lupus erythematosus (SLE)* is an auto-immune inflammatory disorder of connective tissue occurring most frequently in young women. With increased awareness of mild forms has come the realization that for the majority of patients the disease can be controlled without recourse to high doses of corticosteroids.

SLE may be classified as *mild*, with fever, arthritis, pleurisy, pericarditis, headaches or rash; or *severe*, threatening life because of haemolytic anaemia, thrombocytopenic purpura, renal damage, vasculitis or CNS involvement. Mild disease may require no treatment other than hydroxychloroquine, 200 mg daily. Indoor work with light physical demands should ensure regular employment. Severe disease requires immediate corticosteroid therapy, combined with an immunosuppressive agent until the inflammatory process is controlled.

3. *Psoriatic arthritis* has a number of characteristics which differentiate it from rheumatoid arthritis and it is usually mild. In one study, two-thirds of people never required time off work despite suffering from the disease for more than 10 years.[11] Treatment is directed at control of skin lesions and joint inflammation. Task or work modifications are unlikely to be required for all but the most severe cases and for those work should be carefully selected. (See also Chapter 6, p. 106)

4. *Polymyalgia rheumatica* has an incidence of about 5 per 100 000, occurring in people older than 50 years, and in women twice as often as in men. The characteristic symptoms are aching and stiffness of the muscles of the neck, shoulders, and pelvic girdle, worst in the morning.

The onset may be sudden or gradual with fever, malaise, anorexia, loss of weight, moderate anaemia, and erythrocyte sedimentation rate (ESR) raised to over 40 mm/hour. One or two joints may be swollen. The disease responds so well to corticosteroid that relief of symptoms within 24 hours of starting prednisolone confirms the diagnosis. Normal work can soon be resumed and the dose of steroid can be steadily withdrawn over 4–6 months. In 15 per cent, temporal arteritis is present with the risk of irreversible blindness. High doses of steroids under the supervision of an ophthalmologist are required until symptoms are fully controlled and they can then be withdrawn gradually.

5. *Gout* is a recurrent acute inflammation from the deposition of urate crystals in and around peripheral joints. Gout is infrequent before the age of 40 and in women. The age of onset and the risk of gout are related to the serum urate levels. Hyperuricaemia, the biochemical hallmark of gout, is arbitrarily defined as over 7 mg/100 ml in adult males and 6 mg/100 ml in females. Hyperuricaemia may be caused by genetic or acquired disorders of purine metabolism including diuretic therapy, usually with thiazides.

The acute attack causes excruciating pain, coming without warning and often at night, and lasts for a few days. At first one joint is affected, often the metatarsophalangeal joint of the great toe. Later several joints may be involved and attacks last longer. The attacks may become chronic causing joint deformities. Urate crystals are deposited in the kidneys causing gouty nephropathy but less than 5 per cent develop progressive renal failure. Crystals gather in bursae, tendon sheaths, subchondral bone, and subcutaneously; and about 10 years after the first attack may become recognizable tophi.

Immediate control of the acute gouty arthritis is followed by long term control of hyperuricaemia.

Gout can be treated so effectively that activities and work need not be restricted. Gout often affects bartenders, brewery workers, and business executives. They should be advised to limit their alcohol intake, maintain a high fluid intake of at least 3 litres daily and if obese to lose weight.

## 5. Paget's disease of bone (osteitis deformans)

Paget's disease of bone is the most common of the metabolic bone diseases next to osteoporosis, affecting 3 per cent of people over the age of 40, and its frequency increases with age. There is a 3:2 male predominance. Only 5 per cent have symptoms. Affected bones are enlarged, deformed, and warm. Any bone can be involved, a few or many, and those most commonly affected are pelvis, femur, skull, tibia, vertebrae, and humerus.

Pain, stiffness, fatigue, deformity, headaches, and increasing deafness may come gradually. Deafness is one of the most disabling symptoms. Pagetic bone may be painful or pain may arise in arthritic joints, from fractures or from compression neuropathy. Long bones become bowed, the spine kyphotic, and the vault of the skull widens like a soft beret. The spinal cord may be compressed by enlarging bone, excessive vascularity or vertebral collapse. Rarely, in less than 1 per cent of those with symptoms, there may be sarcomatous change in the bone, suggested by increasingly severe pain.

Most patients need no treatment. The indications for treatment are bone pain, nerve compression, or to suppress vascularity before elective orthopaedic surgery. The aim of medication is to suppress bone cell activity.

Most people with Paget's disease are able to continue their usual work, but those having headache, backache, and arthritis should be given mainly sedentary work and enabled to vary their posture. They should be spared climbing stairs and allowed to park their cars close to their workplaces. Concessions may be needed because of deafness.

## Selected references and further reading

1. Smith, R., Francis, M.J.O., and Houghton, G.R. (1983). *The brittle bone syndrome.* Butterworth, London.
2. Stuart, J., Forbes, C.D., Jones, P., Lane, G., Rizza, C.R., and Wilkes, S. (1980). Improving prospects for employment of the haemophiliac. *Brit. Med. J.*, **280**, 1169–72.
3. Barton, N.J., Hooper, G., Noble, J., and Steel, M.W. (1992). Occupational causes of disorders in the upper limb. *Brit. Med. J.*, **304**, 309–11.
4. HSE (Health and Safety Executive) (1983). *VDUs.* HMSO, London.
5. HSE (Health and Safety Executive) (1986). *Working with VDUs.* HMSO, London.
6. HSE (Health and Safety Executive) (1990). *Work-related upper limb disorders*: A *guide to prevention.* HMSO, London.
7. HSE (Health and Safety Executive) (1991). *Safety at work.* HMSO, London.
8. HSE (Health and Safety Executive) (1992). *Display screen equipment.* Guidance on Regulations. HMSO, London.
9. Croft, P., Coggon, D., Crudder, M., and Cooper, C. (1992). Osteoarthritis of the hip: An occupational disease of farmers. *Brit. Med. J.*, **304**, 1269–72.
10. Sheppeard, H., Bulgen, D., and Ward, D.J. (1981). Rheumatoid arthritis—returning patients to work. *Rheumat. Rehab.*, **20**, 160–3.
11. Roberts, M.E.T., Wright, V., Hill, A.G.S., and Mehra, A.C. (1976). Psoriatic arthritis—follow up study. *Ann. Rheum. Dis.*, **35**, 206.

# 11

# Trauma

*D.C. Snashall and L.J. Marks*

## Introduction

This chapter will deal with the effects of direct trauma to limbs, thorax, and abdomen. The effects of direct trauma to the head are dealt with in Chapter 7, and direct trauma to the spine in Chapter 9. The latter part of the chapter will refer to limb deficiencies, whether congenital or acquired (amputation) with reference to exoprosthetic replacement.

## Traumatic injuries

Trauma to a limb can involve damaging several different types of tissue. For simplicity, each tissue layer will be considered in turn, rather than specifically referring to upper or lower limbs unless stated. This is appropriate as the treatment of the individual tissues is broadly similar whether an arm or leg is involved.

Facilitating recovery after trauma requires multidisciplinary teamwork, the more complex the injury the greater the need for such input. Physiotherapists will work in joint range, muscle power, balance and co-ordination. Occupational therapists will advise on activities of daily living and will have a particular role in upper limb injuries, notably sensory re-education after nerve damage. The occupational therapist will also advise on home and workplace modifications, and this role will involve liaison with the social services, Employment Adviser, and occupational physicians.

### Direct trauma

*Skin and subcutaneous tissue*

Skin and the underlying fatty tissue (subcutaneous tissue) can be damaged by direct laceration (puncture, tear or shear) by thermal injury (hot or cold) and by electrical injury. Puncture or laceration of the skin is usually treated by primary repair following adequate cleansing and debridement. Unless there is an underlying medical condition, repair will take place quite rapidly after opposition of the tissue edges. Sutures or steristrips can be removed after about 10 days and minimal time need be lost from work. More extensive damage, where large areas of skin are lost, may require coverage with skin grafts. These may be split skin grafts or full thickness skin grafts, depending on the depth of the injury. The more complex the graft, the more the specialized services of a plastic surgeon are likely to be required.

## Muscle

Muscle may be directly severed, severely bruised or crushed, or be damaged indirectly as a result of trauma to the nerves or blood vessels supplying it. In cases of muscle laceration, it may be possible to restore function by direct suture, providing the blood supply is adequate. In cases of severe bruising or contusion, the muscle compartment may need to be decompressed or the muscle partly removed. Where a group of muscles is profoundly affected, it may be possible to restore function by transferring another group of muscles into the same compartment.

## Tendons

Tendons, unlike muscles, have a poor blood supply and therefore tend to respond less favourably to direct injury. Grafting with synthetic materials is appropriate in some conditions.

## Cartilage

Cartilage is the protective covering over the end of a bone inside a joint. It provides a smooth lining to the joint and in some instances is lubricated by fluid. Cartilage, like tendons, has a poor blood supply and therefore does not repair easily. The result of damage to cartilage may not have any immediate effect, although its loss may lead subsequently to degenerative arthritis (osteoarthrosis). The most common site of cartilage injury is the knee which is covered in Chapter 10, p. 197.

## Blood vessels

Localized damage to blood vessels may possibly be amenable to direct repair by vascular or plastic surgeons. More extensive damage can often be overcome by the use of bypass grafts using either reversed vein or synthetic grafts. If severe trauma is sustained to the blood vessels resulting in complete disruption to the blood supply to the distal limb, then amputation may be required.

## Nerves (see also Chapter 10, p. 194)

Nerves are more commonly damaged in the arms than the legs. Nerves in the hands are commonly damaged in crush injuries, in falls through windows, and in road traffic accidents. The end result depends on a number of factors, including age, associated injuries, involvement of blood vessels, degree of crushing, and speedy access to expert surgical treatment. Wherever possible, primary suture is recommended and results have improved enormously since it was realized that blood vessels must be repaired as well as nerves; in the past it was common to tie off rather than repair a damaged artery, which may itself supply blood to the injured nerve.[1]

There are three main nerves in the arm, the median, ulnar and radial, and damage to these will be considered in turn.

1. *Median nerve lesions.* Division of the median nerve at the wrist results in complete loss of feeling of thumb, index, middle finger and lateral half of the ring finger, and the associated part of the palm below those fingers. As this nerve also supplies some of the muscles of the thumb, the ability to move the thumb across to the little finger is also lost. This loss of movement is rarely a functional problem. Adults do less well than children after nerve suture as, even though touch and pain sensation may be restored, recognition sense (stereognosis) can remain poor. It is possible to re-educate for stereognosis by formal physiotherapy and occupational therapy techniques resulting in good restoration of function. Electronics experts, keyboard operators, sewing machinists and seamstresses, who require sensation for their work, and indeed anyone who requires fine function of the fingers and the ability to recognize textures and objects rapidly, should be referred for formal re-education. This may not be so necessary for patients who are primarily involved in heavy labouring jobs.

2. *Ulnar nerve lesions.* Division of the ulnar nerve in the wrist leads to loss of feeling in the little finger and the medial half of the ring finger and more importantly, paralysis of the muscles that move the fingers apart and close them, bend the hand at the knuckles, straighten the fingers, and control the pinch grip between the thumb and index finger. It is thus a devastating lesion for somebody who requires finely co-ordinated finger movements. Repair of the ulnar nerve in adults does not usually result in independent action of finger movements although a very well-motivated patient may regain this after prolonged training. Power grip, as in gripping a pole or handle is usually retained and therefore, some hand function is possible.

Reconstructive procedures are available to stabilize the knuckle joints. Special splints to avoid stretching these joints can be used in the early stages of recovery. The lack of pinch grip (as used, for example, to hold a key) can be extremely disabling particularly in patients who need to manipulate switches and operate keys. This function can be restored by a tendon transfer operation.

3. *Radial nerve lesions.* Damage to the radial nerve usually occurs in the upper part of the arm following fractures of the humerus where the radial nerve winds round in a groove. The result is a 'dropped wrist' so that the patient cannot lift up the hand or thumb. Grip is substantially reduced if the patient cannot stabilize the wrist in a neutral position. The radial nerve is responsible for very little sensation, nearly all its function being to supply muscles. If direct suture is possible, results are usually good. If however, too much nerve has been lost, or has become embedded in new bone formed around the fracture, then repair may be impossible. In this situation tendon transfer may restore the ability to lift the hand.

4. *Median and ulnar nerve lesions.* Damage to both nerves at the wrist is not uncommon and the result is devastating. Almost invariably most of the tendons and both arteries are cut and this means that all three structures have to be repaired to restore function. Even though modern surgical techniques can give the chance of good functional return, rehabilitation may be prolonged. Restoration of some sensation (for protection as well as recognition) and restoration of the pinch grip, are major objectives. For jobs requiring fine control of both hands, loss of sensation and precise finger movements are a major disability. Careful assessment in a specialist hand unit is necessary with advice from the occupational physician on functional requirements.

5. *Pain in the hand following nerve damage.* Severe pain in the hand (causalgia) can follow *partial* damage to nerves. The patient complains of severe continuous burning pain and an abnormally sensitive response to light touch. The pain may spread outside the anatomical distribution of the damaged nerve because of both physical and chemical factors. These can become more established with the passage of time and therefore *immediate referral to a specialist centre is recommended.* These patients do not respond to analgesics and rest and delayed referral reduces the chance of recovery. Intensive skilled treatment can often materially improve the situation. This may involve use of external stimulators, serial blocks to the sympathetic nerves (to counteract the chemical effects), and intensive rehabilitation to try and restore normal movement patterns. Patients with nerve injuries may also benefit from adaptation of their work equipment, e.g., the use of electronic typewriters and word processors. Such factors can all be considered at the rehabilitation centre.

From the psychological point of view continuity of employment is important even though the individual may have become to all intents and purposes, virtually one-handed.

6. *Brachial plexus lesions.* The brachial plexus is the group of nerve roots which exit from the spinal cord in the neck and weave together, eventually to form the nerves that supply the arm.

In 1987, it was estimated that there were at least 336 individuals with traumatic injuries to the brachial plexus. By far the most common cause of traction injuries to the brachial plexus is motorcycle accidents, when acute depression of the shoulder and acute sideways bend of the neck causes traction on the nerve roots. There are three types of injury which can be distinguished by electromyographic (EMG) techniques:

(i)   traction lesion without rupture of the nerve roots;
(ii)  rupture of the nerve roots; and
(iii) avulsion (tearing away) of the roots from the spinal cord.

Combinations of these injuries are increasingly common.

In a lesion without rupture, the sheath of the nerve is intact but the nerve itself degenerates. Spontaneous recovery after one to two years is possible and the functional result may be quite good. When the nerve root itself is ruptured, there is no hope of recovery unless the nerve is explored and repaired by nerve graft. In avulsion injury, the roots are torn out of the spinal cord and there is no possibility either of spontaneous recovery or repair by grafting. The incidence of ruptures and avulsions has been steadily increasing over the years. This may be related to the decreased mortality from head injuries with modern crash helmets.

These individuals are best referred to a specialist centre as soon as possible to assess whether surgery is indicated or whether the lesion is beyond repair. Grafting of the upper trunks of the brachial plexus may restore elbow function, some movement of the shoulder towards the trunk and protective feeling in the hands. Restoration of the fine movements of the hand is not possible because even if the lower trunks were repairable, by the time the nerve has regenerated to the hand, the muscles of the hand will have atrophied and no longer function.

Severe pain is a problem for the majority of patients with avulsion lesions or high ruptures. The pain is highly characteristic with a constant background pain, described as burning or crushing, and superimposed periodic sharp flashes of pain through the arm. Analgesics are usually ineffective, but *Carbamazepine* is worth a trial. Transcutaneous nerve stimulation or simple distraction techniques seem to be the most effective treatments.

The indications for amputation following brachial plexus lesions are few. It is only advised when the arm becomes a nuisance or the person suffers periodic burns or recurrent injury due to loss of feeling. The psychological effect of losing an arm must not be underestimated. It should also be emphasized that amputation has no effect on the severe central pain.

The youthfulness of the majority, who are predominantly male, coupled with the severity of the lesion and the long-term consequences, calls for a radical appraisal of their work. Clearly, they are unable to return to jobs which traditionally demand two sound arms. The initial absence will be prolonged if the dominant arm is affected, because basic skills are re-learned using the non-dominant arm (dominance transfer). It is here that the rehabilitation skills and mechanical ingenuity of the specialist units have a crucial role to play. Often special functional splints can allow patients to return to work. Occupational physicians may well have to advise if a radical modification of a manual job or a course of retraining is required. This is likely to involve full assessment by an occupational therapist.[2]

7. *Sciatic nerve lesions.* The sciatic is one of two nerves supplying the leg. The other nerve, the femoral nerve is rarely damaged.

The sciatic nerve can be damaged in dislocations of the hip, by direct injury and, rarely, following total hip replacement. A complete lesion of the sciatic nerve results in total paralysis of all the muscles below the knee and therefore, difficulty in walking. Repair of the nerve usually allows the patient to 'point the toes' but the abilities to lift up the foot and turn it out sideways are often lost.

A light splint worn in the shoe can stabilize the foot and allow standing and a fair degree of walking. One of the distressing features of repair of complete sciatic nerve lesions, is the relatively high instance of abnormal sensations and severe burning pain as the nerve attempts to regrow. So much so, that some surgeons are loath to repair the sciatic nerve, believing that the patient is better off with a numb, painless foot than one with feeling and severe pain.

Patients with complete sciatic nerve palsies are clearly unsafe at heights and on ladders, and cannot cope with long periods of standing and walking. Patients with sedentary tasks have less handicap but getting to and from work may present a problem.

*Bone*

Direct trauma to bones results in fractures or breaks. These are classified as simple or closed, when there is no communication between the fracture site and the exterior of the body. A fracture is open or compound, when there is a wound from the skin surface leading down to the site of the fracture. In the latter case, other associated injuries to nearby tissues are more likely.

The normal fractured bone should mend completely in three months if it is properly immobilized. The immobilization may be in a sling, a plaster cast or by external fixation. In some cases internal fixation by open operation using plates, screws or nails to achieve stability is needed. Depending on the person's occupation and site of fracture they may well be able to return to work prior to full healing of the fracture. The two most significant complications of fractures are:

(1)   delayed or non-union: and

(2)   osteomyelitis.

(1) *Delayed or non-union.* Fractures that have still not healed after three to four months may be successfully treated with bone grafts and union achieved. In certain circumstances, however, especially when the fracture is within or near a joint, removal of one of the fragments or its replacement by an artificial joint may be more appropriate.

(2) *Osteomyelitis.* This means infection in the bone. It is a late complication after a fracture, most presenting with pain and persistent discharge from the fracture site. Treatment consists of removing all the infected bone and at times this can require quite radical surgery. Patients may be off work for a considerable number of weeks while bone remodels or bone grafts take, and after that gradual mobilization is allowed.[3]

**Replantation of limbs and digits**

Developments in operating microscopes, instruments, and sutures have allowed very significant advances in microvascular surgery during the last decade. It is possible to rejoin blood vessels with lumen sizes less than 1 mm and accurately re-appose severed nerves. It is very important that the severed tissue is kept cold (lower than 4 °C or packed in ice). Structures containing muscle can be protected from ischaemic damage for 6 hours if kept cold and digits can be preserved for 24 hours. The most important factor for success is the potential for nerve recovery, as there is no purpose in re-attaching an insensate structure. This means avulsion injuries are usually not suitable for replantation. Long term rehabilitation and physiotherapy are always needed and, therefore, the decision to replant must take into account a patient's occupation, pastimes and future prospects. Single digit replants are rarely beneficial in the long term, the exception being the thumb. Children should always be referred as they are the most likely to get a good result. Limb replantation can be successful but the more proximal the injury, the more doubtful the nerve recovery will be.

*Thorax*

The thorax or chest can be considered as a bony cage protecting the enclosed structures, principally the heart and lungs. The 'cage' is formed by the breastbone (sternum) in the front, the ribs at either side, with the spine (backbone) posteriorly. Injuries of the spine are discussed in Chapter 9.

Fractures of the ribs are usually caused by a direct injury, such as a fall against a hard object. The person complains of severe pain made worse by deep breathing. Complications primarily occur if a fragment of a rib is displaced so that it pierces the underlying lung, causing the lung to collapse (pneumothorax) with or without associated bleeding (haemothorax). However, individuals with pre-existing chest disease will be more susceptible to pneumonia even after an undisplaced fracture, because the pain will inhibit normal chest movement. Any lung complications will require specific treatment, but simple undisplaced rib fractures will heal spontaneously.

Fractures of the sternum may occur from direct injury from the front, or vertical compression of the chest with simultaneous fracture of the thoracic spine. In the latter case, the main problem is the spinal fracture and the sternal fracture rarely requires specific treatment. When the sternum is pushed inwards it can cause direct pressure on the heart and lungs, and may need to be restored to its original position surgically.

The term 'stove-in chest' is used when multiple injuries cause a complete segment of the thorax to become detached and 'flail'. This serious injury requires prompt treatment to save life because the underlying heart and lungs are compromised. The flail segment may be controlled by use of a ventilator, but if this is not possible, surgical fixation will be required.

*Abdomen*

The abdomen contains organs which can be damaged by direct trauma. Severe crush injuries cause rupture or tearing. Loss of blood may cause collapse (hypovolaemic shock) and extravasation of urine or faeces can cause infection and peritonitis. Certain organs, such as the spleen, are sometimes removed after severe injury. When the bowel or bladder are injured, temporary diversions, such as colostomy or ureterostomy may be required, which can be reversed later.

The lower part of the abdomen is protected by the bones of the pelvis, which meet at the front in the symphysis pubis and attach to the spine at the back. An isolated fracture of the pelvis seldom causes any problem as there is unlikely to be any significant displacement. When the pelvis is fractured in two places, there is the possibility of displacement and injury to underlying structures. The most common complications are rupture of the urethra or bladder, and occasionally damage to one of the arteries of the leg. If the fracture passes through the roof of the hip joint (acetabulum) this can cause roughening of the joint surface and predisposes to later development of osteoarthrosis of the hip.

Most abdominal and thoracic injuries require surgical exploration with prolonged convalescence depending on the precise nature of damage and the remaining functional disability. Time off work is, therefore, likely to be prolonged and, if recovery is incomplete, it may not be possible for an employee to return to work especially a manual job. Each case will need individual assessment by an occupational physician.

## Amputations and congenital limb deficiencies

The latest national statistics for amputations were available in 1988. These statistics only reflect patients being referred to the Prosthetic Centres in England and therefore, do not give the full incidence of new amputations.

The figures, however, allow some points to be drawn. In 1988, 4472 patients were seen for the first time. Lower limb amputations are more frequent than upper limb amputations, the ratio in 1988 being 27:1. The causes of lower and upper limb amputations are quite different and are shown for 1988 in Table 11.1.[4] Limb deficiencies, or congenital growth anomalies, form a very small percentage of the whole. They may present as a transverse deficiency (like an amputation) or a longitudinal deficiency, which usually presents as a shortened limb with/without an abnormal hand/foot.

In 1988, the overall ratio of male to female amputees was 2.04:1 and this has shown no significant change over recent years. Only 21.3 per cent of patients are in the 20 to 60 age group (working age), 60.3 per cent being between 60 and 79 and 16.2 per cent over 80.

Functionally, the effect of an amputation is on mobility for lower limb amputees and dexterity for upper limb amputees. The extent of disturbance of function will depend mainly on the level of amputation, the more proximal the greater the disturbance. However, it is worth noting that whilst one cannot walk without two legs, it is perfectly possible to do all activities with only one arm. As a rough guide, lower limb amputees will need six months before returning to

**Table 11.1** Amputation by site and cause (1988)

| Lower limb | Percentage | | Upper limb | Percentage | |
|---|---|---|---|---|---|
| Vascular | 65.6 | 87.6 | Trauma | 68.50 | |
| | | | Malignancy | 16.40 | |
| Diabetes | 22.0 | | Vascular | 11.40 | 12 |
| Trauma | 6.2 | | Diabetes | 0.60 | |
| Malignancy | 3.2 | | | | |
| Infection | 1.9 | | Infection | 1.25 | |
| Neurogenic deformity | | | Neurogenic deformity | | |
| – Congenital | 0.8 | | –Congenital | 0.60 | |
| – Acquired | 0.3 | | –Acquired | 1.25 | |
| Total number | 4313 (100%) | | Total number | 159 (100%) | |

work and upper limb amputees three months, although if the dominant arm was amputated rehabilitation may take longer.

**Complications of amputation**

Complications of amputation can be divided into immediate and late, see Table 11.2. Each of these complications can not only delay return to work, but can limit working effectiveness or lead to further absence, with associated social and psychological problems.

In lower limb amputees there is an increased incidence of premature degenerative change in the joints of the contralateral limb, knee more than hip. In upper limb amputees there appears to be an increased incidence of shoulder and neck problems.

In addition to these medical complications there is the inconvenience of relying on a mechanical device which itself requires maintenance and repairs, to provide reliable service. As a result of the McColl report (1986)[5] a number of new prosthetic centres have been established, making the service more accessible. (see p. 217.) However, individuals may still require time off during working hours, to attend for appointments.

**Rehabilitation**

Rehabilitation of the amputee requires multidisciplinary teamwork. Ideally, the team (surgeon, nurses, physiotherapist, occupational therapist, and rehabilitation physician) should assess the individual pre-operatively. The technique of amputation is critical, as satisfactory fitting of a prosthesis starts with the surgeon's fashioning of the stump, which must be viewed as an 'organ of locomotion'. Postoperatively, the amputee will work on general muscle strength, specific

**Table 11.2** The complications of amputation and their management

|  | Complication | Treatment |
|---|---|---|
| **Immediate** | 1. Delayed healing<br>   Infection<br>   Ischaemia | Antibiotics<br>Vasodilators<br>Sympathectomy<br>Higher amputation |
|  | 2. Postoperative<br>   oedema | Stump elevation<br>Exercises<br>Elasticated stump sock<br>Mobilization on an early<br>walking aid |
|  | 3. Phantom pain | Massage<br>Analgesics<br>Carbamazepine<br>Transcutaneous nerve<br>stimulation |
| **Late** | 4. Late changes in<br>   stump volume | Adjust or refit socket |
|  | 5. Stump abrasions,<br>   blisters, corns | Adjust socket |
|  | 6. Infected<br>   epidermoid cysts | Socket fit<br>Stump hygiene<br>? Surgical excision |
|  | 7. Neuromata | Adjust socket<br>Neurectomy |
|  | 8. Stress on other<br>   parts of the body |  |

stump exercises, and be assisted in restoring independence in daily activities. Walking, using an early walking aid under the supervision of the physiotherapist, is commenced 5 to 7 days following amputation. The amputee is usually referred for prosthetic fitting about three weeks after the amputation. Rehabilitation continues following discharge from hospital, until the amputee has achieved maximum functional independence, and in the case of those of working age, has returned to suitable employment (see below).

## Prosthetics

The prosthetist is the person who will tailor the fit of the artificial limb or prosthesis, to the individual. This is a highly skilled job and requires knowledge of traditional materials, such as leather, metal, and wood, as well as an increasing range of modern plastics. Prosthetic joints are becoming more sophisticated; for example energy-storing feet, which incorporate elastic materials which mimic normal gait more closely, and microprocessor-controlled knee units (which automatically control the rate of swing of the calf in relation to the speed of the gait).

Upper limb prostheses can be purely cosmetic, body powered or externally powered. Body powered limbs can be adapted to a wide range of functions and very fine movements can be achieved. Servo-assisted mechanisms can augment weak muscles. Myoelectric prostheses, which are triggered by signals from muscle groups in the residual limb, are increasingly available. At present they still tend to be much heavier than body powered limbs, are less reliable and offer relatively crude hand movement. In complex congenital deficiencies such as those in thalidomide patients, individually designed prostheses may be required.[6]

## Special work problems

A number of general and specific points should be borne in mind when advising both the amputee and employer about working conditions. In general, employers should be made aware that a patient has an artificial limb. It is particularly important that adequate washing facilities can allow the amputee to attend to the limb and stump in reasonable privacy.

Lower limb amputees should avoid working at heights, climbing ladders, and habitually walking over uneven ground. Generally, the more proximal the amputation the more limited the mobility. Lower limb amputees may not be able to stand all day, but equally it is inadvisable to sit all day without periodically getting up and moving around. Bilateral lower limb amputees may need to use a wheelchair if they have stump or prosthetic problems. These employees, therefore, require wheelchair-accessible premises (see below). In the case of upper limb amputation, there is little or no restriction on the clerical worker and manual workers have considerable ability to minimize this type of disability. A full assessment including an employment evaluation, should always be performed before giving a definite opinion.

### Use of walking aids and wheelchairs

Individuals who return to work using sticks or crutches usually experience little difficulty except with heavy spring-loaded doors (e.g., fire doors) and steps/stairs. The latter need to have at least one handrail to ensure safety. Persons using a walking frame would generally find steps/stairs impossible to negotiate unless the depth of step accommodated the frame as well as the individual.

Individuals who require a wheelchair need suitable ramps over all steps and sills. Doorways and corridors need to be of suitable width to allow easy movement with adequate turning space. Particular attention must be given to toilet facilities. If the person has to work on more than one floor, then use of lifts will be needed, with appropriately placed controls. Attention may also be required to desk heights, access to filing cabinets, and other working surfaces or furniture.

## Prosthetic services

In 1984, a working party was set up under the chairmanship of Professor Ian McColl to review the artificial limb and appliance centre services. Their report was published in 1986[5] and as a result, an interim authority The Disablement Services Authority (DSA) was established. This authority was operational from 1 July 1987 to 31 March 1991, at which point the services were transferred to the National Health Service. Prosthetic services became part of rehabilitation medicine and are now provided by consultants in the specialty. Several new prosthetic centres were set up during the time of the DSA to make the service more accessible. New prosthetic companies were encouraged to establish with emphasis on local manufacture and the ability to provide all limb systems. Wheelchair services were, in the main, devolved to district clinics run by occupational therapists, providing assessments for more routine types of wheelchairs. In most regions, specialized wheelchair assessments are still available at the regional centres, most usually for those clients requiring complex or 'specialized' seating.

## Conclusions and recommendations

Despite increasing efforts to improve safety on the road, and legislation on safety at work, traumatic injuries will continue to have an impact on the working population. The majority of individuals, however, will eventually return to work functionally intact.

Medical care following injury and later rehabilitation involving the co-operation of primary care physicians, occupational health services, hospital specialists, remedial therapists, management and fellow workers, can significantly improve the quality of life of those with residual disabilities.

Not to be disregarded is the great improvement of acute trauma services which has led to a greater number of survivors of multiple injuries but who have disabilities as a consequence.

Although most amputations are now for vascular disease in an older population, there are still many individuals of working age who have suffered amputation from trauma or congenital deficiency, who need prosthetic services and support to enable them to continue in employment and enjoy an active life.

## Acknowledgements

The authors wish to acknowledge the contribution on Limb Replantation from P.L. Levick, MS., FRCS., Consultant in Plastic Surgery and Burns at the Birmingham Accident Hospital.

## Selected references and further reading

1. Witherington, R.W. and Wynn Parry, C.B. (1984). Painful disorders of peripheral nerves. *Postgrad. Med. J.*, **60**, 869–85.
2. Wynn Parry, C.B. (1984). Brachial plexus injuries. *Brit. J. Hosp. Med.*, **32**, 130–9.
3. Crawford Adams, J. (1991). *Outline of fractures*, (10th edn). Churchill Livingstone, Edinburgh.
4. DOH (Department of Health) (1989). *On the state of the public health for the year 1988*. HMSO, London.
5. *Review of artificial limb and appliance centre services* (1986). The report of an independent working party under the chairmanship of Professor Ian McColl. Crown Publishers.
6. Ham, R., and Cotton, L. (1991). Limb amputation—from aetiology to rehabilitation. In *Therapy in practice,* Vol. 23. Chapman & Hall, London.

# 12

# Diabetes mellitus and thyroid disorders

## H.G. Vaile and D.A. Pyke

## Introduction

### Diabetes

*Classification*

For practical clinical purposes there are two types of diabetes:

1. Insulin-dependent diabetes mellitus (IDDM), or type 1 diabetes: the cause is not known but it may result from viral damage to pancreatic islet beta cells in genetically susceptible individuals. Auto-immunity may also play a part and islet cell antibodies can be demonstrated in most IDDM diabetics. It can occur at any age, although most of those diagnosed under 20 years of age are of this type.

2. Non-insulin-dependent diabetes mellitus (NIDDM), or type II diabetes: it has a strong genetic component but the cause in most cases is not known. It affects predominantly those over 30 years of age. Approximately three quarters of diabetics are of this type.

*Diabetes and employment*

Despite recent advances in the control of diabetes the condition remains poorly understood and is sometimes feared by employers and even by their medical advisers. As a result, some diabetics still encounter unjustifiable difficulties in finding and keeping work because of their condition. There is a paucity of published scientific data on the work experience of diabetics in general or in particular situations, e.g., in shiftwork, but their underrepresentation in the workforce[1] suggests that there is continuing prejudice against their employment. The risk of hypoglycaemia and visual impairment may legitimately debar poorly controlled insulin dependent diabetics from jobs where safety or vigorous physical effort is an important factor, but diabetics are not invalids and most can work normally and should not be discriminated against in job selection. The British Diabetic Association has published a *Diabetes employment handbook*,[2] a comprehensive and useful guide to the employment implications of diabetes in a wide range of occupations. This helps to fulfil the need for employers to familiarize themselves with the condition and to recognize that the work record of diabetics is good and that they make perfectly satisfactory employees.

## Prevalence, morbidity and mortality

The overall prevalence of insulin-dependent diabetes[3] in the United Kingdom is of the order of 3.5 per 1000 population. It increases with age: for children below the age of 16 the prevalence is around 1.4 per 1000. Most series show some preponderance of males, but this sex difference is not marked. The prevalence of non-insulin-dependent diabetes is 10–12 per 1000. Its annual incidence has been found to be between 10 and 20 per 100 000, the higher figures being found in areas with poor socio-economic conditions.

### Morbidity and mortality of diabetes

The scale of the morbidity of diabetes cannot be estimated accurately, although it is said to be the most common cause of blindness in the working age group. Heart disease and stroke are increased by a factor of two to three; diabetes is the second leading cause of fatal kidney disease, and a diabetic is twenty times more likely to need an amputation than a non-diabetic. It should be emphasized, however, that only a minority of diabetics develop disabling complications. Nevertheless, life expectancy is reduced in all age groups, mainly as a result of renal failure and vascular disease. There is great variation, however, and many diabetics live for 40 years or more after the onset of the disease without developing serious complications. Improved methods of control of diabetes and more effective treatment for end-stage renal failure are likely to improve the prognosis, but some years must elapse before the extent of the benefit is known.

## Clinical aspects affecting work capacity

### Management of insulin-dependent diabetics

There is a large number of insulin regimes varying from once a day injections of long-acting insulin (perhaps with a short-acting insulin) to four injections of short-acting insulin with a long-acting type given last thing at night by conventional pen-injector. A single injection is effective in only a minority of cases. Short-acting with intermediate-acting insulin given twice daily is a popular regime. For insulin-sensitive patients, especially those with a variable lifestyle, three or four injections daily with a pen-injector are often acceptable and effective. Early hopes of success with a continuous insulin infusion by electronically controlled pump have receded somewhat. This treatment involves the permanent wearing of a pump, which miniaturized though it may be, is an impediment, and there is the possibility of failure which can lead to rapid deterioration of diabetic control.

The guideline for insulin treatment is that any treatment which works should be continued. There is no merit in making changes for their own sake. The objectives are always that the patient should feel well, hypoglycaemia should be uncommon, mild and preceded by warning and blood glucose control should be acceptable—in that order.

Flexible regimes with multiple injections make changes arising from shift-work easier to manage.

Insulin was originally produced from pancreatic extracts from animals, at first cattle, later pigs. In the last 10 to 15 years it has been manufactured by genetic engineering, the so-called 'human' insulin. There are minute chemical differences between the various types of insulin. In the great majority of cases these differences do not affect its action. In a few types hypoglycaemia is more frequent, severe or abrupt, in which case a change to another species should be made. Recent anxieties on this account about human insulin have been exaggerated. Although most insulin on the market is now human, porcine insulin is still made and should be used in those cases where human insulin is unsatisfactory.

It is hardly ever possible to achieve consistently normal blood glucose levels in insulin-dependent diabetics throughout the 24 hours and attempts to do so will probably lead to frequent hypoglycaemia. There is nearly always considerable variation in results due to differences in food or exercise or for no known reason. Human bodies are not constant machines and treating them as such, at least as far as blood glucose control is concerned, is likely to lead to frustration, unhappiness, and poor treatment. Blood glucose testing by the diabetic is an important advance but it can have the drawback of undermining confidence and producing worry unless it is seen in context.

## Management of non-insulin-dependent diabetics

Non-insulin-dependent diabetics are managed with diet alone or diet and oral hypoglycaemic drugs. They are frequently obese: the main objective of diet is to reduce body weight, principally by controlling fat intake, although excessive intake of refined carbohydrates is not advisable. High fibre intake seems to be beneficial for all diabetics, as fibre appears to delay glucose absorption and reduce blood glucose excursions. Oral hypoglycaemic drugs are of two types:

1. *Biguanides*, e.g., metformin. Biguanides appear to act by reducing glucose absorption from the gut, reducing glucose release from the liver, and enhancing glucose uptake by the tissues. They are not very potent and they do not cause symptomatic hypoglycaemia.

2. *Sulphonylureas*, e.g., glibenclamide, chlorpropamide, tolbutamide, glipizide. The sulphonylureas act mainly by stimulating insulin release, although they also enhance tissue uptake of glucose. They are more powerful and chlorpropamide and glibenclamide may cause mild hypoglycaemia, especially after unaccustomed exercise, high alcohol consumption, and/or inadequate food intake. This appears to be less common with shorter-acting sulphonylureas, such as tolbutamide or glipizide.

**Recent concepts of control**

With the realization that careful control of diabetes can reduce the risk of long-term complications increasing emphasis is now placed on achieving not only clinical well-being but also near-normal blood glucose levels. Self-monitoring of blood glucose has replaced time-honoured urine testing, especially in younger insulin-treated diabetics. The main advantages of blood testing are that it more accurately reflects diabetic control and is not subject to variations in the renal threshold for glucose; and that it gives information on low blood glucose levels, as well as high, and can thus give warning of impending hypoglycaemia. It is also more aesthetically acceptable to many patients. Blood glucose strips are now included in the drug tariff and are more readily available. Careful regulation of insulin dosage together with blood glucose monitoring should reduce the risk of hypoglycaemia and enable individuals to cope more easily with variations in daily work patterns. It may also reduce the incidence of long-term complications. For these reasons, blood glucose testing should be valuable for some insulin-treated patients who might otherwise experience difficulty in coping with certain types of employment, e.g., shiftwork.

# Special work problems

## The work record of diabetics[4–7]

There has been a great change in recent years concerning the employment of diabetics. Employers used to be frightened of diabetes and diabetics were frightened of employers. Both attitudes were due to ignorance. Now, the general public is better informed about diabetes, as about most other diseases. The result has been wholly beneficial; most employers realize that few occupations should be barred to diabetics. Diabetic employees are better able to manage their condition and less inclined to conceal their diabetes.

Occupations closed to insulin-taking diabetes are those in which a sudden loss of control or consciousness would be dangerous, e.g., airline pilot or large goods vehicle driver. The risk here comes not from the diabetes itself but from its treatment leading to hypoglycaemia. It may be unwise for insulin-taking diabetics to work in jobs where the danger would not be to others but to themselves, e.g., with moving machinery, in foundries, on scaffolding, and fire-fighting. But even here there is room for latitude. Much depends on the exact nature of the work, control of the diabetes, in particular the frequency and abruptness of hypoglycaemic attacks, and the good sense of the patient.

Restrictions on the employment of diabetics treated without insulin are much less. Although hypoglycaemic episodes can occur in those taking suphonylurea tablets (and they can be serious and prolonged) they are rare. If the physician is satisfied with the treatment over a period of time and especially if the patient monitors his own blood glucose level, which is desirable in most diabetics, the risk of hypoglycaemia is remote and will hardly ever be a bar to employment; there are exceptions, e.g., in aircrew, but even that may be a safe occupation for a tablet-taking diabetic and it is certainly safe for someone treated by diet only.

All the comments relate to the *treatment* of diabetes. Clearly, the suitability of a diabetic for employment also depends on his general health. In the case of diabetes this means freedom from sight-threatening retinopathy, severe peripheral or autonomic neuropathy, advanced ischaemic disease or serious renal failure.

With the improved general knowledge of diabetes and attitude towards it, as well as its improved treatment in recent years, the work performance of most diabetics is very good. In general, they suffer from unemployment no more than other people. Even poorly controlled diabetics are only likely to have about one-and-a-half to twice as much time off work and in well-controlled cases the excess is very small, in many cases none at all. This is especially true of non-insulin takers. Good medical treatment and good liaison between physician and occupational health staff are important in controlling diabetes and keeping its effects to a minimum. Compared to the past, present treatment has improved greatly and with better self-monitoring of blood glucose and newer types of insulin and treatment regimes the situation is likely to continue to improve.

## Working patterns and diabetic treatment

There is, in general, no reason why a diabetic on insulin should not do shiftwork. Shiftwork used to be considered a bar to a diabetic taking up nursing;[8] now, provided the person is in other ways suitable, it is not. Most sensible and well-motivated diabetics rapidly learn how to adjust their treatment, especially if they are measuring their own blood glucose levels and using multiple insulin-injection techniques. Thus, shiftwork should not be an automatic bar to the employment of diabetics. One development worth watching, however, is the introduction of shorter and shorter shift cycles, when, for instance, day, evening, and night shifts can follow each other at two-day intervals. This may test the ingenuity of the most intelligent insulin-dependent diabetic. These problems can occur in different types and grades of employment, e.g., supervisors and managers may also be required to undertake shiftwork or work irregular hours.

## Diabetic coma

Many of the more important employment problems in diabetics can be related, directly or indirectly, to the fear of diabetic coma. Strictly, this term applies only to ketoacidosis but is sometimes also used (incorrectly) to cover hypoglycaemia.

**Diabetic ketoacidosis**

This may occur if there is serious loss of control of diabetes, resulting in hyper-glycaemia, dehydration, and acidosis due to the accumulation of ketones. The onset is usually gradual and it is not a cause of sudden collapse at work. It is the cause of significant sickness absence in a small number of individuals.

**Hypoglycaemia**

Hypoglycaemia can cause confusion and loss of consciousness and so it is a much more serious problem from the work standpoint. The majority of insulin-treated diabetics receive ample warning of impending hypoglycaemia, take pre-ventive steps (i.e. take glucose) and experience neither loss of control nor unconsciousness. Yet in some insulin-treated diabetics, hypoglycaemia can develop suddenly and may lead to irrational behaviour, aggression, or even un-consciousness. For this reason many employers have reservations about dia-betics working in potentially hazardous situations, e.g., at heights or near dangerous moving machinery. The majority of insulin-dependent diabetics very rarely experience serious hypoglycaemia and they usually carry glucose tablets, which will rapidly restore the blood glucose level to normal. The risk of hypo-glycaemia has certainly been exaggerated. Nevertheless, it is a factor which has to be considered by employers and occupational physicians when deciding on the placement of diabetics at work and ensuring that they are aware of appropri-ate preventive measures.

It may be important for some diabetics to have regular work breaks when they can carry out blood or urine tests, consume snacks, or take insulin; and it may be sensible to avoid situations where an insulin-dependent diabetic in a responsible position would be working entirely alone for long periods. Oral hypoglycaemic agents rarely cause significant hypoglycaemia and thus non-insulin-dependent diabetics are capable of most occupations. Sulphonylureas can, however, induce mild hypoglycaemia, especially after unaccustomed exercise or if a meal is missed. Because judgement or responses may be impaired, orally treated diabet-ics are currently barred from a few occupations, e.g., flying commercial aero-planes and driving mainline passenger trains, unless they satisfy very stringent criteria with regard to diabetic control. The guiding principle must always be to assess whether or not the development of hypoglycaemia might put the diabetic himself or others at risk. (See p. 228.)

**Complications of diabetes**

A relatively small proportion of diabetics develop long-term complications, usually after many years of diabetes. From the employment viewpoint the most important are cataracts and retinopathy which can lead to visual impairment and blindness; neuropathy, either sensory or autonomic (which may occasionally cause postural hypotension); nephropathy which can lead to renal failure, and foot ulceration which occasionally necessitates amputation. Furthermore, there is an increased incidence of cardiovascular disease in diabetics which can lead to heart attack, strokes, and peripheral vascular disease. Even some treatment may cause problems, e.g., pan-retinal photocoagulation, sometimes used in the treatment of retinopathy, may cause significant diminution in peripheral visual fields. However, few diabetics of working age develop these severe and disabling complications. Recent evidence suggests that careful control of the diabetes from the outset, along the lines discussed above, will reduce their incidence and severity. Those individuals who hold driving licences and develop significant complications should be advised to notify these to the licensing authorities. They are, however, often able to continue driving.

## Superannuation

Difficulty in arranging associated life insurance is sometimes given as a reason for not employing a diabetic. This is not usually a problem in medium or larger sized organizations, where group life insurance schemes can include diabetics without requiring any medical evidence or additional premium. Problems may arise in smaller firms where employees have to be assessed individually, or in larger organizations where the salary of a highly paid executive may rise above the 'free cover level' and attract additional premiums. The attitude of different insurance companies to diabetes can vary considerably. If a diabetic is penalized by a particular insurance company or scheme and this is a major obstacle to his employment, then he should be able to opt out and arrange his own cover with another company, if necessary, paying additional insurance premiums himself. In this context private pension plans are now commonly used by employees whether diabetic or not. The British Diabetic Association can give useful advice on insurance matters (see Appendix 9 for the full address).

## Advisory services

The diabetic specialists, family practitioners, and occupational health services should be able to give advice in cases of employment difficulty. The specialist and/or family practitioner can provide detailed medical information, whilst the occupational physician is best placed to assess the suitability of a diabetic for a particular occupation, or of a particular occupation for a diabetic. Disability Employment Advisers based at Department of Employment Job Centres can advise and help any diabetics with disabilities affecting their work, or disabling complications, to find or keep suitable employment. Careers officers and teachers should be able to advise diabetic school leavers about employment. The British Diabetic Association's Employment Handbook is a comprehensive source of information about the impact of diabetes on some 38 occupations.

## Existing legislation and guidelines for employment

**Road Traffic Acts and diabetes**[9,10] (by Dr John F. Taylor)

*All driving licence applicants and holders*

The UK Road Traffic Acts place an obligation on all applicants and licence holders to declare diabetes to the Driver and Vehicle Licensing Agency, Swansea (DVLA) as soon as they develop any medical condition likely to cause them to be a source of danger to the public driving in pursuance of a licence now or in the future. Persons who make late notifications to the DVLA are not prosecuted. Failure to report the development of insulin-treated diabetes can be used by the motor insurer as a reason to repudiate a motor insurance claim for comprehensive cover of one's own vehicle. However, the Road Traffic Acts compulsorily require the motor insurer to meet third-party motor insurance damage claims. **The Courts, including the Court of Appeal have found that insulin is a drug in terms of Section 4 of the Road Traffic Act and it is an offence to drive under the influence of insulin if the person is adversely affected by it. Insulin-treated diabetics with hypoglycaemia are at risk of being found guilty of driving under the influence of drugs, and in a recent case a driver was fined £600 and banned from driving for 3 years.** Although the statutory responsibility rests with the individual driver to inform the DVLA, it seems probable that the Courts might well find a doctor guilty of negligence and failure in the duty of care, if he failed to advise a diabetic patient on insulin of the legal requirements. Where a patient on insulin is known to be manifestly dangerous, has been told to inform the DVLA and has failed to do so, the doctor after consultation with his defence association may, in the interest of the public at large, have to consider notifying the case himself directly to the DVLA.

Diabetics managed by diet alone need not notify the DVLA unless they develop relevant disabilities, e.g., diabetic eye problems affecting visual acuity or visual fields, or later require insulin treatment.

Diabetics managed by diet and tablets will, subject to satisfactory medical enquiries by the DVLA be able to retain their driving licence until the age of 70, unless they develop relevant disabilities such as diabetic eye problems or a requirement for insulin.

*Vocational driving licences and diabetes*

New applicants on insulin or existing drivers becoming insulin-treated are barred in law since 1 April 1991. Drivers licensed before 1 April 1991 on insulin are dealt with individually subject to a satisfactory annual consultant's certificate from a diabetic clinic.

Vocational applicants and vocational driving licence holders managed by diet and tablets are re-licensed unless they develop relevant disabilities due to complications, e.g., visual, cerebrovascular, cardiovascular, etc. If in the course of the diabetes, insulin treatment becomes necessary, the vocational large goods vehicle (LGV) or passenger carrying vehicle (PCV) licence is revoked. The relevant statutory instruments relating to diabetes and LGV and PCV driving licences are SI 1990 No. 2611 and SI 1990 No. 2612.

## Professional driving and diabetes other than LGV and PCV drivers

Apart from vocational drivers many other individuals drive for a living.

### Taxi drivers, etc.

Local Authorities and the Metropolitan Police license taxi drivers and some local authorities license car hire drivers and minicab drivers. Most apply medical standards similar to those for PCV and LGV drivers as above.

### Police, fire engine, and ambulance emergency drivers

The standard of fitness for emergency police, fire engine, and ambulance drivers is the special responsibility of their employing authorities and most apply the same standards as that required for an LGV or PCV licence.

## Appeal against refusal or revocations

Where a person with diabetes has his licence refused or revoked by the DVLA, there is a right of appeal to the local Magistrate's Court in England, Wales, and Northern Ireland, or to the local Sheriff's Court in Scotland. A person dissatisfied and still refused may seek judicial review by a higher Court.

## Concealment of diabetes

**No driver should conceal diabetes from an employer or from the employer's insurance company. Any person doing so could be found guilty under the Health and Safety at Work Act and could be subject to immediate dismissal without redress to an industrial tribunal.**

Guidance for employers and occupational health services is published both by the British Diabetic Association and the American Diabetes Association and the current situation can be summarized as follows:

1. Diabetics treated with diet alone should be able to undertake virtually any occupation providing they are not suffering from significant and disabling complications of the disease.

2. Diabetics treated with diet and tablets can equally undertake most occupations subject to being free from disabling complications. However, currently they are not permitted to serve in the armed forces or the police. They are not usually permitted to work in air traffic control, pilot transport aeroplanes or work on offshore oil platforms. The criteria relating to mainline train driving have been

relaxed very recently. This occupation is now permitted to diabetics on oral treatment who are well controlled, under regular specialist supervision, who monitor their blood glucose levels and do not suffer from any significant complications, or experience hypoglycaemia. Vocational drivers with uncomplicated diabetes, which is well controlled by diet alone or with oral antidiabetic preparations are usually allowed to continue driving large goods and passenger carrying vehicles subject to not suffering from any significant complications. Merchant seafarers and deep-sea fishermen are allowed to remain at sea subject to regular medical reviews.

3. Diabetics treated with insulin may be prone to hypoglycaemia: in most patients this does not cause problems. They should not, however, work in situations where sudden attacks could endanger themselves or others. For these reasons they are usually not permitted to drive LGVs or PCVs, or enter the fire service,[*] fly aeroplanes, drive trains or continue as seafarers or divers. It may be undesirable for them to work in potentially hazardous surroundings, e.g., at heights or with dangerous moving machinery. They may be barred from certain occupations, such as a railway signalman, because of the risk to the safety of the operation, and diminished vigilance whilst working alone in critical situations for long periods.

## Conclusions and recommendations

Much of the published information on the work record of people with diabetes is old and most of it originated from the United States. Very little information about employment and diabetes has been obtained in the United Kingdom and there is a need for up-to-date surveys. Moreover, information is needed concerning the impact of particular work activities on diabetic control and vice versa. Shiftwork and driving are important examples. Because of the paucity of definitive information, the advice given to diabetics is often arbitrary and decisions are made with little supporting evidence. What published data there are suggest that the sick absence record of well controlled diabetics is comparable to that of non-diabetics. Physicians should take time to inform employers and potential employers factually about the conditions and be careful to dispel any prejudice that might exist.

Although much progress has been made in improving employers' understanding of the problems of diabetics and the sickness record of well controlled diabetics is comparable to that of non-diabetics, there is still some evidence of continuing employment prejudice against diabetics. Regrettably this seems to be due to lingering ignorance and fear of the condition among employers and their medical personnel. A continued effort is necessary to educate employers and persuade them to take a more objective view of diabetics.

---

[*]Individual brigades decide whether serving firemen who develop diabetes are allowed to remain, but diabetes is not an automatic reason for early retirement.

The introduction of finger-prick blood glucose testing and new regimes of treatment which result in improved control, have enabled diabetics to cope more easily with irregular work patterns. It is hoped that these measures will also reduce morbidity.

Careers officers and teachers need to become more knowledgeable about diabetes so that they can give school-leavers accurate advice and enable them to make sensible career plans.

Some pension schemes still exclude diabetics and this is a frequent cause of employment difficulties. Many insurance companies now take a more liberal view of diabetics and so an individual should be able to make his own pension arrangements if rejected by a group scheme. Employers should be encouraged to allow more flexible pension arrangements and this should reduce the occurrence of this distressing problem.

It is essential that each individual case be assessed on its own merits with full consultation between all medical advisers. Diabetes *per se* should not limit employment prospects, because the majority of diabetics have few, if any, problems arising from the condition and make perfectly satisfactory employees in a wide variety of occupations.

## Thyroid disease

Thyroid disease, whether over- or under-function, can be corrected, at least when treatment is started in good time.

### Hypothyrodism

Untreated thyroid deficiency in a baby can cause lasting damage if not diagnosed and treated, but that hardly concerns employment. In adult life hypothyroidism (primary or secondary to hypopituitarism) is often insidious and can easily be missed. The diagnosis may often be made on sight by someone who has not seen the patient for a long time and then notices the change, or who has never seem them before.

During the period of development of symptoms, performance at work (and elsewhere) is likely to be affected—poor memory and concentration; slowing of mental and physical activity are likely to lead to decline of efficiency and even to mental derangement. Unless diagnosis is very severely delayed and the patient lapses into a myxoedematous coma, now an extremely rare event, treatment is simple and effective. Treatment has to be continued indefinitely in most cases but the patient is entirely healthy. The only danger is that someone misguidedly decides that in view of the apparent complete recovery treatment can be stopped. A patient with well-controlled hypothyroidism can lead a normal life in all respects.

**Hyperthyroidism**

Excessive thyroid function (Grave's disease) should present no problem to the occupational physician. Once diagnosed it can be treated, usually by medication, and normality restored.

With the classic features, over-activity, tremor, sensitivity to heat, fast pulse and loss of weight, the diagnosis is not usually difficult, although it must be differentiated from acute and chronic anxiety states. But in some cases, especially older patients, thyrotoxicosis may present as heart disease, commonly sinus tachycardia or atrial fibrillation. If the diagnosis is still not made the patient may present with symptoms of heart failure.

These cases too usually respond to conventional treatment, drugs, radioactive iodine or surgery, and the patient can then work normally without restriction.

## Selected references and further reading

1. Waclawski, E.R. (1989). Employment and diabetes. *Diabet. Med.*, **6**, 16–9.
2. BDA (British Diabetic Association) (1992). *Diabetes employment handbook.* BDA, London.
3. BDA (British Diabetic Association) (1988). *Diabetes in the United Kingdom.* BDA, London.
4. BDA (British Diabetic Association) (1990). *Employing people who have diabetes.* BDA, London.
5. Walker, R. (1993). Employment and diabetes. *Occup. Hlth. Rev.*, **42**, 12–4.
6. BDA (British Diabetic Association) (1987). *Looking for work.* BDA, London.
7. Waclawski, E.R. (1989). Diabetes and employment. MFOM thesis. FOM. London.
8. Bagshaw, E. (1980). Careers for diabetic girls in nursing. *Brit. Med. J.*, **280**, 1227.
9. Frier, B.M. (1992). Driving and diabetes. *Brit. Med. J.*, **305**, 1238.
10. Saunders, C.J.P. (1992). Driving and diabetes mellitus. *Brit. Med. J.*, **305**, 1265.

# 13

# Gastrointestinal and liver disorders

*P.G. Harries and R.J. Wyke*

## Introduction

The gastrointestinal tract and liver are subject to many disease processes, several of which can affect employment and result in large numbers of consultations with general practitioners, referral to hospital specialists, and hospital admissions. Digestive diseases were responsible for 12.4 million (m) days of sickness or invalidity absence in Great Britain between June 1989 and May 1990. Men experienced more lost days (9.5 m) than women (2.9 m). Levels of incapacity were highest in Scotland and lowest in East Anglia. Despite this, there have been very few studies of the influence of diseases of the gastrointestinal tract or liver on work.

Conditions likely to cause employment problems, or risks to individuals and the public, are:

- Gastro-oesophageal reflux and hiatus hernia
- Peptic ulceration
- Acute liver disease
- Chronic liver disease
- Inflammatory bowel disease
- Ileostomy and colostomy
- Gastroenteritis and infestations of the gut
- Functional disorders (non-ulcer dyspepsia, irritable bowel syndrome)
- Coeliac disease
- Chronic pancreatitis

## Oesophageal reflux and hiatus hernia[1]

Oesophageal reflux is experienced at some time by 10 per cent of Americans and, with appropriate positioning during barium meal, most people over 40 can be shown radiographically to have a hiatus hernia. Only a small number of these patients have symptoms and the precise relation between hiatus hernia and reflux is not clear. Morbidity is difficult to estimate but mortality is extremely low.

Oesophageal reflux and heartburn are made worse by bending, especially when this is accompanied by heavy lifting. Symptoms often improve with simple measures such as stopping smoking, weight reduction, wearing looser clothes, and antacid therapy. The use of acid suppressing drugs—$H_2$ antagonists and especially more powerful proton pump inhibitors (e.g., *omeprazole*)— improve symptoms of reflux and heal oesophagitis. Long-term use may be necessary to enable work to be continued. Patients with severe persistent reflux may develop oesophagitis and oesophageal strictures which, if symptomatic, may require dilation under sedation or, in extreme cases, surgery. Surgery is also undertaken to control severe persistent reflux in severely incapacitated cases unresponsive to intensive medical therapy. Time off work will depend on the incision used and type of work and is discussed in Chapter 19.

## Special work problems

The following types of work may produce symptoms in some individuals with these conditions:

(1)   frequent bending;

(2)   lifting and carrying heavy or awkward loads;

(3)   pulling and pushing of heavy loads; and

(4)   work involving stooping, crouching, or working in confined spaces, e.g., maintenance fitters, plumbers.

Although the effects of increases in intra-abdominal pressure and stooping can be reduced by correct lifting or adaptation of the work place, the effect on symptoms is variable.

## Peptic ulceration

### Prevalence and incidence

Peptic ulceration is the most important organic gastrointestinal disease in many Western countries, affecting at some time approximately 10 per cent of all adult males. During the 1970s, there was a fall in hospital admissions and in deaths from peptic ulcer, both of which occur mainly in the elderly patient. The reasons for this change are not clear but it may be due to the influence of modern treatment. Although declining, the resultant sickness absence, morbidity, and mortality are still substantial. In the year 1991–2, 2.7 m days of sickness/invalidity in England and Wales were attributed to ulcers of the stomach and duodenum (the Analytical Services Division of the DSS, Newcastle). Unfortunately, such information may not be based on accurate diagnosis and could include functional disorders of the gut. The risk of developing peptic ulceration is greater for people in jobs with a high level of physical activity than those undertaking sedentary work and is more prevalent in the North of England and Scotland.[2]

Prevalence of peptic ulcers is difficult to obtain as the only accurate way would be to perform endoscopy or barium meals on the whole population. Data from 13 000 autopsies in Leeds, reported in 1960, showed that 13 per cent of men and 5 per cent of women over the age of 35 suffered from duodenal ulceration, and 3.9 per cent and 2.9 per cent respectively from gastric ulceration. Doll and Avery-Jones' survey of factory workers in London (1951) showed that 5.8 per cent of men and 1.9 per cent of women aged 15–64 had peptic ulceration.[3] A study of a static population in Aberdeen (1968) showed that 8 per cent of males aged 15–64 years had peptic ulcers.

During this century the incidence of gastric ulcer has declined and that of duodenal ulcer has risen.

The annual incidence rates for gastric ulcer are 42 per 100 000 in men and 45 per 100 000 in women, while duodenal ulcer occurs in 180 and 85 per 100 000, respectively.[4] There is a tendency for the incidence of peptic ulcers to increase with age.

The incidence of perforation of a gastric ulcer has decreased; this now occurs chiefly in the elderly, and may be associated with ingestion of non-steroidal anti-inflammatory drugs (NSAIDs) which also result in gastrointestinal bleeding.

**Mortality**

During the past 30 years there has been a decline in mortality from peptic ulceration among younger people. In 1990 in the United Kingdom there were 4815 deaths from ulcers of the stomach or duodenum. Mortality was highest in elderly patients, rising from three deaths per million for men and one per million for women aged 15–34 years, to 115 and 55 per million respectively for those aged 55–64 years. There were more deaths from gastric ulcer among women than men, with a ratio of 1.6:1, but deaths from duodenal ulcer were about equal at 0.9:1. Although deaths are related to bleeding or perforation, more than half occur after surgery, especially in the elderly patient with intercurrent illness.[5]

# Clinical aspects of peptic ulceration affecting work

The most common complaint of patients with peptic ulceration is epigastric pain: less common are vomiting (more frequent with duodenal or pyloric ulceration), gastrointestinal bleeding, and perforation. Gastric and duodenal ulcers cannot be distinguished from the history alone and so barium meal radiography or endoscopic examination is necessary to establish the diagnosis. In patients with gastric ulcer, endoscopy has the advantage of enabling cytology and histological specimens to be obtained to exclude malignancy. Only a few hours off work is required for a barium meal radiographic examination, or for endoscopy performed without sedation (not so common in this country). If endoscopy is performed with sedation, and the patient's work involves heavy machinery or driving duties, then normal work should not be resumed until the next day.

The clinical course of duodenal ulceration is one of spontaneous relapse and remission which can vary from a single episode to a progressive disease with few remissions and major complications. The latter include haemorrhage, perforation, or pyloric stenosis, which occur in 1 per cent per year of patients followed, and are more common in the elderly. The clinical course of gastric ulceration tends to be more continuous and is more often associated with weight loss.

Work may be affected by episodes of abdominal pain, consequent loss of sleep, vomiting, and anaemia. The use of $H_2$ antagonists and the newer inhibitors of the gastric proton pump (e.g., *omeprazole*) heal up to 97 per cent of duodenal and 89 per cent of gastric ulcers by 8 weeks and should avoid loss of time from work. A course of medical treatment relieves symptoms and heals ulceration, but does not prevent further ulceration. Ulcers recur in 80 per cent of treated patients within one year, mainly in the first six months, and 25 per cent of these ulcers are asymptomatic. Recent work has demonstrated that relapse of peptic ulceration especially duodenal, is associated with the presence in the stomach of *Helicobacter pylori* (formerly *Campylobacter pylori*).[6] Although $H_2$ antagonists and proton pump inhibitors are very effective at healing peptic ulcers, because the infection remains, relapse is high. Combinations of an ulcer healing drug and an antibiotic to eradicate *H. pylori* are currently being evaluated, and in successful cases the rate of relapse is reduced to less than 10 per cent compared to 65 per cent for cases in which the organism is resistant to treatment.

Surgery should be considered for gastric ulcers which have been shown endoscopically to have failed to heal with intensive medical treatment, as there is a fear of undiagnosed malignancy. With duodenal ulcer, if infection with *H. pylori* is present, this should be eradicated to reduce the risk of relapse. In cases where eradication has failed then the choice is between treating each relapse with a course of medical treatment, or long-term maintenance treatment, and will depend on the individual patient. Hence, the otherwise fit patient who has three or four well-defined relapses of ulceration per year could be managed with a course of treatment for each relapse. On the other hand, long-term maintenance treatment might be more appropriate for patients with continuous symptoms or with short intervals between relapses. Patients with chronic medical conditions, particularly those requiring treatment with NSAIDS or corticosteroids should also receive maintenance treatment. Even on maintenance therapy, approximately 20 per cent of duodenal ulcers relapse within one year.

Surgery is necessary nowadays for the small proportion of patients with duodenal ulcers who develop complications, or have symptomatic ulcers unresponsive or non compliant to medical treatment, or for gastric ulcers which fail to heal. Surgical treatment (Chapter 19, p. 362) may require from six weeks to three months absence from work, depending on the type of operation and the work. The most widely used operation is proximal gastric vagotomy or truncal vagotomy and drainage, with a mortality of 0.5 per cent or less and an ulcer recurrence of under 5 per cent.[5] In comparison, partial gastrectomy has a mortality of 3 per cent and a similar recurrence rate.[5] Long-term complications occur in 3 per cent of patients after proximal gastric vagotomy, compared to 14 per cent for patients treated by partial gastrectomy in whom the dumping syndrome and intractable diarrhoea after eating can have very serious consequences for work. Patients may benefit from eating small dry meals and avoiding drinks containing carbohydrate. Other long-term complications, especially of partial gastrectomy, include anaemia, osteomalacia, and with increasing time a low risk of carcinoma of the gastric remnant.[5]

## Predisposing factors

### Smoking and peptic ulceration

Smoking increases the susceptibility to ulcer diseases, impairs spontaneous and drug-induced healing, increases the risk and rapidity of recurrence and the likelihood of surgery. **Thus, patients with peptic ulcer should stop smoking**.

### Other conditions

Ingestion of aspirin, NSAIDs (see above), and corticosteroids in high dose are generally accepted clinically as predisposing to the complications of peptic ulcer and dyspepsia, but evidence for causing ulceration is not conclusive. Patients with chronic renal failure on dialysis or following transplantation, however, have an increased frequency of peptic ulceration and there is probably an association with hepatic cirrhosis and hyperparathyroidism.

## Special work problems

Generally, patients with peptic ulceration can pursue any type of work. There is no clear relation between peptic ulceration and stress but some patients experience exacerbations of symptoms during periods of stress and some may require long-term maintenance drug treatment or even surgery. A recent study suggests that men with peptic ulcers tend to perceive stressful life events more negatively and may exhibit more emotional distress in the form of anxiety. If a patient works in isolation he may benefit from having other workers around him.

### Shiftwork

Although there has been a steady increase in the number of people working shifts, such work probably does not cause peptic ulcers but may exacerbate symptoms in certain individuals. It has been suggested that a person with a history of digestive tract disorder should be excluded from shiftwork because of irregular meals and other psychological problems, but this seems a rather extreme attitude especially in the context of modern drug therapy. Furthermore, although many shiftworkers report gastrointestinal disturbances, fewer than the expected number of deaths from gastrointestinal complaints were observed among shiftworkers when compared with national rates.[7] Perhaps shiftworkers are a self-selected group and people with significant gastrointestinal problems which tend to deteriorate with disturbed routine seek different work.

A not uncommon problem arises when someone has to work shifts either temporarily as part of in-service training, or due to unforeseen circumstances. Also, the financial rewards for working unsocial hours may make an employee with an exacerbation of peptic ulceration reluctant to change to less well-paid but regular hours. Where peptic ulceration arises in a shiftworker consideration must be given to the advisability of returning to a normal shift, a period of medical treatment or, if repeated relapses occur, maintenance drug therapy or surgery as a last resort.

## Work in remote areas, in particular at sea

The question of work in remote places is difficult, as healed ulcers can recur. The risk is around one complication per 10 patient years but nearly zero for compliant patients on treatment. This suggests that such patients should be considered for maintenance treatment while working in remote areas. Under the Merchant Shipping Regulations, seafaring should not be resumed until patients are free from symptoms without treatment for at least three months, have endoscopic evidence of healing, and are on a normal diet. Where there has been gastrointestinal bleeding, perforation, or recurrent peptic ulceration in spite of maintenance treatment with $H_2$ blockers, or an unsatisfactory operation, the seafarer will be permanently unfit. (See Appendices 3 and 4.)

## Acute liver disease[8]

### Acute viral hepatitis

Hepatitis *A* was responsible for 81 per cent, hepatitis *B* for 5 per cent, and non-A non-B for 14 per cent of notifications of viral hepatitis in England and Wales in 1990.

There is confusion among lay people and some doctors as to modes of transmission and the relative hazard posed by patients with different types of hepatitis, as well as a lack of understanding of the interpretation of serological tests for hepatitis *B* which can result in people being regarded incorrectly as infectious.

## Hepatitis *A* (infectious hepatitis)

This is caused by an enterovirus (HAV) transmitted by the faecal-oral route and affects chiefly children, with only 20 per cent of cases in patients over 16 years of age.

## Prevalence

Children in institutions and adults in communities with poor sanitation, as in developing countries, are at highest risk. Although the prevalence is generally decreasing world-wide there was actually an increase in the United Kingdom from 3.65 cases per 100 000 in 1987 to 14.4 per 100 000 in 1990. Serological evidence of previous infection is found in 45 per cent of adults, and increases with age from less than 20 per cent in people under 30 to nearly 60 per cent in those over 45. Most of them do not give a history of jaundice. Sporadic cases and epidemics are caused by eating virus-containing shellfish or cold food (particularly dairy products) contaminated by food-handlers during the prodrome of acute or anicteric hepatitis.

## Clinical aspects affecting work

Hepatitis is anicteric in 50 per cent of cases and has an excellent prognosis with a mortality of less than 0.15 per cent, no progression to chronic liver disease and no carrier state.

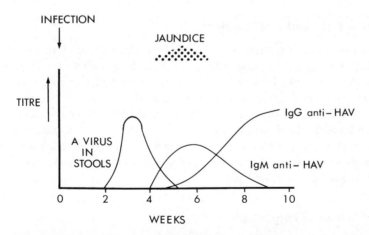

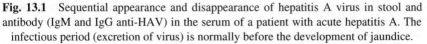

**Fig. 13.1** Sequential appearance and disappearance of hepatitis A virus in stool and antibody (IgM and IgG anti-HAV) in the serum of a patient with acute hepatitis A. The infectious period (excretion of virus) is normally before the development of jaundice.

The incubation period is 21–40 days and the patient is infectious while the virus is in the stools, i.e., from two to three weeks before until not more than eight days after jaundice is apparent (Fig. 13.1). Hence, the period of maximal infectivity occurs before the patient is symptomatic. Patients feel unwell during the prodrome but often improve with the onset of jaundice. Lethargy may continue for six weeks or as long as three months. Diagnosis is based on the detection in the serum of the IgM antibody to hepatitis *A*. The presence of the IgG type of antibody indicates either previous exposure to HAV or passive immunity from immune serum globulin or blood transfusion.

## Special work problems

With the exception of food-handlers, patients can resume or continue all forms of work as soon as they feel fit.

*Food-handlers* must stay off work until jaundice has disappeared, or for one week after the onset of jaundice, whichever is the longer. Those with anicteric hepatitis should remain off work for one week after serum transaminases have reached a peak. It must be recognized that the patient will have been infectious during the asymptomatic phase and special efforts should be made to monitor other staff to detect contact cases. Ideally, staff should report even minor indispositions, so that liver function tests and IgM hepatitis *A* serology can be checked on anyone with suspicious symptoms. This surveillance should be continued for 10 weeks after the index case is diagnosed. It is unnecessary to give unaffected staff immune globulin since this may attenuate symptoms without preventing virus excretion.

### Hepatitis *A* prevention of infection[9]

A vaccine against hepatitis *A* has recently been introduced in the United Kingdom with 2 doses intramuscularly 2 to 4 weeks apart inducing seroconversion in 95 per cent of recipients. It is an alternative to human immune serum for frequent travellers to areas of high or moderate HAV endemicity or for those staying more than 3 months. It is not recommended for use in outbreaks (not yet licensed for under 16-year-olds) and the only occupational group which must be considered for vaccination are sewage workers. In common with administration of immune serum, serological evidence of previous infection (IgG HAV) should be checked before immunizations.

### Hepatitis *B* (serum hepatitis)[8]

This results from the transfer of the hepatitis virus (HBV) in blood, blood products, or body fluids and secretions from an infected to a susceptible individual. Transmission by blood transfusion is extremely rare in this country, but drug addiction, tattooing, acupuncture, dental treatment, and homosexual practices are well-recognized means of transmission.

*Horizontal transmission* from person to person may result from sexual contact or sharing the same razor blade, toothbrush, or syringe. *Vertical transmission* from mother to child is particularly important in highly endemic areas such as the Far East. If the mother is a carrier of hepatitis *B* or suffers acute hepatitis during the third trimester, infection of the newborn infant is likely.

## Prevalence

In England and Wales the number of notified cases of acute hepatitis *B* has fallen from 1313 in 1986 to 564 in 1990. Few cases occur in children and the elderly, with 50 per cent of cases aged 15–34 years. The prevalence of acute hepatitis *B* in adults aged 15–65 years has been calculated at 6 per 100 000 for men and 2 per 100 000 for women.

### Mortality

Mortality from acute hepatitis *B* among adults aged 15–64 is about 0.6 per cent for men and 0.3 per cent for women, and tends to increase with age.

In the United Kingdom, approximately 3 per cent of the normal population have serological markers of previous exposure to HBV. Approximately 10 per cent of patients, mainly men, progress to the carrier state with persisting hepatitis *B* viraemia. World-wide, however, there are estimated to be 200 million carriers, varying from less than 0.15 per cent of the UK population to 15 per cent in the Far East. The risk of becoming a carrier is highest after hepatitis in neonates.

## Clinical aspects affecting work capacity

Acute hepatitis *B* has an incubation period of 3–6 months, with maximum infectivity during the late incubation and prodromal periods (Fig. 13.2). Clinical illness tends to be more severe than in hepatitis *A*, but over half of the infections are mild and often anicteric. In addition to the normal features of hepatitis an urticarial rash and arthropathy, part of a serum sickness-like syndrome, are occasionally seen.

Serological markers of HBV indicate the stage of infection and the degree of infectivity. Serological findings in a typical case of acute type *B* hepatitis and progression to chronic infection are shown in Figs 13.2 and 13.3. The presence in patients' serum of hepatitis *B* surface (Australia) antigen (HBsAg) should be followed by clinical examination for features of acute or chronic liver disease and further tests for other serological markers of hepatitis *B*. The presence of

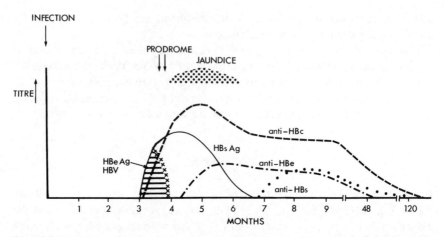

**Fig. 13.2** Relation of serological markers and symptoms of hepatitis to infection with hepatitis B in an uncomplicated acute case. The period of maximum infectivity (shaded area) during which hepatitis B, viral DNA and HBe antigen are found in the serum is mainly immediately before jaundice develops. Note clearance of surface (HBsAg) and e antigens with formation of antibodies (anti-HBe and anti-HBs).

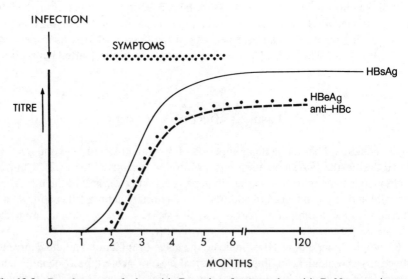

**Fig. 13.3** Development of a hepatitis B carrier after acute hepatitis B. Note persistence in very high titre of surface (HBsAg) and e antigens, and antibody to core (anti-HBc); also absence of antibodies to hepatitis B surface (anti-HBs) and e (anti-HBe) antigens.

antibody to the surface antigen (HBsAb) indicates previous contact with the HBV or vaccination with development of immunity, but the patient is not infectious. High titres of the IgM antibody to core (IgM anti-HBc) denote an acute type *B* viral hepatitis (Fig. 13.2). The finding of hepatitis *e* antigen correlates with a high degree of infectivity, while antibody to *e* shows seroconversion with a low degree of infectivity. From a practical point of view the patient with a resolving acute hepatitis is not infectious once hepatitis *B* surface antigen (HBsAg) is no longer detectable in the blood.

Chronic carriers are those patients who fail to clear the surface antigen from the blood six months after acute hepatitis *B* (Fig. 13.3) and can be subdivided into:

1.  *Simple carriers*: blood contains hepatitis *B* surface antigen in low titre and antibody to hepatitis *e*, but hepatitis *B* virus and DNA polymerase activity are absent. Such cases have a low infectivity.

2.  *Super carriers*: blood contains high titre of hepatitis *B* surface antigen and *e* antigen. DNA polymerase activity, and hepatitis *B* viral DNA are present and the patient is highly infectious.

## Prognosis of carriers

Most carriers are in good health and able to work normally but should be referred to a hepatologist as 70 per cent have histological evidence of chronic liver disease, mainly chronic persistent hepatitis, and 10 per cent have cirrhosis. In the long term they may seroconvert and liver diseases improve, but cases with persistent infection have a high risk of developing cirrhosis and hepatocellular carcinoma, which has a bad prognosis. Strenuous efforts are being made to develop treatments for chronic carriers and make them clear the virus by means of immunotherapy and antiviral agents.

## Time off work

During the acute phase the symptomatic patient will not feel well enough to work and usually rests at home for a period which is normally about twice the time of bed rest.

## Risk of spread of infection

There is no evidence of transmission of hepatitis *B* by casual contact in the workplace, or from contaminated food, water, airborne or faecal-oral routes. Spread of infection is likely only through intimate contact with the patient's blood, or body secretions, as occurs during normal sexual intercourse and some homosexual activities.

**Prevention of hepatitis *B*[9]**

Passive immunity can be provided by hepatitis *B* hyperimmune serum globulin but is only of value if administered prophylactically or within hours of infection (0.06 mg/kg i/m). Such treatment is indicated only for victims of parenteral (needle stick) exposure to HBsAg-positive blood or body fluids, babies born to HbsAg-positive mothers, and sexual contacts of acute sufferers. The former are a particular hazard for health care workers. Blood from the victim and donor should be tested for serological markers of hepatitis *B* but do *not* wait for the result before instituting treatment with hyperimmune globulin. If possible, hepatitis *B* vaccinations should be started at the same time as passive immunization.

Active immunization can be achieved by hepatitis *B* vaccine. The vaccine should be given to people who are exposed regularly to, or at increased risk of contracting, hepatitis *B*; in particular certain health care personnel (Table 13.1). However, vaccination of people at risk is not necessary if their serum contains antibody to hepatitis *B* surface (anti-HBs) or core (anti-HBc) antigen. The cost of vaccination is currently under £35 for a course of three injections, but the costs must be considered in the context of preventing long-term complications and potential liability for compensation. Re-vaccination may be necessary in some individuals after five years, as levels of antibody are undetectable in 15 per cent or inadequate in 27 per cent after this time. Injections should be made into the deltoid muscle and not into the buttocks as there is less subcutaneous fat and a higher antibody response is obtained.

## Special work problems of the hepatitis *B* carrier

The hepatitis *B* carrier is usually in good health and should not be treated as a hepatitis leper or barred from any type of work provided that simple measures are taken. The only risk is of accidental inoculation of his blood or body secretions into other people. Carriers should exercise care to avoid injury to hands, and must appreciate the importance of covering cuts and abrasions.

### First aid

First aid personnel should be reassured that the risk of contracting hepatitis during normal first aid procedures is infinitesimally small. They should be trained in the safe handling of body fluids, including the use of household bleach to disinfect contaminated surfaces, and in the safe disposal of clinical waste.

Concern is sometimes expressed over the action to be taken if carriers cut themselves. Like any normal individual, they should dress the wound and clean up any spilt blood with warm soapy water, then wipe the object or area

**Table 13.1**   General indications for vaccination against hepatitis *B*

*Health care staff*
Surgical and dental staff
Hospital and laboratory staff in regular contact with blood or needles
Necropsy staff
Direct carers of hepatitis *B* carriers, including genitourinary, endoscopy, and accident
  and emergency staff
Staff in oncology, haemodialysis, haemophilia, and liver units
Staff providing maintenance treatment with blood or blood products
Accidental exposure to hepatitis *B* material
Staff on secondment to areas of the world with a high prevalence of hepatitis *B*

*Patients*
First entrants to residential care for mentally handicapped
On maintenance haemodialysis or with chronic renal failure before dialysis or
  transplantation
Requiring multiple blood transfusions or injections of blood products, e.g., haemophilia
Natural or acquired immune deficiency

*Contacts of patients with hepatitis* B
Sexual partners of patients with acute hepatitis *B* or carriers
Other family members in close contact
Infants born to women with acute hepatitis *B* or who are hepatitis *B* carriers, especially
  those with *e* antigen

*Other staff*
Ambulance and rescue services
Staff at reception centres for people from high endemic areas (South-East Asia)

*Others at risk*
Promiscuous homosexuals or prostitutes (male or female)
Intravenous drug abusers

*Lower risk*
Long-term male prisoners
Staff of custodial institutions
Some police personnel

*People living in intermediate[a] and high[b] prevalence areas*
Women
Infants
Children
Susceptible individuals

**In general, people in low-risk careers or those in administrative posts, outpatient
sections, and those working in the community will not require vaccination**

[a] For example, Mediterranean countries.
[b] For example, most of Africa and the Far East.

thoroughly with a solution of household bleach to kill the virus. Food contaminated with blood as a result of the accident should be discarded for both hygienic and aesthetic reasons. With these provisos, the carrier can continue to work in all jobs including food-handling, catering, hairdressing, and teaching but should, of course, not act as a blood donor. Carriers should not be barred from using office equipment, toilets, showers, or eating facilities.

The specific problem of health care workers is more difficult. Staff who are hepatitis *B* carriers are seldom a risk to their patients but should be excluded from renal dialysis and transplantation units. The case of dentists and surgeons requires special consideration, but for the former the wearing of rubber gloves has been shown to prevent transmission to patients. If the chronic carrier develops chronic liver disease with cirrhosis (see below) this may affect his work.

### Non-*A*, non-*B* Hepatitis and Hepatitis *C*[8]

Acute hepatitis without serological markers of hepatitis *A*, hepatitis *B*, hepatitis *delta* virus, cytomegalovirus, or Epstein–Barr virus has been termed non-*A*–non-*B* hepatitis of which 50 per cent is hepatitis *C*. Such cases are responsible for 14 per cent of sporadic hepatitis in England and Wales and 90 per cent of post-transfusion-related hepatitis. Hepatitis *C* is responsible for 95 per cent of hepatitis occurring after transfusion of blood products. Serological tests for hepatitis *C* have only recently become available and blood donors are now routinely screened for antibody to hepatitis *C*. The currently available serological tests for hepatitis *C* do not always indicate an infectious state and there is probably no risk to people in normal social activities and work contact with a serologically positive individual so no particular restrictions are required; but he should not donate blood. Epidemiologically hepatitis *C* resembles hepatitis *B* with an incubation period of about 7 weeks. The hepatitis is usually mild and frequently subclinical but progression to chronic liver disease including cirrhosis occurs in 20 per cent of cases. As with cases of Hepatitis *C*, cases of non-*A*–non-*B* hepatitis pose no threat to others in the course of normal social and work activities so no restrictions are necessary except on blood donation.

## Chronic liver disease[8]

### Cirrhosis

Cirrhosis results from chronic liver injury as a result of which inflammation and necrosis of liver cells leads to fibrosis and nodule formation. There are many causes of cirrhosis (Table 13.2) the most common of which is alcohol, but not all cirrhotics are alcoholics. The crucial consequences of cirrhosis are hepatocellular failure and portal hypertension. These cause serious complications

**Table 13.2**   Some common causes of cirrhosis

Alcohol
Viral hepatitis type *B*, or non-*A*–non-*B*
Chronic active (lupoid) hepatitis
Metabolic, e.g., haemochromatosis
   Wilson's disease
   $\alpha^{-1}$-antitrypsin deficiency
Drugs, e.g., methotrexate
Hepatic venous outflow obstruction
   Budd–Chiari syndrome
Chronic cholestasis, e.g., primary biliary cirrhosis
Cryptogenic

including the development of ascites, encephalopathy, jaundice, gastrointestinal bleeding from oesophageal varices, and malnutrition. Any of these complications can have serious sequelae for work. This section will deal with the problems of patients with cirrhosis, in particular the alcoholic type.

## Prevalence

The prevalence of cirrhosis in the United Kingdom is 15 per 100 000 and 60 per cent are due to alcohol, 30 per cent cryptogenic, and 6 per cent chronic active hepatitis. The mean age of diagnosis of alcoholic cirrhosis is 47 years in women and 52 years in men.

Alcoholism is an increasing problem with 2 million problem drinkers in the United Kingdom, and 28 per cent of men and 12 per cent of women who drink at or above the recommended sensible limits (21 and 14 units of alcohol per week respectively).[10]

Alcoholic liver disease has been increasing in women who develop it at an earlier age than men and have a worse prognosis.

### Prognosis

In the most acute form of liver injury, alcohol causes acute alcoholic hepatitis which is a precirrhotic condition. The overall five-year survival depends on the severity of the liver inflammation and on whether the patient stops drinking: for those who stop drinking it is 74 per cent, compared to 34 per cent for those who continue. There were 1400 deaths in England and Wales in 1990 from alcoholic liver disease, with a ratio of 1.6:1 men to women. Prognosis is worst for women and patients with bleeding oesophageal varices and best for cases with well-compensated liver disease.

## Clinical aspects affecting work

The time off work required for treatment depends on the severity of the liver disease, ranging from none to several months for severe hepatic decompensation, such as occurs in alcoholic hepatitis. Follow-up is likely to vary according to whether the patient is attending an alcohol-dependency clinic or medical out-patients. In the extreme case of a patient at work but undergoing endoscopic injection sclerotherapy to obliterate oesophageal varices, appointments, often with an overnight stay, may be necessary every 2 to 3 weeks for up to 6 months. Such treatment reduces the risk of bleeding and may improve prognosis.

The effect of chronic liver disease, regardless of the aetiology, depends on the degree of hepatic decompensation, in particular on hepatic encephalopathy, ascites, and gastrointestinal bleeding.

*Hepatic encephalopathy.* Mental impairment, reduced physical fitness, and tremor may all reduce work capacity. The development of hepatic (portal-systemic) encephalopathy is usually a feature of severe liver disease or a complication of the now unfashionable operation of porta-caval shunt. Some patients with cirrhosis but without clinical features of encephalopathy have impairment of psychomotor function on testing sufficient to disrupt their everyday life and even render them unfit to drive. This condition has been termed 'latent encephalopathy'. Encephalopathy can be chronic or intermittent and precipitated by a number of causes including a high protein meal, infection, drugs, or bleeding into the gut. Some patients are very susceptible to meals high in animal protein and have to take a special diet and/or lactulose to alter the bowel flora.

*Ascites.* The presence of ascites may limit physical performance both by virtue of the mechanical effect of the large volume of fluid (up to 30 litres) and the associated malnutrition. Fortunately, ascites can usually be controlled with diuretics or paracentesis and hence problems with work can be avoided.

*Bleeding from oesophageal varices.* The prognosis of patients with bleeding from oesophageal varices depends on the severity of the underlying liver disease and on further episodes of bleeding. Recurrence of bleeding occurs in 60 per cent of patients within one year.

*Varices secondary to extrahepatic portal venous obstruction.* Oesophageal varices also occur in patients without cirrhosis, in whom obstruction, e.g., from thrombosis to the portal venous system, results in portal hypertension. Such patients commonly present as children with variceal bleeding which can recur during childhood but becomes less frequent after puberty. They have an excellent prognosis, unlike patients with portal hypertension secondary to cirrhosis.

*Associated conditions.* Other conditions associated with cirrhosis include diabetes mellitus (which is 2–4 times more common than in the normal population), malnutrition, and peptic ulceration (although this association has been refuted by some). Bone disease, especially affecting the back, is a problem for patients with chronic cholestasis, e.g., primary biliary cirrhosis; they may also be troubled by pruritis which can be so distressing and intractable as to result in suicide. In those with alcoholic liver disease, other systemic effects of alcohol (such as on the central nervous system including acute withdrawal; peripheral neuropathy; cerebrovascular accident; or cardiomyopathy) may all affect work.

## Special work problems

Ideally, patients with complications of cirrhosis, that is ascites, encephalopathy, or bleeding from oesophageal varices, should have been managed by a specialist before resuming work. Certain occupations are particularly associated with the *risks of alcoholism*. They include those working in the manufacture, distribution, and sale of alcohol; commercial travellers; seamen and those in the armed forces; and journalists, doctors, and entertainers. To employ someone with an alcohol problem in one of these jobs would seem inadvisable. Whether alcohol is a problem to the individual can be assessed quickly by the use of four 'CAGE' questions (see also Chapter 21):

1.  Have you ever felt you should cut down on your drinking?

2.  Have people annoyed you by criticizing your drinking?

3.  Have you ever felt bad or guilty about your drinking?

4.  Have you ever had a drink first thing in the morning to steady your nerves or get rid of a hangover (eye-opener)?

*Overt encephalopathy* is uncommon but such patients may be a hazard to themselves and others and should not be relied upon for jobs requiring a high degree of vigilance, including driving. The presence of *latent encephalopathy* is more difficult to identify but may have equally serious consequences for work. Individual suitability for driving duties should be discussed with the medical branch of the Driver and Vehicle Licensing Agency (DVLA) (see Appendix 1). Patients who are dependent on alcohol are barred from holding a vocational licence until they have been abstinent for five years and have a normal level of gamma glutamyl transferase.

There is no evidence that *bleeding from oesophageal varices* is precipitated by particular occupations or activities. Patients who have suffered episodes of bleeding from varices will normally have undergone injection sclerotherapy to obliterate the varices by the time they resume work. If treatment has not been completed or undertaken, it would seem prudent for them to avoid jobs involving heavy lifting and contact sports as the associated increase in intra-abdominal pressure might rupture a varix.

Once sclerosis of the varices is completed there is no reason why their work should be restricted, although it would be unwise to travel to remote places where medical services are limited.

Patients with *ascites* may experience difficulty with strenuous work especially lifting, or with bending and stooping.

### Handling of hepatotoxic substances by patients with liver disease

Many substances, including drugs and certain chemicals, particularly solvents which are found in workplaces and are hepatic enzyme-inducers, are known to cause liver damage but by far the most important environmental hepatotoxin is alcohol. Data on these substances are derived from the accidental or deliberate exposure of animals or humans with normal liver function to toxic substances. For obvious ethical reasons, there are virtually no data on the effect of these toxins on patients with liver diseases. Unfortunately, even a knowledge of the mode of action of these substances and the potential influence of liver disease cannot predict accurately the outcome of exposure on the individual patient with hepatic disease. Hepatotoxic substances exert their effect in one of two ways:

1.   By the action of a toxic metabolite, produced by the microsomal enzymes in the liver, which binds to liver macromolecules and results in the necrosis of the cell.

2.   The other chief mode of action is immunological; the metabolite binds to the liver cell and results in a change of antigenicity of the cell membrane with destruction of the cell by the immune system.

Susceptibility to liver damage depends on whether the rate at which the toxic metabolite is formed is greater than the rate of the detoxification, usually by conjugation with compounds such as glutathione. Once the stores of these protective compounds are exhausted, liver necrosis will follow. Chronic exposure to certain substances, such as anticonvulsants, results in induction of the liver microsomal enzymes with increased production of hepatotoxic metabolites. But, paradoxically, these enzyme-inducers may stimulate other pathways for the production of non-toxic metabolites. Although alcohol elevates the levels of hepatic enzymes, the effect on the handling of hepatotoxins is variable and inconsistent. Thus, chronic alcohol exposure can potentiate the toxic effect of paracetamol, while acute exposure protects against paracetamol damage but potentiates carbon tetrachloride hepatotoxicity. It is impossible to predict the result of exposure to hepatotoxic agents of a patient with a normal liver, who is also taking an enzyme-inducing agent.

### Influence of liver disease

There are great variations in the metabolism of toxic substances by patients with liver disease. These are related not only to the severity of the liver disease but also to genetic and environmental factors which result in changes in the activity of liver enzymes. The reduced hepatic mass may result in reduced conversion of the substance to a toxic metabolite and so protect against damage. But protective co-factors and detoxifying enzymes are likely to be reduced and will tend to potentiate liver damage. The outcome of exposure depends on the relative balance between these two effects of the liver disease.

## Guidelines for the employment of workers with hepatotoxins

The previous paragraphs show the unpredictability of hepatotoxins in patients with liver disease and explain the need for restricting the exposure of such people to these substances.

Patients with chronic liver disease or active acute liver disease should not work or be exposed to hepatotoxins. But there are exceptions such as those who have had hepatitis *A*; resolved acute viral hepatitis *B*, or non-*A*–non-*B* hepatitis or hepatitis *C* in whom liver function tests and liver histology have returned to normal; patients with gall stones unless they are jaundiced or have developed secondary biliary cirrhosis which is very rare. All people working with hepatotoxic agents should avoid alcohol and enzyme-inducing agents such as anticonvulsants, in particular *phenobarbitone* and *phenytoin*.

## Inflammatory bowel disease[11]

The most common types of inflammatory bowel disease in the United Kingdom are ulcerative colitis and Crohn's disease, both of which are of unknown aetiology. Inflammation is limited to the mucosa of the colon in ulcerative colitis, while in Crohn's disease the whole of the gastrointestinal tract from the lips to the anus may be affected by transmural inflammation. Both diseases are characterized primarily by diarrhoea, but abdominal pain and the formation of abscesses, gut perforation, and fistulae are features of Crohn's disease.

### Inflammatory bowel disease and employment

Inflammatory bowel disease remains poorly understood by employers and doctors, many of whom remember from their student days the sight of a young patient with extensive, progressive, and disabling Crohn's disease. Such cases are the exception rather than the rule, and most patients with controlled inflammatory bowel disease lead a normal life and work with little sickness absence. Nevertheless, unnecessary concern is expressed over their employment, especially of those with stomas, and employers must learn that most will make perfectly satisfactory employees capable of most occupations.

## Prevalence and incidence

The prevalence of these diseases varies in different parts of the United Kingdom. A survey from Oxford between 1951 and 1960 estimated that there were 80 cases of ulcerative colitis and nine of Crohn's disease per 100 000 population, with an incidence of 6.5 and 1.8, respectively. Crohn's disease is becoming more common, due in part to increased familiarity with the condition: recent estimates put the prevalence at 30 per 100 000 with an incidence of 4–5 per 100 000.

Men and women are equally affected by Crohn's disease, while ulcerative colitis is more common in women. Both diseases can start at any age with a peak from 15 to 40 years and a secondary peak at 55.

### Mortality and morbidity of inflammatory bowel disease

Both types of disease are associated with diarrhoea which can result in intermittent or persistent morbidity the incidence of which is difficult to estimate accurately. The occasional patient experiences one isolated episode only, while, conversely, a fulminating presentation may require early emergency surgery.

### Ulcerative colitis

Patients with ulcerative proctitis have a normal life expectancy but may have considerable urgency of defecation and diarrhoea. Such distal disease may extend to affect the whole colon. Patients with more extensive ulcerative colitis have an increased mortality during the first year after diagnosis, but after this mortality is the same as for the general population. Surgery is necessary for patients who fail to respond to medical treatment and is likely in 1 in 50 patients within five years of the onset of proctitis, 1 in 20 with left-sided colitis and 1 in 3 with total colitis. The most common type of surgery is panproctocolectomy with creation of an ileostomy, which has a mortality of less than 1 per cent in experienced hands. Such patients have a normal life-expectancy with only minor limitations of their work. An alternative to an ileostomy, for patients with ulcerative colitis but not Crohn's disease, may be the creation of an ileoanal anastomosis with a pouch. The advantage is that patients do not require a stoma but usually have to have their bowels open approximately 3 times a day. The surgical morbidity tends to be higher than for the creation of a stoma and more than one operation is required with consequent loss of time from work. Patients with total colitis of more than 10 years duration, especially those in whom disease commenced before the age of 20, have an increased risk of carcinoma of the colon and prophylactic colectomy may be advisable.

## Crohn's disease

### Morbidity of Crohn's disease

The transmural inflammation of the bowel can result in thickening, obstruction, and perforation of the bowel wall, with liability to fistulae or abscess formation. Such complications can cause major morbidity requiring surgery or may be relatively asymptomatic. The natural history of the disease is not related to the age of onset but depends on the extent and site of the lesions. Thus, disease limited to the terminal ileum has a better prognosis than diffuse inflammation of the small bowel. Disease of the colon and rectum will result in distressing symptoms of diarrhoea and urgency, while small bowel disease can have a profound nutritional effect. Exacerbations of the disease occur at variable intervals after presentation, with 70 per cent of patients experiencing relapse within five years.

### Mortality of Crohn's disease

The risk of dying does not increase with duration of disease and is highest for patients whose disease began before the age of 40. Late mortality is only slightly in excess of the expected mortality. Deaths are related to complications of surgery and development of carcinoma of the bowel.

## Clinical aspects of inflammatory bowel disease affecting work

The main problems for patients, irrespective of the type of inflammatory bowel disease, are frequency and urgency of defecation. Urgency is related to inflammation and reduced capacity of the rectum and is as major a problem for someone with proctitis as it is with inflammation involving the whole colon. The urgency and resultant incontinence are very disabling and cause serious restrictions to patients' life and work. The National Association for Colitis and Crohn's Disease (see Appendix 9) issues members with a 'Can't Wait' card which can be presented in shops and places displaying the NACC logo, to help gain access to a toilet.

Most patients with a mild attack of inflammatory bowel disease without constitutional upset can be treated as outpatients and usually without loss of time from work. Treatment of moderate or severe attacks generally requires rest in bed, or in hospital if there is constitutional upset. Time off work for relapses treated medically varies from two weeks to two months.

### Side-effects of medical treatment

Systemic steroids are seldom used long term in the management of patients with inflammatory bowel disease, with the exception of the small number of cases with extensive Crohn's disease of the small bowel. Large doses used in an acute severe attack can cause greater side-effects than in a normal person, owing to the low serum albumin. *Salazopyrine*, used to reduce the frequency and severity of relapse in ulcerative colitis, can cause distressing headaches and rashes but side-effects are less frequent with newer preparations containing only 5-aminosalicylic acid.

### Surgical treatment

Surgical treatment is necessary for patients with ulcerative colitis who fail to respond to aggressive medical treatment or who are at risk of developing carcinoma of the colon. For Crohn's disease, surgery is indicated for the relief of mechanical problems such as strictures or fistulae, or for resection of severely diseased segments of bowel which fail to respond to intensive medical therapy.

### Time off work for bowel surgery[12]

This depends on the type of operation and ranges from two weeks for a minor procedure to up to six months for panproctocolectomy and ileostomy. Employers should be encouraged to be supportive of patients during this time as ultimate return to work is likely. Surgical treatment, especially the formation of an ileostomy, usually restores patients' general health to normal with greater energy, fewer problems at work, and less sickness absence. It is often only after surgery that everyone appreciates just how debilitating the inflammatory bowel disease has been. An ileostomy may require surgical refashioning especially during the first year after its creation but thereafter should be relatively trouble-free. The formation of a pouch and ileoanal anastomosis is more complex and more time off work is necessary.

Patients with ulcerative colitis are usually restored to normal health once the colon has been removed. Crohn's disease, however, is frequently characterized by recurrence of disease despite surgical resection. Thus, 55 per cent of cases develop recurrent disease 10 years after resection of affected bowel. The patient with Crohn's disease affecting long segments of small bowel can be a particular problem, as surgical resection is undesirable. Such cases are uncommon and may require long-term corticosteroid therapy.

### Other conditions associated with inflammatory bowel disease

*Arthritis* occurs in 10 per cent of patients with ulcerative colitis and in 20 per cent with Crohn's disease, tends to affect the lower limbs, and is associated with active bowel disease.

*Sacroiliitis* occurs in 15 per cent of patients with inflammatory bowel disease but is usually not severe and seldom progresses to involve the lumbar and thoracic spine. Unlike peripheral arthritis, sacroiliitis is not related to the extent or severity of underlying bowel disease and can antedate the onset of the latter. These problems may cause some limitation of activity.

*Iritis* (see also Chapter 5, p. 99) is an uncommon (0.5–3 per cent) but serious complication of inflammatory bowel disease, causing painful blurred vision and headaches. It is usually associated with exacerbations of disease and with other extra-intestinal manifestations, such as arthritis and erythema nodosum. Steroid therapy may be required, but colectomy does not always result in resolution.

*Skin problems*, the most severe of which are pyoderma gangrenosum and erythema nodosum, occur in up to 9 per cent of patients, mainly those with ulcerative colitis. Lesions tend to occur on the legs, are associated with active bowel disease in the case of erythema nodosum, and often require steroid therapy.


## Special work problems

Despite the potential for ill health, most patients with chronic inflammatory bowel disease are able to continue to work. One survey found 70 per cent of outpatients to be working with good continuity of employment, over a six-year period of follow-up. Sickness absence was not high, with 70 per cent of patients having lost no time off work in the preceding year. Irrespective of the type of inflammatory bowel disease, patients with an ileostomy took less sickness absence and experienced fewer problems at work, than those without.[12]


### Changes of work due to health and surgery[12]

Premature retirement on account of health is necessary for a few patients (4 per cent), often due to associated conditions (arthritis) rather than to the inflammatory bowel disease itself or surgery. About 50 per cent of patients may find it necessary to change their employment due to their health and about 10 per cent have to modify their work. After surgery many patients are able to resume work often after long periods of sickness absence. Time off work after surgery tends to be longer for patients who undergo panproctocolectomy or ileoanal anastomosis with a pouch than for segmental resections or ileorectal anastomosis. These differences are in part related to the delayed healing of the perineal wound of panproctocolectomy and the more complex nature of the surgery necessary for the creation of a pouch.


### Unsuitable work for patients with inflammatory bowel disease

Most work is suitable for patients with inflammatory bowel disease. Some patients, however, do experience more problems with their disease during periods of increased stress.

The main problems patients experience with work are general fatigue, frequent bowel action, arthritis, and leakage from their stomas. Thus, shiftwork may be a problem to some patients, especially those with active or severe disease. Patients are often the best judge of what work is suitable for them.

General fatigue is a very common complaint of patients with active inflammatory bowel disease. For some patients this may require a change to less strenuous work. Fortunately, energy improves after effective medical or surgical treatment of the diseased bowel.

Frequent bowel action may present problems for patients with limited access to toilets. These include people working out of doors; with restricted toilet access; with restricted mobility due to wearing protective clothing; with severe arthritis; who are production-line workers, especially on paced work.

Hence, it may be important to consider the siting of work to provide easy and adequate toilet access.

Sacroiliitis and arthritis are usually mild but can cause varying degrees of limitation which need to be assessed individually. (See also Chapters 9 and 10.)

### Food-handling and preparation

Once inflammatory bowel disease has been diagnosed and an infectious cause for the diarrhoea excluded, there is no reason why the patient should not work as a food-handler, providing that the normal standards of personal hygiene expected of such a worker are satisfied. Although these patients may always have loose stools, they are usually able to recognize any changes from their normal pattern which would indicate a superimposed gastroenteritis. If this happens the patient should be investigated in the usual way.

### Special facilities

The only provision needed for patients with inflammatory bowel disease is unrestricted access to adequate toilet and washing facilities, which should include some privacy for those with an ileostomy.

### Ileostomy and colostomy

Ileostomies and colostomies are created either as permanent stomas, or temporarily to enable an acute bowel problem to resolve following which the normal route for bowel function is re-established. Such patients have to adjust to their new body image and functions but are generally able to lead a full and normal life. Unfortunately, some of them experience problems and discrimination in obtaining or continuing work, in part due to prejudice and ignorance by both employers and doctors.

In England and Wales there are around 10 000 people with an ileostomy and 250 to 300 permanent stomas are created each year from this population. The majority of ileostomies are created in young people for inflammatory bowel disease. In comparison, there are probably 100 000 people in England and Wales with a permanent colostomy. They tend to be older (peak age incidence 65 years) with a male to female ratio of 1.1:1 and the stoma is often created for cancer of the colon or rectum.

## Clinical aspects affecting work capacity

The capacity of someone with a stoma to work will depend both on the reason for surgery and on his general health after convalescence. Hence, the patient with ulcerative colitis who has had an ileostomy created as part of a colectomy should be returned to full fitness with a near normal life expectancy, while the prospects of a patient with a colostomy for carcinoma of the colon may be less favourable.

Time off work for creation of the stoma ranges from three to six months but in the case of a permanent stoma very little further surgery is usually necessary. Complications include electrolyte imbalance, dehydration, and intestinal obstruction, and, in the long term, an increased risk of biliary and renal stones.

A survey of 1033 members of the Ileostomy Association of Great Britain and Ireland found 79 per cent of women and 96 per cent of men to be working after their operation. Of these, 6 per cent began work for the first time after the operation. Continuity of employment was good.[13]

## Special work problems[14]

While people with an ileostomy or colostomy can be found performing almost every type of work including deep-sea diving (but see Appendix 4), certain jobs are more likely to cause problems. Excessive stooping or bending, especially if accompanied by heavy lifting or carrying loads close to the abdominal wall, and working in a very confined space, may result in leakage from the appliance or injury to the stoma. Modern appliances and a better understanding of optimum siting of the stoma have resulted in the appliance being more stable and less vulnerable. Work in the emergency services, which generally combines the problems of heavy lifting close to the body with the use of restrictive clothing, tends to be difficult for the person with a stoma, although there are a few patients working in this capacity. Miners with stomas who work at the coal face find the hot, dirty, sweaty environment combined with the heavy work and the poor toilet facilities unsuitable.

## Food-handling

The bacterial content of ileostomy effluent is one-twentieth that of normal faeces. Hence, provided the patient has good personal hygiene, the risk of spread of infection should be no greater, and possibly less than in a normal person, and in these circumstances a patient with an ileostomy should not be barred from working as a food-handler. Colostomy effluent has a bacterial content more akin to normal faeces. Patients with colostomies tend to be older, and are sometimes less dexterous, and so the question of food-handling is more contentious but again a decision should depend on the level of personal hygiene.

## Hot environments

Dehydration is a potential problem for anyone with an ileostomy as the stoma results in loss of water and salt such that the total body water is reduced by 10 per cent and salt by 7 per cent, compared to a normal person. People with an ileostomy are thus more susceptible to dehydration when in extremely hot environments or during periods of gastrointestinal upset. Work in hot environments is not contraindicated for the ileostomist, provided that fluid and salt intake are maintained. If the patient is visiting the tropics, he should be instructed on the use of oral rehydration solutions.

## Work in remote places

Concern has been expressed over someone with an ileostomy working in very remote places with limited medical and surgical back-up in case of emergency. This should be taken into account and each case will have to be considered on its merits. Factors to be considered are the reason for the ileostomy, any previous problems, and the length of time since the stoma was created. For example, a person with an ileostomy as part of a panproctocolectomy for ulcerative colitis will not suffer further problems from the colitis, while patients with Crohn's disease may still develop recurrent disease. The need for further surgery to the stoma, regardless of the type of underlying bowel disease, tends to be greatest during the first year after its formation. (See also Appendix 4.)

## Handling of hazardous substances

The handling of toxic chemicals and/or pathogenic material should not be a risk to people with an ileostomy provided that they maintain normal safety standards and safe working practices.

## Air travel

Air travel results in reduced ambient pressure. Gas in the bag expands and unless vented can burst the appliance. People with a stoma should wear an appliance with a flatus valve and avoid aerated drinks before and during the flight.

## Special facilities

The patient with a stoma needs good toilet and washing facilities with privacy so that the appliance can be changed or leakage cleaned up. If a medical department is readily available, staff will help and also help with any problems.

# Gastroenteritis and infestations of the gut[15]

Gastrointestinal infections can result in diarrhoea and ill health which may impair work capacity, but the main concern is the risk of spread of infection, in particular by food-handlers. Fortunately, most of the infections encountered in the U.K. are self-limiting but travellers from abroad may contract more serious chronic infection.

Because of limited space we have dealt only with the most common and with those of particular consequence to the occupational physician. They are: viruses; *Campylobacter* enteritis; *Salmonella* infections; giardiasis; cryptosporidiosis; *Staphylococcus aureus*; amoebiasis; and gay bowel syndrome.

## Viral gastroenteritis

Viruses probably cause more gastroenteritis than bacteria but only a small number of cases are confirmed due to the difficult identification techniques required. In 1991, viruses accounted for 16 000 cases of gastroenteritis of which 13 000 were due to rotaviruses chiefly in children.

Norwalk viruses are probably responsible for 40 per cent of outbreaks of epidemic gastroenteritis. Outbreaks particularly affect families, schools, recreation camps, and cruise ships. Transmission is by eating contaminated food, contact with vomit or faecal–oral routes. Prevention of infection is difficult as transmission of the virus by aerosol or ingestion of contaminated food occurs in the short incubation period and acute stages of the illness.

The patient should stay off work until asymptomatic and, in the case of food-handlers, for 48 hours after recovery.

### *Campylobacter* enteritis[16]

*Campylobacter* (*jejuni* and *intestinalis*) enteritis is now the most common cause of gastroenteritis in adults in Britain and has increased from 12 000 cases in 1981 to 32 600 in 1991. Infection is more common in the summer months.

The most common source of infection is eating inadequately cooked poultry, or food contaminated from poultry by poor kitchen hygiene. After 3–5 days' incubation period, a prodrome is followed by a systemic upset, with abdominal pain, and diarrhoea. Mortality is extremely low, occurring mainly in the young or elderly. Infection is usually self-limiting, although patients may excrete the organism in the stool for up to five weeks. Treatment of severe or persistent infection with *erythromycin* or *ciprofloxacin* is becoming a more common practice although the true place for this approach is not yet clear. Reduced excretion of organisms from treated cases may reduce risk of transmission of infection.

Person to person transmission is only a problem between young children and siblings to parents. **Thus, there is no significant occupational health hazard and even food-handlers can resume work once fit.**

### *Salmonella* infections

In 1991 there were 27 693 cases of *Salmonella* enteritis notified and between 1980 and 1989 *Salmonellae* were responsible for 45 per cent of 294 outbreaks of food poisoning from manufactured food.[17]

Although there are more than 1700 types of *Salmonellae*, from a practical point of view only a relatively small number cause problems for man. *Salmonella typhi* and *S. paratyphi* A, B, and C are primarily human pathogens causing enteric fever. Other *Salmonellae* are primarily animal pathogens causing illness in man usually localized to the gastrointestinal tract; most infections are caused by a small number of different serotypes. The source of most *Salmonella* infection is poultry and agricultural animals, or food contaminated during preparation. Person-to-person spread can occur in closed communities. Watery diarrhoea occurs 12–72 hours after infection, accompanied by abdominal pain, vomiting, and fever. The illness lasts a few days and is usually self-limiting, but in 1–2 per cent of cases septicaemia results in dissemination of infection to other sites, e.g., chest and bone.

Patients who are frail, taking immunosuppressive drugs or who have undergone gastric surgery; those with achlorhydria or on antacid therapy seem to have an increased susceptibility to infection. Fatalities are rare but occur in the young or elderly. Antibiotics are indicated for the patients with septicaemia or focal sepsis. Adults excrete the organism for 4–8 weeks, but can resume work once fit, the exceptions being food-handlers and water workers. Treatment with the new fluoroquinolones (*ciprofloxacin*) clears infection in 50 to 70 per cent of cases.

## *Salmonella typhi* and *paratyphi*

*Salmonella* typhoid and paratyphoid are uncommon gastrointestinal infections in the United Kingdom, and are usually acquired in countries with poor sanitation. Despite widespread recognition by the layman these infections are of little importance to the occupational physician except in the context of food-handlers (see p. 260).

### Immunization against *Salmonella typhi*[9]

This should be considered for travellers to endemic areas and laboratory staff who may handle *S. typhi*. There are now three different types of typhoid vaccine but none provide 100 per cent protection and travellers to endemic areas should still observe scrupulous attention to personal, food, and water hygiene.

## Giardiasis[18]

The protozoan *Giardia lamblia* is common all over the world with a prevalence in the United Kingdom of 5 to 16 per cent and is endemic in several developing countries.

In the United Kingdom during 1991, there were 6279 cases of infection with *G. lamblia*. Infection results from ingestion of mature cysts and although most subjects remain asymptomatic some people, after an incubation period of generally 6–15 (but occasionally up to 75) days, develop diarrhoea often with malabsorption. Many patients have non specific abdominal and general symptoms even after infection has cleared. Excretion of cysts in the faeces is a potential source of infection, especially for food-handlers, although the risk for asymptomatic carriers is probably low. Treatment with *metronidazole* or *tinidazole* results in a cure in 90 per cent of cases. Some cases prove particularly difficult to treat, raising the question of re-infection particularly in an endemic area.

## Cryptosporidiosis[19]

*Cryptosporidium*, an intestinal parasitic protozoan is responsible for 2 per cent of cases of infectious diarrhoea.

In 1991 there were 5163 cases of cryptosporidiosis. Although chiefly affecting children and the immunocompromised there is increasing isolation of this organism from immunocompetent adults. A quarter of cases probably arise from drinking raw milk or close contact with farm animals while the remainder are probably water borne or person-to-person spread and outbreaks are common.

After an incubation period of 3 to 8 days the acute presentation of abdominal cramps and watery diarrhoea lasts 7 days. Severe cases with fever and vomiting occur in 10 per cent of cases especially young men. Some people may have infection with both *Cryptosporidium* and *Campylobacter*. In immunocompetent individuals infection usually resolves in 1 to 3 weeks and asymptomatic carriers are uncommon.

### *Staphylococcus aureus*

Infected food-handlers do not normally play a significant role in bacterial food poisoning except for this variety. This organism may be found in septic lesions and as a commensal in the nose and on the skin. If transferred to food that is not at adequately low storage temperature, the organism will multiply, producing an enterotoxin that is not inactivated by further cooking. If ingested, it will lead to an abrupt onset of severe nausea, vomiting, abdominal cramps, and diarrhoea. The incubation period is short, usually 2–4 hours and the duration of the illness is less than 48 hours. Deaths are usually rare.

### Amoebiasis and gay bowel syndrome

Until 10 years ago amoebiasis was thought to be transmitted by ingestion of contaminated food or water, and was principally a problem of underdeveloped countries with poor sanitation. While the highest incidence is still in South America and southern Asia, in the United States and Europe amoebiasis has become far more common as a sexually transmitted disease, mainly among male homosexuals. When such patients are infected with one or more other enteric organisms including *Giardia lamblia, Campylobacter, Salmonellae*, and *Shigellae*, the condition is termed the gay bowel syndrome. Cysts of *Entamoeba histolytica* are endemic among homosexual males, being excreted by 4 per cent of those attending clinics for sexually transmitted diseases in the United Kingdom. As patients are usually asymptomatic and the amoebae of non-pathogenic types, the place of treatment is controversial. The risk of spread of infection during everyday contact, rather than sexual contact is low. However, there is evidence from the United States of transmission among homosexuals of *Shigella* dysentery and isolated cases of *Salmonella typhi* probably by oral–anal contact. The acquired immune deficiency syndrome (AIDS) is discussed in Chapter 22.

### Food-handlers

The increased production of ready prepared foods and more facilities for eating out mean that food poisoning can affect all sections of the population with serious and even fatal consequences, especially in the very young or weakened individual. In spite of increased legislation, inspection and education, the notifications of food poisoning reported to the Office of Population Censuses and Surveys (OPCS) have increased steadily from 45 253 in 1982 to 53 881 in 1991.

Raw meat and poultry, eggs and raw milk are the foodstuffs usually contaminated with food poisoning organisms. The majority of food-borne infections emanate from the failure to follow good food preparation or manufacturing practices such as proper temperature control for cooking and storage of food, cross contamination from raw to cooked foods and inadequate or inappropriate reheating of cooked foods.

Infected food-handlers account for only a small proportion of food poisoning outbreaks.[20]

### Definition of a food-handler

*A person engaged in the manufacture, storage or transport of food products involving direct contact with the product, or who is engaged in the preparation or serving of food within a catering establishment, canteen or retail food outlet.*

Persons who handle only wrapped, canned or bottled food should not be considered as food handlers. [See Food Hygiene (General) Regulations 1970].

Engineers, maintenance fitters, hygiene, and cleaning workers who come into contact with food-processing machinery or who work in food processing premises should not normally constitute a hazard, provided that adequate hygiene and cleaning regimes are followed. Some employers may, however, wish to extend the application of these health standards to those workers because they are included in the definition of those handling food in the Regulations.[21]

## The Food Hygiene (General) Regulations 1970 (SI 970 WO1172)

These require that food-handlers shall immediately notify their employers who, in turn, must notify the Local Environmental Health Department if suffering from any *Salmonella* infection, amoebic or bacillary dysentery, or any staphylococcal infection likely to cause food poisoning. As many food-handlers fail to notify these illnesses, medical practitioners must be alert to the dangers. Problems frequently arise when individuals contract gastroenteritis, especially on holiday in tropical or semi-tropical areas. In the latter instance, this is often expected by the patient and is not recognized as a potential hazard. Medical practitioners responsible for the health of employees in food factories, hotels, and canteens, should ensure that food-handlers report any episode affecting them or close family contacts before resuming work. Cases should be seen and investigated by the occupational physician, general practitioner or the Local Environmental Health Department.

Food-handlers with vomiting and/or diarrhoea should be excluded from work until they are symptom-free, and have normal formed stools. If there are clinical grounds for believing that they may have or have had, *typhoid, paratyphoid, cholera, amoebic* or *bacillary dysentery, salmonellosis,* or *intestinal worms*, appropriate clearance procedures must be followed (see Table 13.3).

**Table 13.3**   Microbiological surveillance and implications of infections and infestations in food-handlers[22]

| Type of organism | Requirement for resumption of work as a food-handler (criteria for clearance once symptom-free) |
| --- | --- |
| *Campylobacter*<br>*Bacillus cereus*<br>*Clostridium botulinum*<br>*Clostridium perfringens*<br>*Vibrio parahaemolyticus*<br>*Giardia lamblia* | None |
| Cholera<br>Dysentery – amoebic<br>Dysentery – bacillary<br>Enteropathogenic *E. coli*<br>    (outbreaks only)<br>Salmonellosis (excluding<br>    paratyphoid *A* and typhoid<br>    infections)<br>Paratyphoid *B* | 3 consecutive negative faeces specimens at 48 hour intervals |
| Paratyphoid *A* | 12 negative faeces specimens over 6 months |
| Typhoid | Permanently unfit to work as a food-handler |
| Viral gastroenteritis<br>    Rotavirus<br>    Other viruses | <br>7 days after recovery<br>None |
| Worms (threadworm and<br>*Taenia Solium*) | Once treated |
| Hepatitis *A*<br>*Staphylococcus aureus* | 7 days after onset of jaundice<br>Once septic lesions are treated and healed |

## Symptomless contacts of cases of food-borne disease

*Typhoid fever* will have to be investigated in conjunction with the Local Environmental Health Department, the Public Health Laboratory Service, or a consultant microbiologist. Laboratories isolating *Salmonellae* are obliged to inform the Environmental Health Officer who will issue an exclusion order if the individual is a food-handler.

For all other conditions there is no need to investigate unless the contacts develop symptoms. Advice should be given daily to all food-handlers to report any symptoms promptly, and to practise a good standard of personal hygiene.

## Selection of food-handlers

Routine medical examinations for food-handlers are not recommended.[22] Health interviews conducted by occupational health nurses should be done and can usefully elicit conditions which should normally exclude an individual from working as a food handler. These are:

(1)  history of paratyphoid or typhoid disease;

(2)  history of recurrent attacks of gastroenteritis, unless carrier state has been excluded by bacteriological tests (Table 13.3);

(3)  history and presence of persistent and recurring staphylococcal infections of the skin;

(4)  chronic infections of the ears, eyes, nose or throat;

(5)  poor oral hygiene;

(6)  conditions of the upper or lower respiratory tract which cause coughing and production of purulent sputum during normal working hours;

(7)  low standards of personal hygiene, including nail-biters.

Chest radiography and Widal tests are not now considered to be a necessary part of the pre-employment examination, unless there are indications that either is required.

## Meat workers

These are covered by numerous EC Directives which are still being issued. In the UK new regulations are expected to be implemented in late 1994 or early 1995.

The Regulations require workers on recruitment to prove, by a medical certificate, that there is no impediment to such employment. A code of practice to accompany the Regulations explains that whilst a doctor must have overall responsibility for issuing certificates it is ultimately for his or her professional judgement to involve nurses and other medical staff in examinations or allow them to examine employees. A doctor must sign the certificate. Annual renewal certificates will not be required.

Doctors working in the UK food industry consider such certificates to be of doubtful value, and there is no epidemiological evidence that they will reduce the incidence of food poisoning.

## Functional disorders

### Non-ulcer dyspepsia

The widespread use of endoscopy and double-contrast barium-meal radiography has revealed that many people with dyspepsia do not have peptic ulceration. Most of these patients are aged between 20 and 40 years, with a predominance of men. A survey from Sweden estimated that patients with non-ulcer dyspepsia suffered 2.6 times more sickness absence than the general population. Their condition also results in substantial numbers of both in and outpatient consultations, and inappropriate use of anti-ulcer medication. Although some of these patients improve initially on anti-ulcer treatment, this is probably largely a placebo response and may result in psychological dependence. Dyspepsia is more likely to be due to other causes, such as the irritable bowel syndrome and/or gastro-oesophageal reflux, but in a quarter of cases no explanation can be found.

### Irritable bowel (spastic colon) syndrome

This is a disorder of unknown aetiology characterized by abdominal pain, distension, and bowel upset (diarrhoea and/or constipation) in the absence of demonstrable organic disease. It is the most common disorder of the gastrointestinal tract, affecting one-third of the general population, yet only 20 per cent of sufferers seek medical advice. Many doctors do not appreciate the diverse clinical features of the condition which may result in inappropriate treatment for dyspepsia and some patients with severe pain may even have a normal appendix

**Table 13.4** Clinical features of the irritable bowel syndrome

|                                                    | % affected |
|----------------------------------------------------|------------|
| Abdominal pain, often left lower quadrant          | 98         |
| Disordered bowel habit                             | 80         |
| Flatus–distension                                  | 65         |
| Weight usually steady or increasing/modest reduction | 20       |
| Nausea with occasional vomiting                    | 50         |
| Dyspepsia (and occasional dysphagia)               | 25–50      |
| Previous 'normal' appendicectomy                   | 33         |
| Cancer phobia                                      | up to 50   |
| Urinary symptoms: frequency and dysuria            | 20         |
| Gynaecological symptoms                            |            |
|   Dysmenorrhoea                          | 90         |
|   Dyspareunia                            | 33         |

or gall bladder removed without relief of symptoms. In two-thirds of patients, the onset of symptoms is preceded by an anxiety-provoking life situation or an episode of psychiatric illness, such as depression. It seems likely that the syndrome is a normal somatic response to stress rather than a disease. (See Table 13.4.)

## Prevalence

Although only the more severe or chronic cases tend to be referred to a specialist, they account for approximately 50 per cent of gastroenterology outpatient work. There are twice as many women as men amongst those referred.

The onset of symptoms is generally from late adolescence to the late 30s, and is slightly later in men. The syndrome is rare in the over 60s and should only be diagnosed after other causes of gastrointestinal upset have been excluded, especially in the older patient.

The most incapacitating symptoms are diarrhoea and abdominal pain, which are usually intermittent but can have a profound effect on capacity to work. Data on sickness absence, however, are not available.

The response to treatment, especially of those seeking specialist advice, is often transient and variable, with 25 per cent deriving no benefit or even deteriorating. For some patients with food intolerance, dietary manipulation can prove beneficial but for many this is short lived. Reassurance and explanation of the nature of the condition and its relation to stress can be helpful. Severe chronic cases especially with abdominal pain may be helped by hypnotherapy.

The majority of patients manage to work unaffected by the condition but for a small number work may be severely affected by severe or chronic diarrhoea and/or abdominal pain. For patients with frequent bowel action, toilet access can be a problem. Avoidance of excessive stress may be helpful for some patients, although as a group they will tend to worry excessively.

## Coeliac disease

This is due to an allergy to gluten in wheat and results in atrophy of the small bowel mucosa especially the jejunum. Most patients present in childhood with failure to grow and/or diarrhoea, but a small number present as adults. Exclusion of gluten from the diet usually results in complete restoration of normal health. Relapse of symptoms usually occurs only if gluten is inadvertently or deliberately introduced into the diet. Thus, the only restriction for employment of someone with coeliac disease is if they have to consume gluten-containing food as part of their work (i.e. food-taster). Travel is not usually a problem provided that gluten-containing foods are avoided.

## Chronic pancreatitis

Chronic pancreatitis is a rare disorder characterized by chronic severe epigastric pain, steatorrhoea, and diabetes due to damage to the islets of Langerhans. Alcohol is a common cause and has obvious consequences for work. The chronic pain may be so severe as to require opiate analgesia or even pain control by nerve block. Fortunately, with time the condition tends to burn out. There are no special restrictions for work apart from those related to coexistent diabetes mellitus and/or alcoholism (Chapters 12 and 21).

## Conclusions and recommendations

Diseases of the gastrointestinal tract are seldom a hazard to others but if not managed correctly can impair ability to cope with work. Modern drug therapy and or simple adaptations to work especially for patients with gastro-eosophageal reflux should enable them to work productively. New drug regimens hold great promise for cure of peptic ulceration and reduced morbidity.

Once recovered from the acute phase patients with viral hepatitis *A* should be able to resume work without restrictions. A small proportion of patients with hepatitis *B* may progress to chronic ill health but spread of infection results only from intimate contact which should not occur in the normal workplace. Complications of chronic liver disease especially hepatic encephalopathy, ascites, and gastrointestinal bleeding may seriously impair ability to work and usually have a poor prognosis.

Exacerbations of inflammatory bowel disease may result in impaired quality of life but employment record and continuity of work is usually good, so that employers should be encouraged to adopt an optimistic outlook. Surgery for ulcerative colitis dramatically improves health and newer techniques avoid a permanent stoma. The possession of a stoma should not bar patients from most types of work and does not pose a risk of spread of infection provided good standards of hygiene are practised.

Gastroenteritis generally causes more inconvenience than risk, and newer drugs show promise in reducing infectivity and speeding resolution. There is still need for the careful medical management of infected food-handlers.

Functional bowel disorders are extremely common but have a good prognosis and may indicate a reaction to psychological stresses and life events.

### Selected references and further reading

1.  Bouchier, I.A.D., Allan, R.N., Hodgson, H.J.F., and Keighley, M.R.B. (ed.) (1993). *Textbook of gastroenterology,* (2nd edn). Saunders, London.

2. Katchinski, B.D., Logan, R.F.A., Edmond, M., and Langman, M.J.S. (1991). Physical activity at work and duodenal ulcer risk. *Gut,* **32,** 983–6.
3. Doll, R. and Avery Jones, F. (1951). *Occupational factors in the aetiology of gastric ulcer and duodenal ulcer.* MRC Special Report, Series 276. HMSO, London.
4. Langman, M.J.S. (1979). *The epidemiology of chronic digestive diseases,* pp. 9–39. Edward Arnold, London.
5. McCloy, R. and Nair, R. (1993). Surgery for acid suppression in the 1990s. *Baillière Clin. Gastroent.,* **7,** 129–48.
6. Axon, A.T.R. (1991). *Helicobacter pylori* therapy: effect on peptic ulcer disease. *J. Gastroent. Hepatol.,* **6,** 131–7.
7. Taylor, P.J. and Pocock, S.J. (1972). Mortality of shift and day workers. *Brit. J. Indust. Med.,* **29,** 201–7.
8. Sherlock, S. and Dooley, J. (1992). *Diseases of the liver and biliary system,* (9th edn). Blackwell, Oxford.
9. Department of Health, Welsh Office and Scottish Home and Health Department (1992). *Immunisation against infectious disease.* HMSO, London.
10. Royal College of Physicians (1987). *A great and growing evil.* Tavistock, London.
11. Allan, R.N., Keighley, M.R.B., Alexander-Williams, J., and Hawkins, C. (1990). *Inflammatory bowel diseases,* (2nd edn). Churchill Livingstone, Edinburgh.
12. Wyke, R.J., Edwards, F.C., and Allan, R.N. (1988). Employment problems and prospects for patients with inflammatory bowel disease. *Gut,* **29,** 1229–35.
13. Whates, P.D. and Irving, M. (1984). Return to work following ileostomy. *Brit. J. Surg.,* **71,** 619–22.
14. Wyke, R.J., Aw, T.C., Allan, R.N., and Harrington, J.M. (1989). Employment prospects for patients with intestinal stomas: the attitude of occupational physicians. *J. Soc. Occup. Med.,* **39,** 19–24.
15. Public Health Laboratory Service PHL Salmonella Subcommittee (1990). *Notes on the control of human sources of gastro-intestinal infections, infestations and bacterial intoxications in the United Kingdom.* Communicable Disease Report, Supplement 1, PHLS.
16. Pearson, A.D. and Healing, T.D. (1992). The surveillance and control of Campylobacter infection. *CDR Rev.,* **2** (12), R133–R139.
17. Socket, P.M. (1991). Food poisoning outbreaks associated with manufactured food in England and Wales: 1980–1989. *CDR Rev.,* **1,** R105–109.
18. Flanagan, P.A. (1992). *Giardia*—diagnosis, clinical course and epidemiology. A review. *Epidemiol. Infect.,* **109,** 1–22.
19. Casemore, D.P. (1989). Human cryptosporidiosis. In *Recent advances in infection* (ed. D.S. Reeves and A.M. Geddes), Vol. 3, pp. 209–36. Churchill Livingstone, Edinburgh.
20. Roberts, D. (1990). Sources of infection: Food. *Lancet,* **335,** 859–61.
21. Food Industry Medical Officers Working Group. (1987). *Health standards for work in the food industry, food retailing and establishments involved in catering.* Report of Food Industry Medical Officers Working Group. *J. Soc. Occup. Med.,* **37,** 4–9.
22. WHO (World Health Organization) (1989). *Health surveillance and management procedures for food handling personnel.* Report of a WHO Consultation. Technical Report Series, No. 785. (ISBN 92 4120785 X.) WHO, Geneva.

# 14

# Cardiovascular Disorders

*P.J. Baxter and M.C. Petch*

## Introduction

### Congenital and valvular heart disease

Individuals suffering from congenital heart disease will generally be detected in childhood and should seek cardiological advice before entering employment. Employers should not be deterred from taking on young people who have undergone cardiac surgery for the correction of congenital defects in childhood, as many lead a normal life and are capable of full-time employment. Acquired valvular disease (which remains important despite the disappearance of rheumatic fever), endocarditis, cardiomyopathy, and cardiac arrhythmias are responsible for a small but troublesome morbidity and mortality.

Valvular disease, usually degenerative aortic stenosis or mitral regurgitation, is most commonly seen in those beyond working age but the condition of mitral valve prolapse deserves emphasis because it affects some 2 per cent of the population and is perfectly benign; it often presents as an auscultatory finding at a pre-employment medical examination, may be associated with electrocardiographic change, and may sometimes lead to a false diagnosis of significant heart disease.

## Coronary heart disease (CHD)

The greatest scourge affecting the working population is undoubtedly coronary heart disease (CHD). Some CHD is preventable; employers have a duty to support and reinforce community measures by discouraging smoking, encouraging healthy activities during rest and recreational hours, and providing a healthy diet at work.

Some victims of CHD die suddenly and unpredictably from ventricular fibrillation. In the WHO Tower Hamlets study[1] 40 per cent of heart attacks (defined as myocardial infarction or sudden death from CHD) were fatal and 60 per cent of deaths occurred within one hour of the onset of any symptoms. This fact is widely recognized and has naturally affected employers' attitudes towards employees known to be or suspected of suffering from CHD. Heart attacks tend to occur more frequently in the morning, or towards the beginning of shiftwork, as compared with other times of the day.[2] Their onset also tends to be associated with vigorous effort.[3]

CHD usually presents as chest pain, either myocardial infarction or angina; it may also present with symptoms resulting from arrhythmia (including sudden death), or heart failure, or be detected incidentally by electrocardiography. Anyone with chest pain who is suspected of suffering from myocardial infarction should be taken urgently to the nearest coronary care unit where prompt treatment can save lives. After recovery the risk of further cardiac events (i.e., sudden death, recurrent myocardial infarction or need for interventional treatment) is assessed by combination of clinical features and simple investigation (see below). The likelihood of returning to work after a cardiac event is affected by a variety of physical, psychological and social factors.[4]

Effective treatment is now available for many forms of cardiovascular disease. Drug therapy has transformed the management of all manifestations of CHD. The prognosis of patients following myocardial infarction is improved by thrombolysis and subsequent treatment with aspirin. Myocardial ischaemia may be alleviated by nitrites, beta-adrenergic antagonists, and calcium antagonists. The symptoms and survival of patients with heart failure is improved by diuretics and angiotensin converting enzyme inhibitors. Coronary angioplasty is nowadays fairly straightforward and safe and is effective in relieving angina; but it is bedevilled by a high recurrence rate—approximately one-third of patients will experience a recurrence of cardiac pain within four months. Coronary bypass surgery is more complex but is also remarkably safe with most centres reporting mortality rates of around 1 per cent for elective operations. The relief of angina is longer lasting but recurrent angina is again a problem with an incidence of around 4 per cent per annum. Both coronary angioplasty and bypass surgery are indicated for persisting angina, the former is undertaken in those with more localized disease and cannot therefore be expected to improve prognosis, whereas bypass surgery, which is undertaken for those with more extensive disease, has been shown to do so. Coronary bypass surgery can allow patients to resume normal work earlier at a level of fitness higher than that achieved before operation. Improved cardiovascular fitness can also result from cardiac pacing, valve replacement, and cardiac transplantation. Unfortunately, waiting times, particularly for coronary arteriography and bypass surgery, are such that many patients do not return to work. One study showed that of those who had lost more than six months work before operation, fewer (35 per cent) returned to work than those who had lost less than six months.[5]

Rehabilitation programmes are now well established in many hospitals. These enable many patients to make a full physical and psychological recovery following a cardiac event. But some do not. Chronic physical disability from heart disease is unusual, but when present it is due to limitation of exercise tolerance through angina pectoris, dyspnoea, or fatigue reflecting unrelieved myocardial ischaemia and pump failure. There are however other individuals whose persisting disability is psychogenic; recurrent attacks of atypical chest pain, dizziness, constant tiredness, palpitation, and episodic dyspnoea, are not accompanied by objective evidence of cardiac dysfunction. Such individuals deserve sympathy and support. A number of factors, especially fear and a desire to cease work, may be responsible and these are very difficult to correct.

## Prevalence

In developed countries, about one-quarter of all deaths are due to CHD. In England and Wales in recent years there were approximately 180 000 deaths and 130 000 hospital discharges per annum with a diagnosis of CHD. The Royal College of General Practitioners' third national study confirmed the high morbidity.[6] Epidemiological surveys such as the British Regional Heart Study may overestimate the prevalence of CHD, but by using a questionnaire, physical examination, and electrocardiogram, the prevalence was estimated at 24.7 per cent of men aged 40–59 years.[7] The Whitehall study also showed that the incidence was higher in social classes 4 and 5 as compared with classes 1, 2, and 3.[8]

## Clinical aspects affecting work capacity

The risk of sudden disability and death through ventricular fibrillation is the major factor affecting work capacity amongst victims of heart disease. The risk is greatest in the early days following a myocardial infarct and in those with most myocardial damage. The extent of ventricular damage may be judged by the presence of heart failure, gallop rhythm, and estimation of left ventricular function using simple imaging techniques such as echocardiography and radionuclide ventriculography. The presence of residual areas of myocardial ischaemia is the second determinant of prognosis in the longer term and is a manifestation of more extensive coronary disease. This may be judged by a recurrence of cardiac pain or the development of angina pectoris which may be confirmed by exercise testing. An exercise test may also reveal cardiovascular incapacity in other ways, viz. exhaustion, inappropriate heart rate and blood pressure responses, arrhythmia, and electrocardiographic change, especially ST segment shift. In practice, the exercise test in combination with an experienced clinical opinion, has superseded the coronary angiogram in assessing fitness for work. This is reflected in the guidance material relating to vocational drivers (see Annex). Individuals who are free of symptoms and signs of cardiac dysfunction and who can achieve a good workload with no adverse features, have a very low risk of further cardiac events. This applies particularly to younger individuals whose employers need have little hesitation in taking them back to work. An ability to reach stage 4 of the Bruce protocol on a treadmill is judged to place an individual at such low risk of further cardiac events that vocational driving may be permitted. The DVLA guidelines are the result of careful deliberation by an Honorary Medical Advisory Panel and could be applied more widely to other groups of workers whose occupation may involve an element of risk to themselves or others should that individual suffer cardiovascular collapse. Most employees, however, are not required to demonstrate such high levels of cardiovascular fitness and lower levels would be acceptable for those in more sedentary and low-risk occupations.

Subjects with continuing severe disability, sinister arrhythmias, or poor left ventricular function should generally be advised to retire, whatever the cause of their cardiac disease. This also applies to any subjects with a progressive cardiac disorder, e.g., dilated cardiomyopathy. In contrast, subjects with good ventricular function, a stable cardiac rhythm, and minimal disability will usually fare well and should be encouraged to work. If the cause of the disability was corrected by surgical treatment, e.g., valve disease, then a return to work 2–3 months after surgery can be expected.

Following myocardial infarction, assessment of prognosis along the lines outlined above is recommended: those with no complications and good exercise tolerance may return to work in 4–6 weeks. A few will take longer.

Patients with CHD and persistent angina despite medical treatment should be assessed with a view to coronary bypass surgery. Return to work, when possible, is usually 2–3 months after the operation. Following less traumatic procedures, such as the implantation of a pacemaker or coronary angioplasty, return to work is much quicker, sometimes 48 hours following angioplasty. In all cases, when work is resumed, the levels and duration of activity should be increased progressively; returning to work implies a level of sustained activity well above that achieved by most who are recovering at home or who are undertaking hospital rehabilitation programmes.

Psychological difficulties may be experienced even by those with no signs of cardiac damage. Anxieties of both the patient and wife have been shown to affect the ability of men surviving myocardial infarction to return to work; half may have some anxiety or depression and, of those, half may have severe symptoms persisting, if untreated, a year later.[9]

In general, physical activity is good for the heart. The degree of physical activity must take into account patients' previous fitness and the results of exercise testing, etc. Patients with stable angina pectoris can safely work within their limitations of fitness but should not be put in situations where their angina may be readily provoked. Although it may be possible to be dogmatic in giving advice about physical work, guidance about the psychological stresses associated with managerial duties must be individually tailored. Personality has little influence on survival following myocardial infarction. The existence of patterns of coronary-prone behaviour is well embedded in Western business culture but the results of epidemiological and clinical studies remain conflicting as to whether the entity has a role in the aetiology of coronary heart disease. Nevertheless, modification of hectic work patterns marked by long hours, competitiveness, time urgency, and aggression (so-called type A behaviour) as part of other stress reduction measures may be beneficial.[10]

Transient cardiac arrhythmias (e.g., extrasystoles) are extremely common and do not usually indicate heart disease. They may be provoked by a variety of substances, e.g., coffee. Assessment by a cardiologist is recommended for those with persisting symptoms. A few individuals will suffer recurrent paroxysms of tachycardia which necessitate drug treatment; for some, an opportunity to withdraw from work and rest for a short period may be required. Symptomatic bradycardia is usually treated by permanent cardiac pacing.

Uncontrolled high blood pressure carries the risk of sudden disabling illness (e.g., stroke), yet may be silent until the onset of catastrophe. Screening for hypertension by occupational health staff is to be encouraged. Some antihypertensive drugs may provoke a tendency to faintness, but most nowadays are safe.

Peripheral vascular disease may cause intermittent claudication which limits the victim's mobility. Medical treatment is relatively unsatisfactory, although surgical treatment may be very successful. The prognosis depends upon any associated coronary disease. The presence of an aortic aneurysm also indicates arterial disease and a liability to vascular catastrophe.

These groups of patients should be carefully assessed, both clinically and by non-invasive investigations, with particular attention being paid to the likelihood of cardiac involvement. Raynaud's phenomenon, on the other hand, is a benign, albeit distressing, complaint. Underlying disorders, e.g., collagen disease, should be excluded; vibrational trauma from work with chain-saws or pneumatic hammer devices, must be avoided. Sufferers should work in a warm environment and be allowed to wear gloves and heated socks if indicated.

## Special work problems and restrictions

For most forms of heart disease the general rule is that activities causing no undue symptoms can be undertaken safely. Artificial restrictions are, therefore, unnecessary.

Most problems with work occur in patients with coronary heart disease. Not everyone will be able to go back to their own work after a coronary event. In light engineering it has been observed that after one year about half those returning were fully fit, requiring no job change.[4] The remainder had some limitation of fitness; half required a job change. About one-tenth of all those returning to work had severe limitations of fitness requiring a change of work. Work responding to emergency calls may place unacceptable demands on the cardiovascular system and such duties should be avoided. Heavy physical work, the need to climb up and down stairs, rapid and tight pacing of repetitive operations, such as component assembly, technical skill, and the stress of responsibility will all be relevant.

In most situations a full working day must be managed from the day of restarting. Tiredness which will often be more burdensome initially usually resolves over the subsequent days or weeks. It may be helpful to arrange temporary shorter hours, perhaps curtailing both ends of the day, so as to avoid rush-hour travelling. This recommendation can usually be accomplished by a defined time through which the hours can be extended towards the full working day. By defining this time period, the perceived stress on colleagues and working arrangements is notably less than leaving the period open-ended.

The stress of managing or supervising may be significant and consideration will need to be given to the time necessary to catch up with events that the employee will have missed while being away, and to allow a gradual resumption of responsibilities. Consideration should be given to the requirements for overtime, meetings that occur early or late in the day, and the managerial responsibility that may be exercised. For all these, shortening the hours of work temporarily signals to the organization that the employee is not yet fully recovered, and perhaps encourages those who have been managing in the employee's absence to continue to do so for a further period of time.

Psychological stress may arise from a variety of circumstances peculiar to the patient, his relatives, friends (and others), or his particular working circumstances. These factors are usually the source of discouragement and may delay recovery. In the present climate of employment many individuals will take the opportunity to cease work and hope to obtain favourable financial terms; many will be disappointed.

In some jobs sudden collapse would be disastrous and the likelihood of a further sudden illness such as a ventricular arrhythmia needs careful assessment. Airline pilots, mainline train drivers, and those at sea in merchant shipping, are rarely allowed to resume their employment following a myocardial infarction. The same applies to policemen, fire brigade officers, and others on active duty. Formerly, vocational drivers, i.e., those holding large goods vehicle (LGV) and passenger carrying vehicle (PCV) licences, rarely regained their licences following the development of heart disease and then only after extensive testing including angiography.

This situation has now changed, partly because recent data from other European countries which have not had the UK restrictions, have shown that the risk of sudden collapse at the wheel as a result of cardiovascular disease is an extremely rare cause of road accidents. The rate of all medical events at the wheel was 4 per 1000 serious accidents and most of these were due to other illnesses, e.g., epilepsy. The other reason for the change has been the growing body of evidence which indicates that exercise testing has good predictive value so that those at low risk of cardiovascular collapse can be identified by a combination of clinical factors and treadmill testing as outlined in the Annex to this chapter.

There is a further problem with this sort of regulatory medicine. Those at high risk of collapse can be identified once their disease has declared itself. But silent coronary disease is extremely common and most cardiac events occur in those who appear to be fit. Many cardiac events in vocational drivers, as in others, cannot therefore be predicted. One solution to this problem is to attempt to screen employees for 'silent' myocardial ischaemia.

Screening may be justifiable in certain groups of individuals and has been adopted by the US Air Force for example. The usual screening measures are a clinical examination and an exercise test. Experience has shown that exercise induced electrocardiographic ST segment change in an asymptomatic individual is common and has a variety of causes; only about one-third will turn out to have coronary disease on angiography.[11] Screening for asymptomatic CHD in this way cannot therefore be routinely recommended because of the high incidence of false positive results. Simple clinical features such as age, male sex, history of chest pain, smoking habit, or a strong family history of premature CHD, are a better method of assessing apparently asymptomatic individuals. If there is a strong clinical suspicion of CHD and a certain diagnosis is essential, then coronary angiography should be undertaken. This policy, however, would only be justifiable in those with very high-risk occupations. In the past, myocardial perfusion imaging using thallium has been recommended for this group of individuals, but the improved safety and ease of coronary angiography, coupled with the significant number of inconclusive results from myocardial scintigraphy,[12] means that angiography is preferable.

The weights to be lifted regularly in manufacturing industries have tended to reduce in recent years and can usefully be considered on the scale indicated by the US Department of Labor 1981.[13] (See also Chapter 1, p. 16). Only the very fit and confident might reasonably attempt heavy work, such as lifting 50–100 lb (23–45 kg). Many employees may manage quite comfortably medium work, such as lifting 25–50 lb (11–23 kg) perhaps at the rate of one a minute, providing they do not have any other physical limitations. The presence of support for the weights and keeping them at waist height, eases the strain considerably and if the task only requires the weights to be slid along benches or roller tracks, then the strain can be considered to be reduced by some 50 per cent. Those with moderate to severe restriction may need to be confined to a maximum of 10 pounds (4.5 kg) or an equivalent degree of force on levers, turning wheels, and similar machine controls. In any work organization there may be a few jobs requiring light-weight detailed work or simple checking which are suitable for those who are quite severely disabled. Some patients have sufficient skills to learn inspection tasks which may be physically much less stressful.

Other opportunities may be found in material and production control, progress chasing, recording, indexing, etc., which may allow continued work in basically fairly heavy industries. Exercise requirements well above normal, such as foundries and forges, may well be reasons for debarring the employment of patients with or without shortness of breath or angina.

Rapid and tightly controlled pacing of work such as on assembly lines has not been shown to be a precipitating factor for myocardial infarction and should not inhibit a normal return to work after a heart attack. If employees were managing satisfactorily before their infarction they may well manage afterwards, if they are not severely disabled by shortness of breath or angina. Returning to their own work, where social support is provided by former rather than new colleagues, may be less of a problem then trying a new task.

Similar arrangements apply to shiftwork and to the permanent requirement of those in supervisory and management work to cope with responsibility. If all has been well before the illness, returning to the same job may be the least stressful option. Permanent night-working can be easier if it has been managed well previously. At night, organizations tend to function more routinely with less interference from peripheral parts of the organization. The co-operation amongst members of a team may well be higher and productivity can appear better. Those who have shortness of breath or angina find it an advantage to be able to rise from their bed during the day when the weather may be warm, or at least the house warm, to have some contact with their family and to travel to and from work in quieter times than their day-shift colleagues. New work can bring new situations, different personalities, different tasks and different sorts of components, all of which can be difficult to cope with even without the presence of heart disease. But working reduced hours on a temporary basis may be all that is required.

## Toxic substances

Work involving exposure to certain hazardous substances may aggravate pre-existing coronary heart disease and careful consideration should be given to patients who are returning to jobs involving exposure to chemical vapours and fumes. Methylene chloride, a main ingredient of many commonly used paint removers, is rapidly metabolized to carbon monoxide in the body and in poorly ventilated work areas, blood levels of carboxyhaemoglobin can become elevated enough to precipitate angina or even myocardial infarction. A blood carboxyhaemoglobin level of 2–4 per cent has been shown to be associated with impairment of cardiovascular function in patients with angina pectoris. The World Health Organization[14] recommends a maximum carboxyhaemoglobin level of 5 per cent for healthy industrial workers and a maximum of 2.5 per cent for susceptible persons in the general population exposed to ambient air pollution; this level may also be applied to workers whose jobs entail specific exposure to carbon monoxide, e.g., car park attendants, furnace workers, etc. There is a good correlation between carbon monoxide levels in the air with blood carboxyhaemoglobin, in accordance with the Coburn equation, and the WHO guideline level of 2.5 per cent implies an 8 hour occupational exposure average, well below the current occupational exposure standard of 50 ppm. In fact, to ensure that the 2.5 per cent carboxyhaemoglobin level is not exceeded, the ambient carbon monoxide concentration should not be higher than 10 ppm over an 8 hour working day: equivalent to exposure to the current occupational exposure standard (50 ppm) for no more than 30 minutes.

Occupational exposure to carbon disulphide in the viscose rayon manufacturing industry is a recognized causal factor of coronary heart disease but the mechanism remains unclear. Reports of sudden death from angina are well recognized in dynamite workers, particularly after a period of 36–72 hours away from work and following re-exposure, an effect almost certainly related to direct action of nitroglycerine on the blood vessels of the heart or peripheral circulation. Persons with clinical evidence of coronary heart disease should avoid occupational exposure to these substances.

Solvents, such as trichloroethylene or 1,1,1-trichloroethane, may sensitize the myocardium to the action of endogenous catecholamines resulting in ventricular fibrillation and sudden death in workers receiving heavy exposure in poorly ventilated workplaces.[15] Chlorofluorocarbons (CFCs) are still widely used as propellants in aerosol cans and as refrigerants—CFC-113 has been implicated in sudden cardiac deaths and CFC-22 has been reported to cause arrhythmias in laboratory workers using an aerosol preparation. Certain industrial workers will need proper assessment of their workplace by an occupational physician with an occupational hygienist, so that they can be advised on their suitability for work handling chlorinated hydrocarbon solvents or involving exposure to gases.

There are no formal medical requirements for workers who have to enter confined spaces where there may be hazards of oxygen deficiency or a build up of toxic gases. Persons with heart disease or severe hypertension may need to be excluded. Certain occupations may require the use of special breathing apparatus either routinely (e.g., asbestos removal workers), or in emergencies (e.g., water workers handling chlorine cylinders). The additional cardiorespiratory effort required whilst wearing a respirator, combined with the general physical exertion that may be required, usually means that persons with a previous history of coronary heart disease are excluded from such work.

### Hot conditions

Working in hot conditions may prove difficult for some patients with heart disease. High ambient temperatures or significant heat radiation from hot surfaces or liquid metal, added to the physical strain of heavy work, will produce quite profound vasodilatation of muscle and skin vessels. Compensatory vascular and cardiac reactions to maintain central blood pressure may be inadequate and lead to reduced cerebral or coronary artery blood flow. The resulting weakness or giddiness could prove dangerous.

### Travel

Following a cardiac event such as myocardial infarction, individuals should convalesce at home and not travel and should then be assessed by their physician at 4–6 weeks. Those with no evidence of continuing myocardial ischaemia or pump failure can then travel freely within the United Kingdom for pleasure, e.g., holiday. Business and overseas travel is more problematical because the physical and psychological demands are greater. Additional difficulties for the overseas traveller include the uncertain provision of coronary care facilities in some countries and the justifiable reluctance of insurance companies to provide health cover. Such travel is best deferred until three months have elapsed and any necessary further investigations and treatment have been carried out to ensure cardiovascular fitness.

Overseas travel for those with continuing cardiovascular unfitness need not be ruled out. Utilizing the airport services for disabled travellers can ease a passenger through customs, passport control, etc., at major airports like Heathrow. Modern aircraft can be very comfortable. The cabins are kept at a pressure equivalent to 6000 feet (2000 metres) so that those with angina are not likely to experience an attack; and all developed countries have a coronary care service which is often better than that in the United Kingdom. Businessmen with continuing cardiac disorders may therefore fly to Europe and North America with very little risk. But flights in unpressurised aircraft, work in undeveloped countries or in remote areas of the world, and work in a hostile environment (both climatic and political) is best avoided.

Cardiac deaths are uncommon in trekkers or workers at high altitude (8000–15 000 ft—2440–4570 m.). The increase in cardiac output at altitude will exacerbate symptoms in those who already experience symptoms at sea level, but asymptomatic individuals with coronary heart disease are unlikely to be at special risk.

Ordinary driving may be resumed after one month provided that the driver does not suffer from angina which may be provoked at the wheel. Vocational driving may be permitted at three months, subject to a satisfactory outcome from non-invasive testing (see the Annex). Ordinary driving licence holders do not need to notify the DVLA, Swansea if they have made a good recovery and have no continuing disability, but vocational drivers must notify the DVLA. Insurance companies vary in their requirements but most policies are temporarily invalidated by illness.

## Implanted cardiac pacemakers devices

The presence of an implanted pacemaker device to maintain regular heart action is entirely compatible with normal or even strenuous exercise. The underlying heart condition for which the pacemaker was implanted may, however, impose its own restrictions. If the heart is otherwise healthy, then it is reasonable for strength and endurance to be explored gradually and for activity to be progressively increased. Effort tolerance is more likely to be maintained in patients fully dependent on pacing if they have a generator that preserves atrioventricular synchrony. Pacemakers are generally implanted by physicians using local anaesthesia. Recovery is rapid. Modern pacemakers are very reliable and long-lasting. All pacemaker patients remain under the care of a cardiac centre and are generally reviewed at annual intervals. Depending upon usage a pacemaker generator may need to be replaced after about 10 years.

The indications for cardiac pacing are widening as the efficacy of this form of treatment improves; some paroxysmal tachycardias can be controlled by pacemaker therapy and automatic implantable defibrillators are now available, although at present they are relatively expensive and, in the United Kingdom, few have been implanted. Modern pacemaker technology allows pacing of atria and ventricles, variation in the output of the generator, facilities for telemetry, etc.

Virtually all pacemakers have the capacity to sense and be inhibited by the patient's own heart rhythm. Somatic muscle action potentials, e.g., pectoralis major, can occasionally interfere with the pacemaker, causing temporary cessation of pacing which may induce faintness. Usually the interference will be brief and the pacemaker will revert to a fixed-rate mode which will prevent symptoms.

In theory, cardiac pacemakers are vulnerable to extraneous electrical interference but in practice most pacemakers have good discrimination. Industrial electrical sources such as arc welding, faulty domestic equipment, engines, anti-theft devices, airport weapon detectors, radar and citizen-band radio, can all potentially affect pacemakers but, in general, the patient has to be very close to the power source before any interference can be demonstrated, and the pacemaker abnormality is confined to one or two missed beats or reversion to the fixed mode. The number of documented cases of interference in the United Kingdom is less than three a year.[16,17]

If pacemaker patients are expected to work in the vicinity of high-energy electric or magnetic fields capable of producing signals at a rate and pattern similar to a QRS complex (e.g., on some electrical generating and transmission equipment and welding) then formal testing is recommended. The cardiac centre responsible for implanting the pacemaker will usually provide a technical service for this purpose, thus enabling the risk of interference to be defined precisely. Nuclear magnetic resonance (NMR) imaging machines may be found in certain chemical laboratories and hospital radiological departments. Patients with pacemakers should not be subjected to NMR imaging. Persons with pacemakers are generally advised to avoid work which may bring them into close contact with strong magnetic fields. If a pacemaker patient should experience untoward symptoms while near electrical apparatus then he should move away. In the event of collapse the patient should be moved but other causes for the collapse should also be sought. Pacemaker patients carry cards which identify the type of pacemaker, the supervising cardiac centre, etc. Further advice is readily available from the British Pacing and Electrophysiology Group (see Appendix 9 for the address).

Other implanted devices include antitachycardia pacemakers and the automatic implantable cardioverter defibrillator (AICD). The latter is gaining popularity because it is indicated for those patients with heart disease who have experienced ventricular fibrillation and for whom other treatments are ineffective. Patients with AICDs commonly have severe underlying heart disease and may well not be able to work. But if they can work then this should be in a safe environment because the AICD takes 20 seconds or so to charge and during that time the patient may lose consciousness.

## Cardiac surgery

Replacement of the aortic and mitral valves by mechanical or biological prostheses is a common and safe procedure. Patients generally recover rapidly and resume work fully 2 to 3 months after the operation. Those with mechanical valves need to take anticoagulants indefinitely and are thus at slightly increased risk from bleeding. (See also Chapter 19, p. 367) Sudden failure of mechanical valves is extremely uncommon. Some biological valves undergo slow deterioration some years after implantation.

Coronary artery bypass grafting also allows most patients with ischaemic heart disease to resume work within 2 to 3 months of surgery. Most patients are relieved of their angina and for many the prognosis is improved. Patients who are able to work before surgery should generally be able to work afterwards, and restrictions that may have been appropriate previously should no longer be relevant. Similarly, many who could not work before surgery because of their disability should be able to do so afterwards. Unfortunately, surgery constitutes a rather dramatic event that may prompt over-protective attitudes amongst family members, friends, employers, or even medical advisers. Many individuals who could and should return to work fail to do so for this reason rather than because of continuing incapacity. No special restrictions are usually necessary after return to work.

Coronary graft stenosis and occlusion, however, leads to recurrence of angina at a rate of about 4 per cent per annum. This is seldom severe but may affect long-term occupational planning. The criteria for fitness to resume vocational driving after coronary artery bypass grafting are set out in the Annex.

Cardiac transplantation may allow dramatic improvement in working capacity but recipients do have to be maintained on immunosuppressants and other drugs. For advice about work the transplantation centre should be consulted.

## Other cardiac interventions

Coronary angioplasty is indicated for patients with angina and one or more localized coronary stenoses. The procedure is undertaken using local anaesthetic via the right femoral artery. The initial results are highly successful but about 2 per cent will be unsuccessful and need emergency bypass surgery. Groin haematomas are unusual. Patients usually return to work one week later. Angina recurs in about one-third of patients within the first three to four months due to re-stenosis. A second angioplasty carries very similar benefits and risks. Other percutaneous intracardiac procedures are proving increasingly successful. Balloon valvotomy is the treatment of choice for pulmonary stenosis and is indicated in some, generally younger, patients with mitral and aortic stenosis. Certain cardiac arrhythmias, viz., those that depend on an accessory conduction pathway, can be eliminated by radio frequency ablation using transvenous electrode catheters. These, and other therapeutic catheterization techniques, will undoubtedly gain more widespread acceptance. Hitherto, the numbers of patients are small and any employment problems should be referred to the patient's cardiologist.

## Hypertension

Untreated hypertension carries the risk of sudden disability from heart attack or stroke; discovery of this condition may require cessation of some employment where a serious accident risk exists. For controlled hypertension the risks must be carefully assessed in the context of the individual's work. When considering the need to continue in employment, well-controlled hypertension may be risk-free, especially if control is by diet only or with small doses of a mild diuretic. Control with more powerful drugs may carry the risk of side-effects, such as hypotension with resultant giddiness and fatigue, and limited effort tolerance. Central nervous system side-effects may affect judgement and the performance of skilled tasks. But modern antihypertensive therapy with beta-adrenergic and calcium antagonists, diuretics, and angiotensin-converting enzyme inhibitors is remarkably free from side-effects.

Patients with controlled hypertension can expect to manage most varieties of working activity. Frequent postural changes occasionally prove troublesome due to altered central and peripheral vascular responses. Very heavy physical work and exposure to very hot conditions with high humidity may result in postural hypotension. Such work should not be attempted if these ill-effects might prove dangerous either to health or because of the associated accidental risk. Provided blood pressure readings can be maintained under satisfactory control and are checked regularly, heavy goods and public service vehicle driving is allowed.

## Other circulatory problems

Postural hypotension and syncope occasionally trouble the young and fit and may also be recognized as a complication of neuropathy affecting autonomic nerves, as may occur occasionally in diabetes (see Chapter 12). The circumstances and frequency of postural hypotension would need to be assessed against job requirements and environment.

Cerebrovascular disease may produce disturbances of consciousness and other neurological effects (see Chapter 7).

Impaired circulation to the limbs will result in an increased risk of claudication, especially in cold and wet, risk of damage to skin (frost-bite), and poor recovery from accidental injury to skin and deeper structures (see Chapter 10, p. 200). Raynaud's phenomenon can be provoked by the use of vibrating tools and work processes that transmit vibration to the fingers. Common situations are the use of power-saws, pneumatic chisels, and rough grinding of metal objects. Clearly, those with symptoms should avoid such work.

Outdoor work and work in cold stores or cold test rooms (some with moving air increasing the chill factor) may prove unsafe if peripheral circulation is significantly restricted and may also provoke angina. The risk of frost-bite and gangrene would be high in cases where a serious circulatory restriction existed.

Cuts and bruises from accidental contact with furniture, machinery, etc., or from dropped objects, may not heal at all well in the presence of circulatory restriction, and there could be a risk of the onset of gangrene and the subsequent need for disabling operations. Limbs at risk need adequate protection continuously while at work.

Varicose veins of the legs present similar problems; accidental injury may lead to severe blood loss and protection is essential. Work routines involving standing still are difficult to cope with but some walking is helpful. Sitting for long uninterrupted periods may aggravate ankle swelling and, if the hip and knee are awkwardly flexed, there could be some risk of vascular thrombosis. (See also Chapter 10, p. 201)

## Conclusions and recommendations

The high incidence of coronary heart disease remains a major problem for the UK workforce. The technical advances of the past few decades have permitted greater accuracy of diagnosis, and hence prognosis. Improvements in treatment, medical and surgical, have allowed much higher expectations of recovery and ultimate fitness. Those with other heart conditions have shared in these improvements and expectations.

It is possible to give clear recommendations for patients returning to normal active life and work. These recommendations help not only patients and their doctors, but also employers, who should understand what is happening to their employees to be able to assist them in their return to work.

The possibility of sudden loss of consciousness through a cardiac arrhythmia represents the most difficult disability to accommodate, but improvements in workplace safety allow many people to be suitably employed.

Limitation of exercise tolerance may prevent patients managing their transport to and from work. For many, the work itself can be organized to avoid undue extra stress. Developments towards automation and robotic manufacturing promise to reduce the physical content of a day's work, perhaps improving the opportunities for continued working by those disabled with cardiac conditions.

ANNEX

**Cardiac Fitness for Vocational Driving**

*Revised guidance notes for drivers of Large Goods and Passenger Carrying Vehicles (LGV/PCV), and other professional drivers from the Secretary of State for Transport's Cardiovascular Advisory Panel.*

A person who has suffered or suffers from a disqualifying condition in Section A–H shown in **bold capitals**, and/or is within the recommended period of unfitness should be advised to notify DVLC and cease driving their vehicle. If able to meet the qualifying conditions in the relevant (re)licensing section(s) an application usually will be successful and the driver permitted continued entitlement to drive. If unable to meet the qualifying conditions in the (re)licensing sections the licence with be recommended to be refused or revoked.

*A.* **CORONARY HEART DISEASE**

(i)    Angina pectoris or heart failure (whether or not maintained symptom free by the use of medication.

(ii)   Within 3 months of:
       Myocardial infarction or any episode of unstable angina.
       Successful coronary artery bypass grafting
       Successful coronary angioplasty.

(Re)licensing normally will be permitted 3 or more months after successful rehabilitation following the events in (ii) above, if there are no other disqualifying conditions, provided the applicant or driver can complete safely at least the first 3 stages of the standard Bruce treadmill protocol or equivalent, off cardioactive treatment for 24 hours and during the test remains free of symptoms and signs of cardiac dysfunction. The licence normally will be **refused** if he develops pathological ST segment shift during or after the test, fails to achieve or maintain a rise in systolic blood pressure, develops sustained ventricular tachycardia or other malignant arrhythmia or develops symptoms attributable to peripheral vascular disease which limits the investigation.

If the identity of the chest pain is in doubt an exercise test should be carried out as above. Those with a locomotor disorder who cannot comply should notify DVLA.

**Coronary Angiography is not required**. If it has been undertaken, the Licensing Authority will be recommended to refuse the application or revoke the licence if it demonstrates:

(i)    Impaired left ventricular function, i.e., an ejection fraction < 40% or,

(ii)   Significant (i.e., > than or −30% reduction in intraluminal diameter) occlusive disease in the left main coronary artery, or significant (i.e., > than or −50% reduction in intraluminal diameter) occlusive disease in the proximal part of the left anterior descending artery, i.e., proximal to the origin of the first septal and diagonal branches, or in two or more major coronary arteries.

## B.  DISEASES OF OTHER ARTERIES

(i)  Confirmed peripheral vascular disease (including aortic aneurysm, with a transverse diameter of 5 cm or more, either thoracic or abdominal) with clinical evidence of myocardial ischaemia.

(ii)  Dissection of the aorta.

(Re)licensing normally will be permitted in (i) above if there has been satisfactory surgical repair of the aneurysm, provided there are no other disqualifying conditions, and no clinical evidence of myocardial ischaemia. Patients with peripheral vascular disease without clinical evidence of myocardial ischaemia will be (re)licensed, provided there are no other disqualifying conditions.

### *Licence duration: Requirement for periodic review*

An applicant or driver who has been permitted to hold LGV or PCV entitlement with a history of coronary heart disease or other arterial disorder will normally be issued with an annual entitlement subject to satisfactory medical report(s). The driver should be assessed at least every 3 years or as recommended by the investigating physician, and should remain free from other disqualifying conditions.

## C.  HYPERTENSION

At the time of the examination for the licence or while the licence is held

(i)  The casual blood pressure is 200 mmHg systolic or over, or 110 mmHg diastolic or over, or

(ii)  With established hypertension, blood pressure readings consistently 180 mmHg systolic or over, or 100 mmHg diastolic or over.

(iii)  Medication causes symptoms which will affect driving ability.

(Re)licensing normally will be permitted provided the above conditions are not present, and there are no other disqualifying conditions.

## D.  ARRHYTHMIA

1. If within the past 5 years, any significant disturbance of cardiac rhythm has occurred, i.e., bradycardia due to atrioventricular block (including congenital heart block) or sinus node disease, or a supraventricular (including atrial flutter and fibrillation), junctional or ventricular tachyarrhythmia

(Re)licensing normally will be permitted on the basis of clinical opinion if:

(i)  The arrhythmia or its medication has **not** caused within the past 2 years or is **not** likely to cause sudden impairment of consciousness or distraction of attention during driving.

(ii)  There is no documented significant structural abnormality present on echocardiography.

(iii)  The exercise test is satisfactorily completed as in A above. (NB in this situation cardioactive treatment need *not* be discontinued).

**NB Ventricular premature beats** occurring singly or as couplets do not necessarily constitute a reason for revoking or refusing a licence unless any other disqualifying condition is present.

    2. A pacemaker has been implanted.

(Re)licensing normally will be permitted provided there is no other disqualifying condition, the pacemaker was inserted to prevent bradycardia and the person is symptom free and attends a pacemaker clinic at least annually. Annual review of the licence will be required.

    3. A cardioverter-defibrillator device has been implanted.

### E. ELECTROCARDIOGRAPHIC ABNORMALITY

The electrocardiogram shows pathological Q waves in three leads or more, or left bundle branch block (LBBB), (A pathological Q wave is defined as having a duration of 40 milliseconds or more and a depth of at least a third of the succeeding R wave).

    (Re)licensing normally will be permitted provided there are no other disqualifying conditions provided the exercise requirements in paragraph A are fulfilled. **Pre-excitation may be ignored unless associated with a history of arrhythmia**.

### F. VALVULAR HEART DISEASE

Acquired heart valve disease is present, with or without valve surgery.
(Re)licensing normally will be permitted provided within the past 5 years there is no history of cerebral ischaemia, no history of embolism, no persistent or intermittent arrhythmia, and no documented significant persisting hypertrophy or dilation of the left or right ventricle. Regular review may be required. (NB anticoagulant treatment does not constitute a bar to the holding of a licence.)

### G. CARDIOMYOPATHY

(i)    Established cardiomyopathy (i.e., dilated, hypertrophic or restrictive) or heart muscle disease

(ii)   Heart or heart/lung transplantation.

### H. CONGENITAL HEART DISORDERS

(Re)licensing normally will be permitted provided there are no other disqualifying conditions whether or not (reparative or palliative) surgery has been undertaken for mild pulmonary stenosis, atrial septal defect, small ventricular septal defect, bicuspid aortic valve and mild aortic stenosis, patent ductus arteriosus, coarctation of the aorta with mild gradient and no systemic hypertension, and anomalous pulmonary venous drainage.

    Complex congenital heart disorders are likely to disqualify.

    Marfan's syndrome and allied disorders with aortic root dilatation normally will disqualify.

A complete list can be obtained from the DVLA Medical Branch (See Appendix 9 for the address).

## Selected references and further reading

1. Tunstall-Pedoe, H., Clayton, D., Morris, J.N., Brigden, W., and MacDonald, I. (1975). Coronary heart attack in East London. *Lancet*, **2**, 833–8.
2. Muller, J.E. *et al.* (1985). Circadian variation in the frequency of onset of myocardial infarction. *NEJM*, **313**, 1315–22.
3. Mittleman, M.A., Maclure, M., Tofler, G.H., Sherwood, J.B., Goldberg, R.J., and Muller, J.E. (1993). Triggering of acute myocardial infarction by heavy physical exertion. *NEJM*, **329**, 1677–83.
4. Nagle, R., Gangola, R., and Picton-Robinson, I. (1971). Factors influencing return to work after myocardial infarction. *Lancet*, **2**, 454–6.
5. Clark, D.B., Edwards, F.C., and Williams, W.G. (1983). Cardiac surgery and return to work in the West Midlands. In *Cardiac Rehabilitation*, pp. 61–70. Proceedings of the Society of Occupational Medicine Research Panel Symposium, London.
6. Royal College of General Practitioners (1986). *Morbidity statistics from general practice 1981–2*. Third National Study. HMSO, London.
7. Shaper, A.G., Cook, D.G., Walker, M., and Macfarlane, P.W. (1984). Prevalence of ischaemic heart disease in middle-aged British men. *Brit. Heart J.*, **51**, 595–605.
8. Rose, G., and Marmot, M.G. (1981). Social class and coronary heart disease. *Brit. Heart J.*, **45**, 13–9.
9. Cay, E.L. (1983). The influence of psychological problems in returning to work after a myocardial infarction. In *Cardiac rehabilitation*, pp. 42–60. Proceedings of the Society of Occupational Medicine Research Panel Symposium, London.
10. Friedman, M., Thorensen, C.E., and Gill, J.J. (1986). Alteration of type A behaviour and its effect on cardiac recurrence in post myocardial infarction patients. Summary results of the recurrent coronary prevention project. *Amer. Heart J.*, **112**, 653–5.
11. Froelicher, V.F. *et al.* (1977). Angiographic findings in asymptomatic aircrew with electrocardiographic abnormalities. *Amer. J. Cardiol.*, **39**, 31–8.
12. Schwartz, R.S., Jackson, W.G., Celio, P.V., Richardson, L.A., and Hickman, J.R. (1993). Accuracy of exercise Th[201] myocardial scintigraphy in asymptomatic young men. *Circulation*, **87**, 165–72.
13. US Department of Labor (1981). *Selected characteristics of occupations defined in the Dictionary of Occupational Titles*. US Government Printing Office, Washington DC.
14. WHO (World Health Organization). (1979). *Carbon monoxide*. Environmental health criteria, No. 13. WHO, Geneva.
15. Boon, N.A. (editorial) (1987). Solvent abuse of the heart. *Brit. Med. J.*, **294**: 722.
16. Gold, R.G. (1984). Interference to cardiac pacemakers—how often is it a problem? *Prescribers J.*, **24**, 115–23.
17. Sowton, E. (1982). Environmental hazards and pacemaker patients. *J. Roy. Coll. Phys.*, **16**, 159–64.

# 15

# Respiratory disorders

*D.A. Scarisbrick and D.J. Hendrick*

## Introduction

While an individual's skin presents a surface area of up to 2 square metres to the environment, the gas-exchanging membrane of the lungs is exposed to environmental insults over an interface some 100-fold greater. This makes the lungs uniquely vulnerable to environmentally induced diseases, and this is reflected in a wide variety of common respiratory ailments despite the presence of formidable defence mechanisms. Respiratory diseases may consequently pose many special problems at work, and these will differ according to the nature of the disorder and the nature of the workplace.

## Prevalence

Prevalence of a disease is the proportion of a given population which is affected at a given time. It is usually expressed per 100 000 population, but with diseases of high prevalence, such as asthma, percentages may be more useful. Its numerical value depends on the incidence of the disease (the rate at which new cases occur), its natural history (whether it resolves or persists), and its effect on survival. Thus, diseases of low incidence may still show high prevalence if they persist and do not reduce life-expectancy. This has been true of pneumoconiosis in many mining communities, and it is broadly true of asthma. Conversely, lung cancer occurs with high incidence in heavy smokers aged over 50 years, but it quickly resolves (if there is successful surgery) or it leads rapidly to death. Its prevalence among the same population at any particular time is therefore much less remarkable.

In Britain, respiratory diseases account for 14 per cent of working days lost through ill health by employed men (about 38 million annually) and for 11 per cent lost by employed women (about 5 million annually). 'Influenza' accounts for 4 million (9 per cent) of these days, although for about 44 per cent of the total number of spells of respiratory sickness.[1] The discrepancy is attributable to the relatively short periods (4–6 days) associated with influenza. Most lost days are attributable to emphysema, chronic bronchitis, and asthma. In the 16–64-year-old working population, respiratory diseases account for 18 per cent of general practitioner consultations, and 10 per cent of all hospital admissions.

They also account for 10 per cent (82 000) of the men and 5 per cent (7000) of the women aged 16–64 years who receive invalidity benefit because they are too disabled to work. Approximately 63 000 individuals of working age die annually because of respiratory diseases.

The SWORD (Surveillance of Work-related and Occupational Respiratory Disease) project has been set up in an attempt to produce an informal national register of the incidence of work-related respiratory disease. The project has shown that, currently, the most commonly observed occupationally induced lung disease in Britain is asthma, accounting for 25–30 per cent of the 2000 annual reports.[2] This is the consequence of exposures to many different causative agents. By contrast, asbestos alone continues to cause a variety of different respiratory diseases (benign pleural disease, mesothelioma, asbestosis, lung cancer), and these together account for 45–50 per cent of SWORD reports. Thus, the majority of currently recognized occupational respiratory problems are related to either asthma or asbestos. Inhalation accidents, building-related disorders (e.g,. sick building syndrome and humidifier fever), infectious diseases, and extrinsic allergic alveolitis together account for about 20 per cent, i.e., for all but 5–10 per cent of the remainder.

## Clinical aspects affecting work capacity[3]

### Lung function

The chief function of the respiratory system, exchange of oxygen and carbon dioxide, takes place in the parenchyma of the lung—the huge 'sponge' of air spaces, known as alveoli, where air and blood are separated only by the thin alveolar–capillary membrane. For gas exchange to occur, air must pass freely through the many branching airways between the trachea and the lung parenchyma. This to-and-fro movement constitutes ventilation, and its effectiveness can be assessed by specific tests of ventilatory function. These can be usefully distinguished from tests of parenchymal function which assess the effectiveness of oxygen absorption from air in the alveolar space to blood in the capillaries.

Ventilatory function is most readily assessed with a spirometer, which records simultaneously the volume of air expired and the time elapsing during a full forced expiratory manoeuvre (Fig. 15.1). The forced expiratory volume in the first second ($FEV_1$) reflects speed of airflow, and the forced vital capacity (FVC) quantifies the total volume change from full inspiration to full expiration. These measurements are highly dependent on age, height, and sex, and they are usually expressed as a percentage of a predicted (i.e., normal) value obtained from reference tables. There is still a wide range of normal variability when account is taken of these factors, and some caution must be used in interpreting a single slightly low value. Serial measurements of ventilatory function over a period of

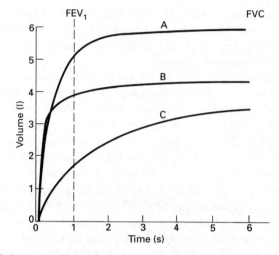

**Fig. 15.1** Spirograms illustrating obstructive and restrictive patterns of abnormal ventilation. A, normal spirogram; B, restrictive defect; C, obstructive defect.

time are more useful in assessing the significance of slightly low values and they are invaluable in recognizing excessive longitudinal decline. $FEV_1$ normally declines by some 10–30 ml/yr from the time when lung growth ceases in the mid-20s.

Two main patterns of ventilatory abnormality can be identified from spirometric recordings—obstructive and restrictive (Fig. 15.1). Obstruction occurs in asthma and emphysema and is characterized by reduced expiratory flow. $FEV_1$ is diminished more than FVC, giving a characteristic and diagnostic low $FEV_1/FVC$ ratio.

The restrictive pattern of ventilatory impairment is a consequence of failure to inflate the lungs fully, and this causes an overall reduction in lung volume. Such impairment occurs with diffuse inflammatory and fibrotic diseases of the lung parenchyma such as fibrosing alveolitis, extrinsic allergic alveolitis, and asbestosis. These increase the stiffness of the lungs and limit inflation without impairing expiratory flow rates. Pleural disease, chest wall deformities and certain muscle and diaphragm disorders may cause a similar effect. The FVC is consequently reduced, but the $FEV_1/FVC$ ratio remains normal or even increases.

The peak expiratory flow rate (PEFR), can be measured with simpler and cheaper peak flow devices but is much less informative. As with spirometry, measurements require a maximal forced expiration made from full inspiration. Serial measurements of PEFR can be very useful in detecting changing ventilatory function, particularly the variable obstructive defect of asthma and the work-related changes typical of occupational asthma.

Parenchymal function is best assessed by measurement of the gas transfer factor of the lung for carbon monoxide (TLCO). It measures the ability of the lungs to absorb carbon monoxide (and by inference oxygen) from a single breath-hold. The carbon monoxide absorption rate per unit volume of ventilated lung (TLCO divided by alveolar volume) is known as the gas transfer coefficient (KCO) and provides a useful measure of parenchymal function when TLCO is reduced simply as a consequence of diminished lung volume.

The degree of impairment of lung function is only one of a number of factors which determine work capacity. Psychological factors, such as motivation and mood are also important. With mild degrees of impairment (e.g., $FEV_1 > 60$ per cent predicted), the results of lung function tests correlate poorly with symptoms and the results of exercise tests. However, symptoms become inevitable with greater degrees of impairment. Most subjects with $FEV_1$ in the range 40–60 per cent of predicted have symptoms on strenuous exertion, and with an $FEV_1$ of less than 40 per cent of predicted heavy manual work becomes very difficult to sustain.

Chest radiographs are used widely in the surveillance of workers exposed to potentially fibrogenic dusts, e.g., coal, silica, and asbestos. Clinically important exposures to these agents should no longer occur, but radiographs are nevertheless invaluable in monitoring the effectiveness of dust-control measures (the proof of effective prevention is the absence of disease). They can also provide useful diagnostic information in suspected cases of lung cancer, asbestos-induced pleural disease, mesotheliomas, and a number of other focal lung diseases. The possible benefit of using chest radiographs to screen asymptomatic subjects for lung cancer does not justify the cost nor the radiation risk. The position is similar for tuberculosis. The prevalence has declined so much in Britain that radiographic screening of asymptomatic subjects without recent close contact is no longer cost-effective.

Modern imaging techniques have shown plain radiographs to be relatively insensitive in recognizing the early signs of many lung diseases, but cost (and the radiation involved) make more sensitive techniques, such as computerized tomography, unsuitable for surveillance purposes.

## Specific clinical problems

### Influenza

Acute upper respiratory tract infections with fever and aches and pains are common and are often called 'flu'. These episodes are usually self-limiting with recovery in less than a week. Their importance lies in their ubiquity and therefore the volume of sickness absence they generate.

True influenza is a more serious illness and absences of up to two weeks can be expected. The disease is highly infectious during the first two days and tends to occur in epidemics. These can be predicted by public health surveillance services (e.g., the Public Health Laboratory Service in Britain).

Influenza may be complicated in previously healthy subjects by tracheobronchitis or pneumonia (viral or bacterial), and in such cases recovery may be delayed and longer periods of sickness absence may result. However, full recovery can be expected and there is unlikely to be any lasting impairment of function preventing the employee returning to his or her occupation.

Influenza may cause serious exacerbations in subjects with pre-existing lung disease such as asthma, chronic bronchitis, and emphysema. In these cases it is important that adequate convalescence is allowed before a return to work is attempted. Prophylaxis with influenza vaccines is particularly desirable in these groups and may be useful in some occupational groups at high risk (e.g., health care workers, teachers, and child care workers) and in small closed communities (e.g., offshore oil rigs). Its benefit in other situations is uncertain.

## Pneumonia

Community acquired acute bacterial pneumonia is most commonly caused by *Streptococcus pneumoniae*. Those affected are often house-bound for one to two weeks. Full fitness might not be regained for up to six weeks—or longer if there are complications such as a lung abscess or an empyema. Pneumonia with the same clinical picture but caused by *Legionella pneumophila* is often acquired from hot water systems, forced draught cooling towers or air conditioning systems. Clustering of cases (which may involve occupational populations) should help identify the source.

In previously healthy subjects full recovery from pneumonia is likely but an adequate period of convalescence should be allowed before permitting a return to work.

## Tuberculosis

Pulmonary tuberculosis is the most common chronic respiratory infection in Britain with 4000–4500 new cases annually. About half of these infections occur in people of working age. The disease remains an important cause of morbidity and even mortality when diagnosis is delayed or patients are poorly compliant with treatment. It usually presents non-specifically with weight loss, fever, sweats, cough, and breathlessness. In most cases it is not highly infectious and two weeks treatment using modern antituberculosis chemotherapy generally renders the affected individual non-infectious, although cure requires regular treatment for at least 6 months.

It is not usually necessary to restrict the work of individuals under treatment for tuberculosis once the initial 2–3 weeks of chemotherapy have been completed. When health care workers are in contact with particularly vulnerable groups, such as immunosuppressed patients or young children, however, it is desirable to show that the sputum is sterile on culture before a return to work is approved. The management of health care workers with active pulmonary tuberculosis requires collaboration between the chest physician, the occupational physician, and management.

Health care workers are at increased risk of contracting tuberculosis, especially in areas receiving large numbers of immigrants from the Indian subcontinent. The excess risks are not great and are largely confined to those who work in pathology departments, chest clinics, or AIDS units. For such workers appropriate screening and surveillance programmes should be provided through occupational health services to minimize the risk, and BCG vaccinations may be offered when appropriate.

The rate of decline in the prevalence of tuberculosis has slowed in recent years and this has been partly attributed to the increase in prevalence of HIV infection. Not only has pulmonary tuberculosis become common in patients with AIDS, but their contacts with individuals without HIV infection has increased the reservoir of tuberculous infection in the population at large. This has become a problem of great importance in Africa, and is also emerging as a major public health issue in industrialized countries. (See also Chapter 22.)

## Asthma

Asthma is a disease which affects about 5 per cent of the adult population. It is characterized by episodes of airways obstruction and by undue responsiveness of the airways to a variety of non-specific stimuli, such as exercise, cold air, dust, smoky atmospheres, emotion, and diurnal body rhythms. In sensitized subjects common allergens may also be relevant. These stimuli trigger bronchoconstriction and the symptoms of intermittent wheeze, chest tightness, cough, and breathlessness.

Ventilatory function measurements are often entirely normal between attacks and a single normal value cannot be used to exclude the diagnosis. Conversely, after many years of activity asthma may be associated with obstruction which is very poorly reversible,i.e., is fixed and indistinguishable from other causes of chronic airways obstruction.

Because of the wide range of asthmatic activity occurring in the general population, it is rarely sensible to make a decision on fitness for work solely on the basis of the diagnosis alone. The large number of eminent and successful sportsmen with asthma is testimony to this. Decisions are more appropriately made from an estimate of its severity. This can be judged from symptoms, spirometry, PEFR monitoring, and even measurements of airway responsiveness using histamine or methacholine tests.

The asthmatic worker might experience difficulties at work in dusty or smoky atmospheres, when there are exposures to extremes of temperature, or when sudden strenuous exercise is called for. These responses are largely predictable from an assessment of the day-to-day severity. Occasional episodes are usually well tolerated or are easily treated with inhaled bronchodilators. Problems might arise if an inhaler is not available or cannot be used, for example because a respirator is being worn. Shiftwork should pose no major problem because circadian rhythms depend on sleeping patterns rather than time of day, although some workers may have difficulty adapting to rapidly changing shift rotas.

## Occupational asthma[4]

Approximately one-third of all cases of asthma arise for the first time in adult life, when it is important to consider whether it might have been caused by hypersensitivity to an inhaled agent at work. Some 400 causative agents have been described and as new ones continue to be reported almost monthly, virtually no environment can be assumed to be entirely risk-free. The most important causes in the U.K. in recent years are listed in Table 15.1.

Early recognition followed by quick cessation of exposure is important because continuing exposure over a year or so often results in persisting active asthma irrespective of continued exposure. The recognition that a new case of asthma is occupational in origin is not always easy, however. Indeed, the problem often presents at a stage when the diagnosis of asthma itself is not clear, and repeated respiratory tract infections are suspected. Work involving exposure to dust, fumes, or low temperatures often causes wheezing in asthmatic individuals irrespective of whether or not the asthma is occupational in origin, and these non-specific reactions should not be allowed to confuse a diagnosis of occupational asthma. Features which point to specific hypersensitivity and hence to true occupational asthma are summarized in Table 15.2. PEFR measurements showing improvements at weekends or on holidays are useful pointers to the diagnosis.

A diagnosis of occupational asthma has important implications for the livelihood of the affected worker and, perhaps, the economic viability of the industrial process. In 1993, Gannon and co-workers[5] reported that while removal from exposure after diagnosis of occupational asthma led to improved symptoms and lung function, there was appreciable loss of income for the average affected worker. The diagnosis should not be made lightly and referral to a special centre is often necessary, particularly if inhalation challenge testing with the suspected asthmagenic agent is contemplated. Such a centre may also be able to organize serial measurements of airway responsiveness. These may be invaluable in suggesting a causal relationship between worsening asthma and periods at work.

When there is a high risk of occupational asthma, surveillance programmes are now mandatory in the U.K. under the Control of Substances Hazardous to Health (COSHH) Regulations. Symptoms, use of medication, and medical diagnoses should be recorded before employment and at regular intervals thereafter, particularly symptoms which appear to be work-related. Questionnaire data should be interpreted with some caution as the symptoms of mild asthma are

**Table 15.1**  Major causes of occupational asthma

| | |
|---|---|
| *Animal* | Arachnids (storage mites*) |
| | Crustaceans (crabs, prawns) |
| | Laboratory insects* and rodents* |
| | Pancreatic extracts |
| | |
| *Vegetable* | Beans (castor*, green coffee, soy*) |
| | Colophony (soldering flux)* |
| | Flour/grain dust* |
| | Ispaghula (psyllium)* |
| | Papain* |
| | Wood dusts* |
| | Tea dust* |
| | |
| *Microbial* | Proteolytic enzymes* |
| | Mixed organisms (humidifiers, oil mists) |
| | |
| *Pharmaceutical* | Antibiotics* |
| | Cimetidine* |
| | Cephalosporins* |
| | Ipecacuanha* |
| | Methyl dopa |
| | |
| *Chemical* | Aluminium smelting |
| | Azodicarbonamide* |
| | Isocyanates* |
| | Epoxy resin hardeners (acid anhydrides*, certain amines*) |
| | Glutaraldehyde* |
| | Formaldehyde |
| | Nickel |
| | Persulphates (hairdressers)* |
| | Platinum salts* |
| | Reactive dyes* |
| | Fumes from stainless-steel welding* |

* Prescribed agents for compensation in Britain. In addition occupational asthma shown to be attributable to any respiratory sensitizer is a prescribed disease.

often non-specific. Limited reassurance should be taken from normal spirometric measurements, and measurement of airway responsiveness may be needed if an at-risk worker reports suspicious symptoms but has normal spirometry.

Consideration also has to be given to excluding asthmatics from occupations where there is a recognized risk of occupational asthma. There is little evidence that those with pre-existing mild asthma or a history of asthma as a child are

**Table 15.2**    Recognition of occupational asthma

---

1.   Onset (or appreciable worsening) of symptoms after commencing current job.

2.   Improvement during weekends or holidays; and corresponding worsening on return to work.

3.   Exacerbations with accidental heavy exposures.

4.   Presence of a recognized asthma inducer in the workplace; or other respirable dusts, fumes, gases, or mists, derived from organic matter or reactive chemicals.

5.   Suspicion that undue number of fellow workers are affected.

---

more likely to develop occupational asthma than others, although intuition suggests that this would be likely. The additional insult of occupational asthma on top of pre-existing non-occupational asthma might lead to disproportionate disability, but possibly the strongest argument for excluding asthmatics is that pre-existing asthma makes occupational asthma much more difficult to recognize if it does arise.

Atopy (the tendency to develop IgE-mediated allergic reactions) and asthma are closely associated in childhood but less so in adults, and atopy does not seem to be an important predisposing factor in the majority of cases of occupational asthma. There is little justification for excluding atopics from workplaces where there is a risk of occupational asthma, unless there is a strong history of allergy to a closely related agent, e.g., to domestic pets in those seeking to work with laboratory animals. Even in situations where atopy does pose some risk for occupational asthma (e.g., platinum refining), smoking is a more important risk factor and the arguments for excluding smokers from the workplace are much more compelling.

Once sensitization to a substance has taken place very low concentrations (even below the exposure control limit) may be sufficient to stimulate an asthmatic response. Therefore, sensitized workers may have to be redeployed to alternative work away from the offending substance, in order to avoid the risk of developing irreversibly impaired lung function, or even an acute life-threatening attack, following heavy accidental exposure.

## Chronic obstructive airways disease (COAD)[6]

The nomenclature of chronic obstructive diseases of the airways is a source of considerable confusion. The term COAD is most appropriately applied to irreversible airflow obstruction associated with cigarette smoking, but the term is also used more loosely to include chronic bronchitis. In the more restricted sense it is largely attributable to widespread narrowing of the small peripheral airways, either because of intrinsic disease (bronchiolitis) or because of loss of extrinsic elastic support (emphysema), although narrowing of the larger airways may play some role. However, it should be recognized that minor degrees of reversibility are common in COAD and, conversely that long-standing asthma may produce obstruction which is largely irreversible. Emphysema can be diagnosed with reasonable certainty if there is fixed airflow obstruction with over-inflated lungs and reduced carbon monoxide gas transfer (TLCO). In asthma, the TLCO is unimpaired.

The term chronic bronchitis refers to excessive mucus production in the bronchial tree resulting in a chronic productive cough. It does not imply airflow obstruction, though this may coexist if there is extensive bronchiolar disease or emphysema. Chronic bronchitis without airflow obstruction does not cause disability or reduce the capacity to work. Occupational exposures to dust and fumes commonly cause chronic bronchitis (industrial bronchitis) and they probably cause COAD in addition through bronchiolar involvement.

COAD is common. It affects some 5–8 per cent of men and slightly fewer women, and accounts for approximately 10 per cent of all deaths in the 50–70 age range. It is currently the fifth most common cause of death in Britain. The minority of smokers who are particularly vulnerable to the effects of cigarette smoke show annual declines in $FEV_1$ of the order of 100 ml/yr or more, and they can be detected in early and middle adult life by screening programmes (e.g., 5-yearly measurement of $FEV_1$). If they stop smoking at this time, a continuing excess loss of ventilatory function (and disabling COAD) can be avoided. Once symptomatic COAD develops, and asthma is excluded with a trial of corticosteroids, the prospects for any significant improvement are negligible. At this stage, acute infective exacerbations become common, and result in episodes of temporary incapacity. **Smokers of 20 or more cigarettes per day lose twice as much time from work as non smokers**. Incapacity increases as lung function continues to decline, and this may impose inevitable restrictions on fitness to work particularly for manual and outdoor jobs. However, significant limitation is often delayed until after retirement. The relationship between exposure to mineral dust and chronic bronchitis and COAD is discussed in the section on pneumoconiosis (p. 297).

## Lung cancer

Primary lung cancer is the most common malignant disease in the Western world, causing 12–15 per cent of deaths in the 50–70 age range. At least 95 per cent of lung cancers occur in current or former cigarette smokers, the risk of developing the disease being proportional to the cumulative level of consumption. Four main histological cell types are recognized—squamous cell, adenocarcinoma, large cell undifferentiated, and small (oat) cell carcinomas.

Typical presenting symptoms of lung cancer include expectorating blood, breathlessness, a persisting productive cough, weight loss, and malaise. The

**Table 15.3**   Reported causes of occupational lung cancer

| | |
|---|---|
| 1. | Acrylonitrile |
| 2. | Arsenic |
| 3. | Asbestos |
| 4. | Beryllium |
| 5. | Bischloromethyl ether (BCME) and chloromethyl methyl ether (CMME) |
| 6. | Cadmium |
| 7. | Chromium and chromates (hexavalent) |
| 8. | Coking fumes |
| 9. | Mineral oils |
| 10. | Mustard gas |
| 11. | Nickel |
| 12. | Radiation |
| 13. | Silica (in the presence of silicosis) |

affected individual may feel relatively well at the time of diagnosis but without treatment deterioration is generally rapid. The average survival without treatment is 10–12 months with non-small-cell carcinomas and only 2–3 months with small-cell carcinomas. Small-cell tumours are usually responsive to chemotherapy and current regimens usually induce a remission lasting one to two years during which time the patient might feel well enough to continue at work, if it is not too physically demanding and provided the patient can have regular time off for surveillance and treatment. If a non-small-cell tumour is localized and can be removed surgically, there is approximately a 50 per cent chance of a complete cure and a successful return to work after some 4–6 months convalescence. When an employee is returning to heavy manual work after successful treatment for lung cancer his capacity for physical exertion must be assessed by the occupational physician. Graduated return to full activity may be appropriate, and in some cases job modification or redeployment may be necessary.

A number of occupational agents are known to be carcinogenic (Table 15.3), the most important of which is asbestos. When lung cancers arise in workers with such exposures it may be impossible to distinguish the rare but truly occupational cancer from the majority which are coincidental and attributable to cigarette smoking alone. The issue is complex because important multiplicative interactions may occur between the smoking and occupational risks. Thus, the overall risk when there is occupational exposure to a carcinogen such as asbestos, chromium, or coke-oven fumes, may be relatively trivial (an increase over the non-occupational risk of, say, 1.5-fold) unless the worker is also a smoker. Increasing a low risk by 1.5 times still leaves the non-smoker with a comparatively low risk, but the same multiplying factor to a smoker whose existing risk is already increased, say, 40-fold produces a new total of about 60-fold (a net further increase which is equivalent to 20 times the normal non-smoking and non-occupational base risk). The actual multiplying factor will, of course, vary with the carcinogenic potency of the agent and the cumulative dose level sustained.

Passive smoking may increase the risk of developing lung cancer by up to 50 per cent and **employers are increasingly being seen to be responsible for the risk to the health of non-smokers exposed at work to tobacco smoke generated by others**. This has led to the introduction by a growing number of companies of formal smoking policies in the workplace. This important health initiative is of potential benefit in encouraging smokers to give up, as well as for the protection and comfort of other workers. It is likely to lead to a major reduction in sickness absence.

### Pneumoconiosis

Pneumoconiosis is a term used to describe the characteristic chest radiological appearances resulting from the inhalation of mineral dust. Pathologically, pneumoconiosis includes innocuous dust accumulation and dust-induced fibrosis affecting, primarily, the interstitium and gas exchanging regions of the lungs. Iron, tin, carbon black, and barium compounds are examples of substances whose dusts are not fibrogenic and which produce 'benign pneumoconiosis'. Coal, quartz (silica), and asbestos are the commoner substances producing fibrosis, i.e., coalworkers' pneumoconiosis (CWP), silicosis, and asbestosis respectively. These conditions, especially silicosis and asbestosis, are often associated with loss of lung function.

Pneumoconiosis typically arises after decades of relevant exposure and is recognized in life from the appearances of chest radiographs. The types of pneumoconiotic opacity and their profusions have been classified and illustrated by the International Labour Organization (ILO) using a set of standard chest radiographs.[7]

Simple pneumoconiosis is defined by scattered small opacities on the chest radiograph. They may be rounded or irregular in outline, and three levels of profusion are described by 'Categories 1–3'. Shadows larger than 10 mm in diameter represent complicated pneumoconiosis, otherwise known as progressive massive fibrosis (PMF).

The small rounded shadows of simple silicosis and CWP represent foci of dust within the lungs and localized minor fibrotic reactions to them. They are not associated with symptoms and they cause little impairment of pulmonary function. Affected workers consequently are not incapacitated. They have, however, shown themselves to be susceptible to developing pneumoconiosis, implying that continued exposure is likely to carry a disproportionate risk of progression. Simple pneumoconiosis is therefore an important identifier of the risk of developing PMF. The higher the category of simple pneumoconiosis the greater is the risk of PMF. Once PMF has begun it is likely to progress, even if further exposure to dust is avoided. It may eventually cause severe impairment of lung function, disability, and even premature death. Silica is far more fibrogenic than coal, and simple silicosis more often progresses after cessation of exposure even in the absence of PMF. Furthermore, it carries with it an increased risk of mycobacterial infection and, possibly, lung cancer.

Because of their increased risk of PMF, workers who have developed simple CWP or silicosis should not continue to be exposed to the causative dust. In the coal mining industry in the United Kingdom, miners who develop Category 2 simple CWP must be offered employment in workplaces where the dust concentrations are less than 3 mg/m$^3$. On the other hand, there is no medical reason why those working with the non-fibrogenic dusts, and who have developed radiological signs of dust retention may not continue at work, because their pulmonary function is unaffected and there is no risk of PMF though efforts to reduce dust concentrations must be maintained.

Dust suppression and other preventive measures have been very successful in recent years, and the prevalence of CWP among current coal miners (although not retired miners) is small. Early retirement of coal workers due to impaired lung function is usually the result of COAD (and smoking) rather than pneumoconiosis, although there is evidence that chronic occupational exposure to mineral and other dusts may itself induce COAD. The importance of this effect, which is independent of pneumoconiosis, has been disputed, but on the advice of the (British) Industrial Injuries Advisory Council in 1992, chronic bronchitis and emphysema in coal miners have been prescribed for disablement benefit purposes, subject to certain conditions.

Asbestosis is pneumoconiosis attributable to the inhalation of asbestos fibres. It is generally more disabling and life-threatening than silicosis or CWP, even though PMF very rarely occurs. The typical radiological appearances are of small irregular opacities, mainly in the lower zones of the chest radiograph. Lung function becomes impaired at an early stage and progression is to be expected even after exposure has ceased. Unlike silicosis and CWP, which have no specific clinical signs, asbestosis can be recognized clinically by basal inspiratory crackles and sometimes by clubbing of the fingers, together with lung function abnormalities of ventilatory restriction and impaired gas transfer.

The importation of asbestos is now strictly controlled and the material is only used in applications where no satisfactory alternatives exist, e.g., in the manufacture of brake and clutch linings. However, the effects of high levels of exposure in the past, particularly in shipyard and insulation workers, are still being seen with depressing frequency, and there is a continuing occupational risk associated with the need for asbestos to be maintained safely or removed.

The pneumoconioses are prescribed diseases under the Social Security Administration Act (1992) and diagnosis and assessment for compensation is carried out by special Medical Boards of the Benefits Agency on behalf of the Department of Social Security (DSS). Disablement benefit is payable in respect of Category 2 or more silicosis and CWP, and for any category of asbestosis. Claimants who are dissatisfied with the decision of the special Medical Board may appeal to a Medical Appeal Tribunal which is independent of the DSS and has the power to alter the decision.

## Asbestos-induced pleural diseases

In addition to pneumoconiosis and lung cancer, asbestos inhalation may lead to disorders of the pleura (the thin membrane covering the lung and lining the chest wall). The most common pleural effect is the formation of discrete plaques. Although often striking in their appearance on the chest radiograph, especially when calcified, they are rarely symptomatic, they rarely impair lung function, and they do not lead to mesothelioma. Asbestos-induced pleural effusions and the subsequent development of diffuse pleural thickening may have greater consequence, particularly if present bilaterally. There may then be significant ventilatory restriction, which may progress and become seriously disabling.

More important is the emergence of mesothelioma, which is a cancer originating from the pleura or the peritoneum (the similar membrane which lines the abdominal cavity). It is a very rare tumour in individuals without apparent exposure to asbestos, and in practice, 90 per cent or more are thought to arise as a direct consequence of exposure to asbestos. The latent period from exposure onset to tumour development is characteristically long, usually a matter of 30–50 years. The current incidence in U.K. of some 500 cases a year consequently reflects the exposure levels of the 1940s, 1950s, and 1960s. The incidence is still rising, due to the increasingly widespread use of asbestos during and immediately following World War II, and a peak is not expected until the 2000–10 decade.

Like most malignancies, mesothelioma causes general ill health, loss of energy, and weight loss. More specifically, it usually causes undue breathlessness and chest pain. There is currently no satisfactory treatment, and death usually occurs within one to two years of the diagnosis being made.

## Extrinsic allergic alveolitis

A number of substances (dusts, gases or aerosols) may cause allergic reactions in the lung after an initial asymptomatic or latent period of exposure. Although most of these sensitizers act on the conducting airways producing asthma, a few penetrate more deeply and exert their effects in the gas-exchanging region. This results in extrinsic allergic alveolitis (also known as hypersensitivity pneumonitis). The acute episode of allergic alveolitis consists of systemic 'flu'-like symptoms of fever, aches and pains, and general malaise, associated with dry cough and undue breathlessness, usually beginning 2–10 hours after the onset of exposure. The classical signs are fever and crepitations at the lung bases. Mild attacks usually resolve over a few hours without the need for specific treatment, but severe attacks may last for some days and require corticosteroid therapy.

In contrast to the acute form of the disease, some subjects encounter repeated exposure without obvious immediate effect, only to develop a slowly progressive loss of exercise tolerance because of undue breathlessness due to progressive pulmonary fibrosis.

**Table 15.4**  Major causes of extrinsic allergic alveolitis

| Agent | Source | Common name |
|---|---|---|
| **Microorganisms** | | |
| *Aspergillus clavatus* | Whisky maltings | Malt worker's lung |
| *Aspergillus fumigatus* | Vegetable compost, hay/straw/grain | Farmer's lung |
| Thermophilic actinomycetes* (e.g., *Faemia rectivirgula* and *Thermoactinomyces vulgaris*) | Mushroom compost | Mushroom worker's lung |
| **Miscellaneous** | | |
| Bacteria/fungi amoebae/nematode debris | Air conditioners/ humidifiers/tap water | Humidifier lung, ventilation pneumonitis |
| **Animals** | | |
| *Birds* | Bloom/excreta | Bird fancier's lung |
| *Mammals* | | |
| Pituitary (cattle, pig) | Pituitary extracts | Pituitary snuff taker's lung |
| Urine (rodents) | Urinary protein | Rodent handler's lung |
| **Chemicals** | | |
| Isocyanates | Plastics industry | |

Most causes of extrinsic allergic alveolitis are occupational in origin and associated with the handling of mouldy vegetable produce. Table 15.4 provides a list of the principal causative agents in Britain, of which farmer's lung provides a classic example. Most cases could be prevented by drying vegetable material before storing. This avoids the growth of contaminating microbes. Respiratory protection may also be necessary. If affected workers are unable or unwilling to avoid exposure they should be kept under surveillance with regular chest radiographs and lung function tests. Eventually a change of occupation may become inevitable.

Extrinsic allergic alveolitis due to occupational causes is prescribed under the Industrial Injuries Legislation, and affected workers qualify for the payment of disability benefit.

**Work in abnormal environments**

Employees are occasionally required to work in environments of abnormal atmospheric temperature, pressure or gas content. Hot or cold conditions, unless extreme (i.e. accidental), rarely cause respiratory problems except in the case of asthmatic workers.

Problems associated with reduced atmospheric pressure are more common. Air travel usually involves depressurization to a cabin altitude of 6000 ft (1830 m) and a reduction in atmospheric oxygen pressure. This has little effect in healthy travellers but if there is pulmonary disease, the fall in oxygen tension may cause symptoms of hypoxia. Travel to high-altitude cities or jobs may cause similar problems. Therefore, employees with respiratory disease should be assessed and advised before undertaking work involving air travel or work at high altitudes.

## Pneumothorax

Pneumothorax is a condition in which air leaks into the pleural space (the potential space between the pleural membranes covering the outside of the lung and the inside of the chest wall), thereby allowing the elastic lung to recoil and deflate. It may occur following trauma to the chest wall, or spontaneously due to rupture of a bulla or enlarged airspace in the lung. Such airspaces may be congenital or they may develop in emphysema. Occasionally, an air leak will occur when a cancer infiltrates the chest wall. Typically, pneumothorax occurs suddenly so that symptoms develop abruptly, but occasionally the symptomatic onset is insidious.

Small leaks usually heal spontaneously and quickly, and the lung may not deflate fully. Such an event may not even produce symptoms. The air within the pleural space will then be slowly reabsorbed by blood flowing through the capillaries in the adjacent lung and chest wall. More commonly there is some pain, often pleuritic; sometimes there is a little bleeding into the pleural space; and if there is major collapse of the underlying lung there may be undue breathlessness—particularly if both lungs are already diseased. In these circumstances the air should be aspirated from the pleural space, and the patient needs admission to hospital.

Rarely, pneumothorax may prove life-threatening and there is considerable urgency for the insertion of a chest tube and aspiration. If the ruptured air space develops a valve-like action, each new breath will lead to more air being trapped in the pleural space and to an increase in volume of the pneumothorax. This progressively diminishes the space available for ventilating the other lung, and this becomes increasingly compressed. In an emergency a simple stab wound (ideally, with a medium-bore needle) will allow the pneumothorax air, now under excess pressure, to escape. This requires a confident diagnosis (perhaps a previous history of pneumothorax, coupled with diminished or absent breath sounds over one hemithorax, which is tympanitic rather than dull to percussion, and shift of the mediastinum to the contralateral side), since in the absence of pneumothorax the procedure will puncture underlying lung. Ideally, there will be time to obtain a diagnostic chest radiograph. Even more rarely, pneumothorax may occur spontaneously on both sides concurrently, and in these exceptional circumstances death may occur within minutes unless a chest tube is promptly inserted on one side and the pneumothorax evacuated by pump or underwater drain.

Because of these risks, individuals suffering recurrent spontaneous pneumothoraces on two or three occasions are generally subjected to surgical obliteration of one pleural space. This effectively attaches the underlying lung to the chest wall and prevents any possibility of further pneumothorax on that side. It also makes subsequent lung surgery on that side more difficult, and so the procedure is only performed when the risk from recurrent pneumothorax is deemed to be significant. Most spontaneous pneumothoraces do not require such management, however, and in most cases affected workers may return speedily to work. Convalescence should be extended until complete resolution has been demonstrated on an expiratory chest radiograph (a minor persisting pleural collection of air may not be seen readily on a conventional inspiratory film) if the job involves moderate or heavy exertion or if air travel is contemplated.

For divers, caisson workers, and commercial or military flyers, who may face major and rapid decompression in the course of their work, the occurrence of even a single spontaneous pneumothorax is a matter of considerable concern—and is generally an indication for a change of job. Recurrent spontaneous pneumothorax in such circumstances may become rapidly life-threatening because any trapped air will expand. It is likely to be a good deal more disabling than a spontaneous pneumothorax occurring in a more usual work environment, and the affected worker (who may have responsibility for the lives of others) may find himself critically beyond the reach of emergency aid. (See also Appendices 2 and 4.)

## Existing legislation and guidelines for employment

Under the Health and Safety at Work Act, etc., 1974, and in response to European Community Law, a number of regulations have been introduced in the United Kingdom designed to reduce the risk of occupational ill health. Most respiratory hazards are covered by the Control of Substances Hazardous to Health (COSHH) Regulations (see below), but the management of Health and Safety at Work Regulations 1992 apply to certain situations not covered by the COSHH Regulations, notably underground in coal mines, and have the effect of extending the application of COSHH to those situations. Certain work-related respiratory conditions are prescribed under the Social Security Administration Act 1992.

### Control of Substances Hazardous to Health (COSHH) Regulations 1988

The COSHH Regulations place a duty on employers to assess every working situation to determine whether the use of any substance constitutes a risk to the health of employees. Where a risk of ill health exists, and where there are medical tests which can identify pathological change at an early stage when remedial action can be taken, such tests must be provided. The Regulations also require that the risk of ill health must be controlled by appropriate means, such as elimination of the harmful agent, enclosure of the process, exhaust ventilation or the provision of respiratory protection.

Workers exposed to respiratory sensitizers with the risk of occupational asthma and extrinsic allergic alveolitis should be subject to periodic assessment by means of a questionnaire and/or measurements of ventilatory function. Such surveillance procedures may not, however, be fully satisfactory, as indicated earlier. Workers exposed to fibrogenic mineral dusts may be screened for the earliest signs of pneumoconiosis by periodic chest radiographs.

## Control of Asbestos at Work Regulations 1987

These regulations make similar provisions for the medical surveillance of people working with asbestos. Such workers must be examined every two years by an Employment Medical Adviser or an appointed doctor. The examination required is clinical, with a chest radiograph and pulmonary function tests.

## The Coal Mines (Respirable Dust) Regulations 1975

Under the Mines and Quarries Act 1959, these regulations require the operator of a mine to control the exposure to dust of his employee, to provide periodic screening by means of chest radiographs, and, in the case of those men who develop the earliest signs of pneumoconiosis, to offer relocation into areas of low dust exposure. See also the reference to the Management of Health and Safety at Work Regulations 1992 above.

## The prescribed diseases

The Social Security Administration Act 1992 prescribes diseases which are accepted as being occupational in origin, together with the relevant occupations and working conditions. Workers who wish to claim Disablement Benefit must apply to the Benefits Agency of the Department of Social Security (DSS) who will, after investigating the occupational exposure arrange for a medical examination at a Medical Boarding Centre. If granted, Disablement Benefit may be paid in full, or in cases of partial disability, as a percentage of the maximum.

Having made the diagnosis of the prescribed disease and made a recommendation as to the level of disablement and therefore the appropriate award of benefit, the Medical Board may make recommendations to the claimant and his or her employer as to the conditions under which they should work.

A summary list of the prescribed respiratory conditions and the relevant occupations is given in Table 15.5. A comprehensive account is beyond the scope of

**Table 15.5**  List of prescribed diseases of the lungs (from the Department of Social Security)

| Code | Disease |
| --- | --- |
| B5 | Tuberculosis |
| B6 | Extrinsic allergic alveolitis |
| B10 | Chlamydiosis (avian or ovine) |
| C14 | Poisoning by nickel carbonyl (pneumonitis) |
| C17 | Poisoning by beryllium or its compounds (berylliosis) |
| C18 | Poisoning by cadmium (pneumonitis and emphysema) |
| C22b | Primary lung cancer in nickel production |
| D1 | Pneumoconiosis |
| D2 | Byssinosis (airway obstruction in cotton workers) |
| D3 | Mesothelioma of pleura or peritoneum |
| D7 | Asthma |
| D8 | Primary lung cancer (associated with asbestosis or bilateral diffuse pleural thickening) |
| D9 | Diffuse bilateral pleural thickening (due to asbestos) |
| D10 | Lung cancer (other causes than D8) |
| D11 | Primary lung cancer (associated with silicosis) |
| D12 | Chronic bronchitis and emphysema in coal miners |

this chapter, but further information can be found in DSS leaflets NI 2 (Prescribed diseases except certain respiratory conditions), NI 3 (Pneumoconiosis and byssinosis), and NI 237 (Occupational asthma). Additional information for doctors is contained in the DSS booklets, 'Notes on the diagnosis of prescribed diseases' (HMSO 1991), and 'Pneumoconiosis and other prescribed respiratory diseases' (NI 226 1989).

## Conclusions and recommendations

Acute respiratory illnesses may cause short term sickness absence followed in most cases by recovery. Employment problems relate mainly to chronic lung diseases, some of which may be direct consequences of exposure to harmful agents or conditions in the workplace. Although a variety of complex mechanisms and pathological processes may be involved, assessment of an individual's fitness for work is generally a simpler matter. It depends essentially on whether the various elements of pulmonary function are adequate and whether there is any restriction, through breathlessness, of capacity to undertake the level of physical exertion required by the job in its particular environment. Rarely, cough alone may be sufficiently distressing to the worker (or his or her fellow workers) to limit effective work capacity.

Individuals with certain diseases (e.g., asthma and COAD) may need to be protected against occupational factors, such as irritant dusts and fumes or cold air, which may provoke acute but transient exacerbations even if the disease itself is not primarily a consequence of the occupational environment. More importantly, individuals with occupationally induced hypersensitivity diseases, such as asthma and alveolitis, require particularly high levels of protection in order to avoid acute exacerbations and progressive irreparable damage. They may need to be redeployed to exposure-free areas.

Employers and their employees must be fully aware of and take appropriate precautions against those respiratory diseases of occupational origin (such as pneumoconiosis, mesothelioma, and lung cancer), which are predictable consequences of undue levels of exposure at work but have long latencies and for which there is little or no treatment. There is a duty on the employer to eliminate the risk of these conditions, and where appropriate, to provide medical surveillance to monitor the preventive measures. Some respiratory diseases (e.g., *Legionella* infection or gassing), may arise less predictably as the result of accidental circumstances. For these the responsibility of prevention must lie also with the employers and their medical and engineering advisers.

Although much has been learned, the occupational environment is changing continually and new occupational hazards are arising with surprising frequency. The continued alertness of general practitioners, hospital doctors, occupational health staff, managers, and the workers themselves is essential to control existing hazards and to recognize new ones.

### Acknowledgements

We are pleased to acknowledge a major contribution to this chapter from Dr S.C. Stenton, Lecturer in Medicine, Department of Medicine, University of Newcastle upon Tyne.

### Selected references and further reading

1. Social Security Statistics (1989.) London, HMSO.
2. Meredith, S.K., Taylor, V.M., and McDonald, J.C. (1991) *Occupational respiratory diseases in the United Kingdom 1989*. Report to the British Thoracic Society and the Society of Occupational Medicine by the SWORD project group. *Brit. J. Indust. Med.*, **48**, 292–8.
3. Brewis, R.A.L., Gibson, G.J., and Geddes, D.M. (1990). *Respiratory medicine*. Baillière Tindall, London.
4. HSE (Health and Safety Executive) (1991). *Medical aspects of occupational asthma*. Guidance note MS25. HMSO, London.
5. Gannon, P.F.G., Weir, D.C., Robertson, A.S., and Burge, P.S. (1993). Health, employment and financial outcomes in workers with occupational asthma. *Brit. J. Indust. Med.* **50**, 491–6.

6.  DSS (Department of Social Security) (1992). *Chronic bronchitis and emphysema.* Report, Social Security Administration Act 1992, Industrial Injuries Advisory Council, Cmnd. 2091. DSS, London.
7.  ILO (International Labour Organization) (1980). *Guidelines for the use of ILO international classification of radiographs of pneumoconiosis*. ILO, Geneva.

# 16

# Renal and urological disorders

*C.A. Veys and R. Gokal*

## Introduction

Advances in the treatment of end-stage renal failure using hemo- and peritoneal dialysis, and the success of kidney transplantation itself have not only improved the quality of life for patients, but opened up new avenues for their employability. Better management of urinary infections and calculi, prostatic obstruction, incontinence, and other complications of urinary tract disease enable the attending physician or surgeon to predict less time lost from work and better capability for doing it. The impact of renal and urinary tract disorders on work attendance and performance has been scantily reported in the literature. Only about 3 million(m) days of certified sickness absence are recorded equally for both men and women for GU tract conditions out of a grand total of 290 m days lost for men, and 100 m days lost for women from all causes. Whilst these are small proportions, much of the loss occurs in the population of working age. There are, however, few overall contraindications to undertaking gainful employment for those suffering from renal or urological disorders, and now there is plenty of opportunity for encouraging both an early return to work and continuing in the same job.

The kidney has the vital function of excretion, and controls acid-base, fluid, and electrolyte balance. It also acts as an endocrine organ. Renal failure, with severe impairment of these functions, results from a number of different processes, most of which are acquired although some may be inherited. Glomerulonephritis, which presents with proteinuria, haematuria, or both, may be accompanied by hypertension and impaired renal function. In occupational terms, a link between working in industries related to hydrocarbon products and a resultant higher prevalence of glomerular and tubular disorders has recently been suggested.[1] Pyelonephritis with renal scarring is the end result of infective disorders. Additionally, systemic diseases, such as diabetes, hypertension, and collagen disorders, can affect the kidney. Polycystic kidney disease is the most common inherited disorder leading to renal failure. Chronic renal failure implies permanent renal damage which is likely to be progressive and eventually requiring renal replacement therapy.

The renal tract can also be affected by problems of an anatomical nature, such as stones, strictures, obstruction, and tumours; disorders of this sort involving the urinary tract are the province of the urologist.

## Prevalence, morbidity, and mortality

### End-stage renal failure

End-stage renal failure is reached when the glomerular filtration rate is irreversibly reduced to less than 5 ml per minute. Without renal replacement death is inevitable. The main causes of renal failure are glomerulonephritis (30 per cent), diabetes mellitus (20 per cent), hypertension and vascular disease (20 per cent), polycystic kidney disease (10 per cent), and pyelonephritis (10 per cent). Renal replacement therapy can be achieved in one of three ways.

(1)  *haemodialysis* performed at home, in hospital, or in specialized minimal care units;

(2)  *peritoneal dialysis*, the most common form of which is continuous ambulatory peritoneal dialysis (CAPD), done at home or at work as a self dialysis technique; and

(3)  *renal transplantation* (cadaveric, or living relative).

In the United Kingdom, there are currently 60 new patients accepted for renal replacement therapy per million of population per year. This is well below the uptake in other EU countries. The number of patients on therapy in the United Kingdom (December 1990) was 330 per million of the population in contrast to over 400 in the other European countries.[2]

### Morbidity

The main reasons for hospital admission in patients on peritoneal dialysis are peritonitis or catheter-related problems; for haemodialysis patients, vascular access problems predominate. Hospital admission is much more common in patients with systemic disorders such as diabetes and cerebrocardiovascular disease. Patients receiving dialysis or having a first transplant need frequent outpatient visits at first, but eventually stabilize to fewer visits (every two to three months for dialysis patients, and every four to six months for transplant patients).

The Department of Social Security in its publication of general statistics for 1991[3] lists the number of spells of certified incapacity, nationwide, for various diseases. For diseases of the genito-urinary system (ICD-9, Nos 580–629) during the quinquennium 1986–90, these averaged 7500 spells annually for males, and 13500 annually for females. An analysis covering April 1985–March 1990 indicated that at ages above 20, spells averaged 1–2000 in each 10-year age-grouping in males; for females between the ages of 20–50, spells numbered 2–3000. Between 1985 and 1990 for each sex, the number of days of certified incapacity due to sickness from GU causes averaged about 3 million annually. In contrast, all causes of incapacity accounted for 290 m days in males and 100 m days in females. Days lost for GU tract diseases rose from 200 000 in 20–29-year-old men to 800 000 in those aged 60–64 years. In women, a peak of 900 000 was reached in 30–39-year-olds, remaining at 800 000 in 40–49-year-olds, but falling thereafter.

## Mortality

In 1990, there were 1858 male and 2061 female deaths (all ages) from glomerulonephritis, nephrotic syndrome, and chronic renal failure (DSS, ICD-9, Nos 580–9). Even though most of these (90 and 97 per cent in men and women, respectively) occurred in the population over retirement age, much of the associated morbidity would have been incurred during the working years. These totals represent 53 per cent of all deaths from the diseases of the genito-urinary system.

In Europe, patients maintained on haemodialysis and CAPD have a similar survival of approximately 60 per cent at 5 years and 30 per cent at 10 years measured from the start of dialysis. Survival, however, is age-related and is higher in younger age groups; it is also higher for home haemodialysis patients. The 5 year survival of cadaveric transplant patients is 65 per cent, but it is better in those with a transplant from a living relative. Kidney survival from cadaveric transplantation is 50 per cent at 10 years after the first year.[2] Death, as well as some morbidity, is related to premature atherosclerosis, hypertension, and vascular disease.

## Urinary tract infections

Symptoms that relate to urinary infection are very common, but of serious importance only when there is an underlying anatomical abnormality. A small percentage of women suffer from repeated infections and remain symptomatic in spite of antibiotic therapy. Anatomical abnormalities (such as ureterovesical reflux, or obstruction) are associated with repeated infection, which can eventually lead to chronic renal failure later in life.

Although many infections are symptomless, there is much morbidity from this condition. The size of the problem is difficult to ascertain. Up to 50 per cent of females have symptoms at some stage in their lives. Occurrence is much less frequent in males but rises sharply after the age of 60 due to lower urinary tract conditions, especially prostatic problems. Infection of the kidney and of the urinary tract killed half as many men (711) as women (1440) in 1990, with most of the deaths occurring over the age of 55 years. In terms of morbidity, it has been estimated that between 12 to 60 per 1000 consultations in general practice are from symptoms suggesting a urinary tract infection[4] while an estimated 45 days per 100 persons per year are lost from work from this cause.

## Urinary tract calculi

The predominant composition of idiopathic renal calculi is calcium oxalate. Urolithiasis of the upper urinary tract is a fairly common condition in the United Kingdom, with a prevalence of 3.5–4 per 100, but the incidence appears to be on the increase. The peak incidence in males occurs at the age of 35 years. Renal stones cause much morbidity, but with the widespread availability of lithotripsy, extensive renal surgery can be avoided in most cases and as a consequence time off work is considerably reduced. Deaths occurring as a direct result of all renal tract calculi (in the pelvis, ureter, and bladder) are generally few. In 1990, only 112 (male) and 160 (female) deaths were coded to this cause in England and Wales.

## Tumours of the renal tract

Adenocarcinoma of the kidney is the commonest adult renal tumour. In the bladder, more than 95 per cent of tumours are urothelial in origin. Only about 4–5 per cent are occupational in origin from former association with the chemical, dye-stuffs, rubber, cable, and other industries, or from occupations where exposure to carcinogenic aromatic amines or polycyclic aromatic hydrocarbons has occurred.

In England and Wales during 1990, bladder cancer (DSS, ICD-9 No. 188) killed twice as many men (3299) as women (1602) in all age groups. Most of the deaths were in those over the age of 55 years. As a cause of death it was the fifth most common tumour for men and the eleventh for women; it accounted for 4.4 per cent of all male cancer deaths and 2.4 per cent of all female cancer deaths. However, only a minority of the male (522 or 16.2 per cent) and female deaths (87 or 5.4 per cent) occurred in the population of working age. Carcinoma of the body of the kidney (DSS, ICD-9, No. 189) caused fewer deaths—1431 men and 871 women during 1990.

Overall, there has been a slight but steady increase in the number of both registrations and deaths from bladder cancer over the last decade. The rise has been more marked in males than females and for incidence more than mortality. Undoubtedly improved final prognosis and extended survival times have in part accounted for the increase, but a change in nomenclature which previously excluded papilloma has also contributed. New cancer registrations in 1986 (latest figures available) were 6781 for males and 2081 for females in England and Wales. The relative five year survival rate has risen from 38.7 per cent in 1963 to 63.4 per cent in 1984, and the ratio of new registrations to deaths in a given year is now more than two.

## Prostatic disease

Benign prostatic hyperplasia (BPH), is the most common prostatic problem after the fourth decade; 50 per cent of men have BPH when they are 51–60 years old. At the age of 55, 25 per cent notice some decrease in force of their urinary stream. At age 40 (surviving to 80) there is a cumulative incidence of 29 per cent for prostatectomy.

# Clinical aspects affecting work capacity

## Complications and sequelae of renal disease

These include hypertension, haematuria, and proteinuria. The discovery of asymptomatic haematuria, whether macroscopic or microscopic, and not related to urinary tract infections, requires further investigation. Initially, microscopy and culture should be undertaken. If this is negative then nephro-urological investigations are necessary to ascertain any underlying pathology before making decisions about treatment and employment.

Proteinuria needs to be quantified and if it is more than 0.3 gm/24 hours referral for further nephrological investigation will be required.

### Hypertension

Hypertension is a common sequel of renal parenchymatous disease, but is itself a cause of chronic renal failure in 8–10 per cent of cases. Antihypertensive therapy, together with salt and water restriction is usually necessary. The condition can sometimes be difficult to control and the drugs used may themselves cause side-effects, which may affect fitness for work in certain jobs. This is discussed more fully in Chapters 3 and 14.

## Transplantation

In successful renal transplant patients, renal function returns to normal, as does the haemoglobin level. These patients can thus lead a normal life to all intents and purposes, but need daily immunosuppressive therapy (*prednisolone, azathioprine, cyclosporin A*). Because of this, the transplant patient is more prone to common infections. Patients on prolonged immunosuppressive therapy have a slightly increased risk of developing non-Hodgkin's lymphoma and possibly bladder cancer as well.

Following a transplant, frequent outpatient visits are needed for the first 3–4 months to monitor renal function and to treat rejection episodes, which are more likely in that time. Most employers will understand this, and will be sympathetic and willing to accommodate the delay if the reasons are explained.

## Chronic renal failure and dialysis

Impaired renal function leads to a progressive anaemia with haemoglobin values around 8–10 g/dl. Consequently, patients may be chronically tired and more quickly fatigued, which can impair work performance. However, the availability of recombinant human erythropoietin has made symptoms of anaemia a thing of the past, with substantial improvement in well-being and employment prospects.[5] In spite of regular dialysis, the biochemistry at no time returns to normal; at best, dialysis therapy imparts a renal function equivalent to a glomerular filtration rate of 5–7 ml/min. Dietary modifications of protein, fat, carbohydrate, sodium, potassium, phosphate, and vitamin intake, and restriction of fluid intake are therefore necessary. With control of dietary and fluid intake and adequate dialysis it is unusual to experience uraemic symptoms (nausea, vomiting, itching, cramps, and diarrhoea) but some surveillance at work may be opportune.

Several complications other than anaemia can affect dialysis patients. In a minority, disordered metabolism of vitamin D, parathyroid hormone, calcium, and phosphate can lead to osteodystrophy, which can present with bone pain, proximal myopathy, and, rarely, pathological fractures. Vascular disease is a more common problem, with angina, hypertension, peripheral vascular complications, and cardiovascular accidents. These set-backs are more marked in the elderly and in those with other systemic disease.

For the younger patient with good family and hospital support, and without other serious medical problems, dialysis now offers the chance of increased longevity and a much better prospect of employment. Physicians advising on fitness for work and on specific employment must actively seek out ways and means whereby a successful job placement can be achieved, rather than just looking for the contraindications. They should also take every opportunity to educate not only patients but employers and medical colleagues alike into a more positive approach.

With flexibility, adaptation, careful planning and support, and a change of attitude on the part of employers, many more dialysis patients could work successfully. The aim should be to adapt both ways; the work to the patient's needs and the patient's treatment regime to the work, whichever direction best achieves a satisfactory outcome.

It should be recalled that haemodialysis has now kept patients alive for up to 20 years, with 60 per cent of those aged 15–34 surviving at least 10 years. Peritoneal dialysis appears to be good as a long-term treatment; but either treatment increases the chance of longevity and decreases the likelihood of serious morbidity. Although the final goal is a successful renal transplant, which offers the opportunity of a full and normal working life, dialysis treatment itself is fully compatible with many types of employment. It is worth re-emphasizing that the time off needed to learn to cope independently with haemodialysis is no more than that required for a medium to major operation, and should therefore be considered as sympathetically.

Medical surveillance at the workplace and close liaison with personnel and management can help to maintain satisfactory work performance for employees with renal or urological disease. Complications can be watched for, remedial action taken, and any further adjustments to the job can be anticipated. Such surveillance also benefits patients with hypertension complicating renal pathology, and those with urinary tract infections, or renal tract tumours.

## Dialysis routines

Dialysis improves many of the signs and symptoms of uraemia by removing solutes, water, and toxins which accumulate as a consequence of inadequate kidney function. Either peritoneal (PD) or haemodialysis (HD) are effective, both relying on a semipermeable membrane which separates blood from a dialysis solution (the dialysate). Removal of fluid (ultrafiltration) is by osmosis in PD (glucose is the osmotic agent), or by applying transmembrane pressure in HD. Selecting the dialysis routine and adapting this to the requirements of the job can be the vital factor in deciding whether a patient is successful in gaining or keeping employment. It is here that co-operation between renal unit staff (particularly the specialist nurse), family practitioner, and occupational health staff can reap most reward.

### Haemodialysis (HD)

Patients must undergo dialysis three times a week for 4–8 hours on each occasion. For those working full-time, home dialysis is done in the evenings and at weekends, while those dialysing in hospital during the day may only be able to manage part-time employment on non-dialysis days. It is not unusual for a haemodialysis patient to feel 'washed out' after a session of dialysis. This is related to the rapid removal of fluid and uraemic toxins (disequilibration). Although this usually passes off completely by the next day, it may linger and affect the patient's performance at work. Machine failure at home may also mean a return to hospital dialysis, requiring more time off work.

After starting haemodialysis, patients may be unable to work for some 3–4 months while undergoing training for home therapy.

### Continuous ambulatory peritoneal dialysis (CAPD)

This entails 3–4 daily exchanges of about 2 litres of fluid drained in and out of the peritoneal cavity, each taking about 30 minutes to perform and being spaced out over the day. This usually means that at least one exchange must be done at work; this can often be conveniently fitted into the lunch break, but needs to be performed in a suitably clean and private area.

Automated peritoneal dialysis is a modification of the routine, in which all the exchanges of fluid are done at night using a cycler machine, thus obviating the need for day-time exchanges. The apparatus is expensive, but can help those (e.g., salesmen and representatives) in occupations that involve much day-time travel. CAPD is flexible enough to allow an individual to do most types of work and is unlikely to cause problems in employment. The training period required for peritoneal dialysis is usually about two weeks, so work can start quite soon.

## Special work problems

Although few figures are published, the hospitalization rate for dialysis patients is about 10–15 days per patient year of treatment.[6] This would be the minimum time off work, as the figures do not include outpatient visits.

For dialysis patients, fatigue and a tendency to tire quite quickly make heavy manual and other physically demanding work unsuitable (see Table 16.1 and p. 317 *et seq.*), but the position is much improved since the advent of erythropoietin therapy.[5] Apart from problems posed by fatigue, patients may also have visual impairment related to diabetes or hypertension, which may dictate special provisions and added surveillance.

Patients undergoing dialysis live a stressful life. Although most patients adjust to their dialysis regimes, some may have psychological problems related to dialysis itself. Additionally, the altered quality of life, and other problems such as loss of libido and impotence, understandably cause further stress. Such patients may thus over-react to any small difficulties in their work situation. Nevertheless, there is no doubt that satisfactory rehabilitation can be achieved by those who learn to adapt to their condition. Whilst employment is one objective parameter of the quality of life, it is a difficult one to assess, because it is related to social circumstances; reimbursement for unemployment; 'employability' reflected in employer-related bias against dialysis and transplant patients, and the concept of placing housewives in an unemployed category.

### Social security provisions

There are social security provisions for working while sick for patients undergoing haemodialysis or plasmapheresis [Regulations 3(3) and 15 of the Unemployment, Sickness and Invalidity Benefit Regulations 1983]. Patients not capable of holding a full-time job may do limited work with a doctor's encouragement. This is known as Therapeutic Earnings for which a doctor's supporting letter and agreement from the Department of Social Security is required before entering the scheme. If invalidity benefit is also being claimed, there is an earnings limit—currently (1993) £42 in any week.

Patients who can work at least 16 hours a week, but whose medical condition puts them at a disadvantage in getting a job may now be able to get Disability Working Allowance (introduced in April 1992) to supplement their earnings. This provision is 'means tested' so advice is needed before making a claim,

**Table 16.1** Haemodialysis (HD) and continuous ambulatory peritoneal dialysis (PD), and types of employment

| (Unsuitable) Contraindications | (Possible) Relative contraindications | (Suitable) No contraindications |
| --- | --- | --- |
| Armed forces (active service) | Catering trades* | Accountancy |
| | Farm labouring* | Clerical/secretarial |
| Chemical exposure to renal toxins | Heavy goods vehicle driving* | Driving (unless other medical problems) |
| Construction/building/ scaffolding | Horticultural work | Law |
| Diving | Motor repair (care with fistula in HD patients) | Light assembly |
| Firemen | | Light maintenance/ repair |
| | Nursing* | |
| Furnace/smelting | | |
| | Painting and decorating* | Light manufacturing industry |
| Heavy labouring or heavy manual work | | |
| | Printing* | Medicine |
| Mining | | |
| | Refuse collection* | Middle and senior management |
| Police (on the beat) | | |
| | Shiftwork | |
| Work in very hot environments | | Packing |
| | Welding* | |
| | | Receptionist |
| | | Retail trade |
| | | Sales |
| | | Supervising |
| | | Teaching |

*Notes*: For patients on haemodialysis, shiftwork and extended hours may present problems requiring greater adaptation. Some patients have learnt to dialyse while asleep using the built-in warning devices on the machine.

If occupations in the second column entail much heavy lifting, or manual work, they may be unsuitable.

* Not contraindicated in haemodialysis.

which, however, will not normally require any additional medical support on the first claim. Those on regular haemodialysis or plasmapheresis which prevents them working for 2 or more days in any 6 consecutive days (excluding Sundays) are allowed to claim sickness benefit for those days.

## Urinary tract infections

Most episodes are short-lived and respond well to therapy. Those with repeated episodes, however, may succumb to chronic illness with backache, dysuria, and frequency of micturition, in spite of long-term antibiotic therapy. These problems can be difficult to manage and may result in frequent absences from work. Tuberculous infection of the urinary tract is being seen again more often, but employment can continue because therapy is usually administered as an outpatient procedure.

## Renal tract calculi

The newer treatments of percutaneous nephrolithotomy, and especially extracorporeal shock-wave lithotripsy for urinary tract stones, now offer the prospect of dramatically improving the previous picture of long periods off work and poor attendance. The average inpatient stay for extracorporeal shock-wave lithotripsy is 3–7 days, with minimal postoperative discomfort, and generally a resumption of normal activity within a day or so after discharge.[7]

Those with a strong history of stone formation should be encouraged to increase their fluid intake liberally if they want to accept overseas postings in tropical climates and to maintain a high intake during their stay, especially when undertaking strenuous outdoor work. Fitness for furnace or other very hot work must be carefully assessed because of the relative dehydration and increased tendency for stone recurrence, which should be easily prevented by increased fluid intake.[8]

It is interesting to note that urinary stone formation is increased in male marathon runners,[9] lifeguards in Israel,[10] hot-metal workers,[11] British Naval Officers, and ship-board engineers and cooks.[12] Whilst the underlying causative factors are partly socio-economic (associated with affluence), occupational factors, such as a high ambient temperature, chronic dehydration, and physical inactivity because of sedentary work are also implicated.

## Urinary incontinence and retention

Improved incontinence devices, more thorough investigation and improved therapy with anticholinergic drugs have greatly assisted sufferers to stay at work. Urinary diversion procedures for incontinence are becoming more acceptable. The specialist continence nurse adviser can help to improve work attendance by giving advice, reassurance, practical help, and support. The value of intermittent self-catheterization for helping patients with poor bladder emptying, urinary retention, and incontinence, or even voiding difficulties, often associated with a neuropathic or hypotonic bladder, is underestimated.[13] The technique is still much under-used but, as awareness grows, it will be more frequently applied at the place of work. Those who learn the technique can become dry, gain more social acceptance, and by establishing effective drainage, protect their kidneys from the effects of back pressure and urinary infection.

Disabled patients in wheelchairs learn to catheterize themselves and so improve their morale, quality of life, and increase their ability to attend at their place of work. Clean and private provisions at the workplace will enable the technique to be properly and hygienically undertaken.

## Renal failure and employment

Many patients with end-stage renal failure remain unemployed because of the problems potentially imposed by their demanding treatment regimes, and the need to undergo haemodialysis in the renal unit or at home during the day. Their real difficulty is to find suitable work when they are available for it. Sometimes a rearrangement of dialysis regimes will give the flexibility needed for a particular job. Patients who are not able to continue in their original work may need further training once treatment has been started.

Some dialysis patients are faced with the additional burden of frequent trips to the clinic or renal unit for treatment and review, and this may pose further problems for their employability. If reasonable adaptation cannot be made, a special rehabilitation programme should be considered in conjunction with the social worker and the Disability Employment Adviser (DEA). Further details of help with return to work through the Employment Service are given in Chapter 2, p. 37 *et seq.*

Many employers, although sympathetic, misunderstand what can be achieved by patients with chronic renal failure, and this by itself may preclude successful employment. There is thus a real need first to educate both doctors and employers about the work capabilities of such people, and to encourage a positive attitude in the patients themselves. The close co-operation of all concerned (the renal unit, the patient, the general practitioner, occupational health staff, and the employer) is often needed to effect a successful placement. The occupational physician is usually best placed to catalyse the necessary adjustments. There is sometimes a dilemma in advising a patient to become a Registered Disabled Person, because some patients feel strongly that they are not really disabled. Pressing for registration as a disabled person in these circumstances can thus have an adverse psychological effect without the compensatory advantages.

The work record of those who have received a successful transplant is especially good. A transplant cannot now be accepted as a valid reason for denying employment, or of restricting work content, for transplant patients are capable of virtually any normal work. A useful simple guide for employers, patients, and their doctors has been published.[14]

Thus the main problems surround those on dialysis. The special needs of these patients and their capabilities are less well understood and, thus far, little studied. A recent joint study from the Manchester and Oxford renal units,[15] found that there was a sharp decline in the percentage of those working some

6–12 months after the start of CAPD (44 per cent from 73 per cent), or of HD (42 per cent from 83 per cent) compared to those in employment before therapy commenced. The figures however seem to support better employability of successful renal transplant patients.[16]

In the United States, sharp differences have also been found in vocational rehabilitation in end stage renal therapy patients:[17]

|  | Male (%) | Female (%) |
| --- | --- | --- |
| Transplant | 70 | 33 |
| CAPD | 35 | 15 |
| Hospital haemodialysis | 19 | 11 |

These statistics do not take into account patient selection, which favours fitter patients for transplant, and usually means that high-risk patients receive peritoneal dialysis or centre haemodialysis. It is worth pointing out that one of the most arduous jobs is performed by housewives, and there are many women on dialysis coping with both a home and a family quite successfully. In essence, data from published series show that only about half the patients able to work are actually in employment.

## Other urinary tract conditions and employment

Two situations arise with respect to the employment of someone with renal tract cancer. For the patient with an existing tumour who is seeking employment, the extent of the pathology and the patient's general condition dictate employability, remembering that the relative five-year survival rate is now over two-thirds. On the other hand, someone who develops a tumour and is already in employment, perhaps in one of the relevant former at-risk industries, may be included in a urinary cytology screening programme. There are particular advantages for them continuing their surveillance scheme at work in conjunction with the urologist's regular reviews, because an early warning of cytological change can herald recurrence and thus initiate early further treatment. Local treatment using bladder instillation therapy has proved helpful in some cases. On leaving work, or on retirement, a postal cytology service can ensure the necessary continuity.

There are few contraindications to employment for those with renal stones, but arduous outdoor work in tropical climates is likely to be unsuitable. Patients with repeated urinary tract infections may well lose time from work, but this should not be a bar to employment. Those with a urinary diversion may work, but should be kept under review to detect the early onset of possible complications. Patients with indwelling catheters can work, and those with prostatic obstruction and incontinence should be encouraged to continue at work, especially if intermittent self-catheterization can be utilized. The advice of an occupational physician or nurse is particularly helpful in the management of these cases.

*Shiftwork*

Shiftworking is not generally contraindicated for patients with renal or urinary tract disorders. Neither is shiftwork an absolute contraindication to employment for dialysis patients, because their treatment can often be rescheduled to fit in with a regular shift rota. Rapidly rotating shift systems can be more difficult to accommodate because of their constantly changing patterns, especially for patients on haemodialysis.

## Existing legislation and guidelines for employment

The essential and relative employment contraindications for dialysis patients are shown in Table 16.1. Patients in irreversible renal failure are unsuited for work as firemen, police on the beat, rescue personnel, or the armed forces on active service, because of the high energy demands, extended hours, and the flexibility required for emergency duty imposed by these jobs. Similar restrictions may apply to particularly stressful jobs demanding a very high degree of vigilance (e.g., air traffic controllers). Jobs combining both a high radiant heat burden and high physical activity may also be contraindicated. Patients in end-stage renal failure on dialysis are not suitable for underground working, for diving or other work in hyperbaric conditions such as tunnelling under pressure. They are also unlikely to meet the standards required for merchant shipping which may require lengthy periods at sea and in tropical and sub-tropical climates. Additionally, most seafarers nowadays will need to join and leave ships by air travel. (See also below.)

Although air travel is not contraindicated for those undertaking CAPD regimes, it imposes extra difficulties and the added inconvenience of carrying supplies of the dialysate solution. Also in the context of travel abroad, the reduced dosage required for drug prophylaxis against malaria for those in renal failure should be recognized.

Because of prolonged absences from home, fatigue, and the many hours spent at the driving wheel, heavy goods vehicle driving may also be precluded. (See also below.) Again, the physical demands of loading and unloading wagons and constant climbing in and out of cabs, may preclude similar work in transportation such as removals, warehouse storage, or dockyard labouring.

Patients who are students when dialysis starts will certainly experience an interruption in their studies and may fall behind their contemporaries. Their long-term future and the suitability of a particular course should be considered in relation to the proposed dialysis regimes. Nevertheless, firm encouragement to continue should be given, for much can be achieved with motivation and support, and there is always the chance of a kidney transplant.

Usually there are no restrictions to employment for persons with only one kidney which functions well.

It is essential for those on peritoneal dialysis to avoid work in dirty or dusty environments, and also work which requires heavy lifting or constant bending. Tight or restrictive clothing should not be worn. Patients also need a clean area for performing their midday fluid exchange, as it is essential to prevent infection. The suitability, both of the type of work and of an area at the workplace for the exchange, should preferably be assessed on site by the renal unit specialist nurse, in conjunction with the occupational health staff and the employer.

Patients on haemodialysis need to be within easy reach of a dialysis facility, so work involving much distant travel and frequent periods away from home may not be suitable.

Those with a successful transplant can lead a normal life at home and at work. The work situation should, however, carry no undue risk of blows or trauma to the lower abdomen, for the transplant site must be protected. The arteriovenous fistula at the wrist can be injured by sharp projections or tools, and cutting instruments need to be carefully handled using suitable protective clothing.

If there are canteen facilities, it can be helpful to ensure that the necessary low salt and high/low protein foodstuffs are readily available.

Those with incontinence, repeated urinary infections, ileal conduits, or catheterization need good toilet facilities and nearby access. Ileostomy bags may be compressed by low benches, or desks, or the sides of bins or boxes. Excess bending, crouching, or poor seating may inhibit the free flow of urine in the bag, or damage it, causing leakage.

Mining, tunnelling, quarrying, or foundry work is contraindicated for these patients including those using intermittent self-catheterization because a clean and private place is required to effect catheter changes, or bag-emptying. Most other jobs, however, can accommodate this requirement.

### Seafarers

Restrictions on the employment of persons suffering from diseases of the genito-urinary tract are imposed by the Merchant Shipping (Medical Examination Regulations) 1983, SI: 1983 808, which require a statutory examination for fitness to work (see Appendix 3). The Amendment Regulations 1990, SI: 1985 enable an approved medical practitioner to suspend or cancel a medical fitness certificate under certain circumstances, i.e., when the seafarer was not able to meet the appropriate standard, or if the certificate was incorrect. The medical standards for service in the tropics, or other conditions of high ambient temperature, would not be met by those with recurrent urinary tract infections, stone formation, urinary obstruction, renal transplant, or intractable incontinence.

### Drivers

Patients on peritoneal dialysis could seek an exemption under the Motor Vehicle (Wearing of Seat Belt) Regulations 1982, SI: 1982 Regulation 5, or under the

Motor Vehicles (Wearing of Seat Belts in Rear Seats by Adults) Regulations 1991, SI: 1991 No 1255, by obtaining a valid medical certificate from a registered medical practitioner. However, the hazards of not wearing a seat belt must be weighed against any relatively minor inconvenience and restrictions. Adaptations to seat-belt mountings can often solve any problems.

### Advisory services

The staff of renal units, general practitioners, occupational health services, the Employment Service's Disability Employment Advisers, and the Employment Medical Advisory Service should variously be able to advise on all employment matters. The approach is usually spearheaded by members of the renal unit team; physician, specialist nurse, social worker, home dialysis administrator, and transplant co-ordinator. An occupational health physician or nurse is uniquely qualified to assess the suitability of a patient with renal or urinary tract disease for a particular job, as well as on the ways and means to adapt it. The advice, guidance, and contacts of the social worker attached to renal units will be indispensable. Several associations offer useful advice and support, and their addresses and phone numbers are given in Appendix 9.

### Holidays

Most patients on peritoneal dialysis can take a holiday without restrictions, but haemodialysis patients either need to make special arrangements for a dialysis facility at the holiday centre, or arrange for the use of portable machines. Such provisions need to be planned well beforehand.

## Conclusions and recommendations

Because of the great advances in dialysis and the good results of renal transplantation, most people with renal failure can now achieve significant rehabilitation, and often a degree of independence and quality of life sufficient to allow useful, gainful, and active employment.

Employers must be actively encouraged to take on those with renal tract disease who are quite fit for work, but who may otherwise experience minor inconveniences (like catheterization) or experience more frequent short absences from work. Prejudice, however, still abounds, and occasionally difficulty in arranging associated life insurance cover, or joining superannuation schemes is given as the reason for not employing someone in end-stage renal failure. It should be made clear to employers that none of the causes of renal failure are contagious, and so there is no risk to other workers. Thus apart from the renal condition itself those with renal failure should be regarded in the same way as anybody else. A successful transplant restores the recipient to full health with the same capability as his or her contemporaries.

There are now few absolute contraindications to the successful employment of those with renal or urological disorders.

## Selected references and further reading

1.  Yaqoob, M., Bell, C.M., Stevenson, A., Mason, H., and Percy, D.F. (1993). Renal impairment with chronic hydrocarbon exposure. *Quart. J. Med.*, **86**, 165–74.
2.  Brunner, F.P. *et al.* (1991). Combined report on regular dialysis and transplantation in Europe 1990. *Nephrol. Dial. Transplant.* **6**, (suppl. 4), 5–28.
3.  DSS (Department of Social Security) (1992). *Social Security Statistics 1991.* Tables D1. 11–16, pp. 153–70. HMSO, London.
4.  Cattell, W.R. (1992). Lower and upper urinary tract infections in the adult. In *Oxford textbook of clinical nephrology*, (ed. S. Cameron *et al.*), Vol. 3, pp. 1676–99. Oxford University Press.
5.  Canadian Erythropoietin Study Group (1990). Association between recombinant human erythropoietin and quality of life and exercise capacity of patients receiving haemodialysis. *Brit. Med. J.*, **300**, 573–8.
6.  Gokal, R. *et al.* (1987). Outcome in patients on continuous ambulatory peritoneal dialysis and haemodialysis: 4 year analysis of a prospective study. *Lancet*, **ii**, 1105–9.
7.  Wickham, J.E.A. (1993). Minimally invasive surgery. Treatment of urinary tract stones. *Brit. Med. J.*, **307**, 1414–17.
8.  Pin, N.T., Ling, N.Y., and Siang, L.H. (1992). Dehydration from outdoor work and urinary stones in a tropical environment. *Occup. Med.*, **42**, 30–2.
9.  Milvy, P., Colt, E., and Thornton, J. (1981). A high incidence of urolithiasis in male marathon runners. *J. Sports Med.*, **21**, 295–8.
10. Better, O.S. *et al.* (1978). Studies on the pathogenesis of increased incidence of nephrolithiasis in lifeguards in Israel. *Clin. Res.*, **26**, 126.
11. Ferrie, B.G., and Scott, R. (1984). Occupation and urinary tract stone disease. *Urology*, **24**, 443–5.
12. Blacklock, N.J. (1965). The pattern of urolithiasis in the Royal Navy. *J. Roy. Nav. Med. Serv.*, **51**, 99–111.
13. Consumers' Association. (1991). Intermittent self catheterisation. *Drug Therapeut. Bull.*, **29**, 37–9.
14. *MIMS: Pocket guide to chronic renal failure.* (1991). Haymarket Medical Publications, London.
15. Auer, J. *et al.* (1990). The Oxford–Manchester study of dialysis patients. *Scand. J. Urol. Nephrol.*, **131**, (suppl.), 31–7.
16. Gokal, R. (1993). Quality of life in patients undergoing renal replacement therapy. *Kidney Int.*, **38**, (Suppl. 40), S23–S27.
17. Simmonds, R.G., Anderson, C.R., and Abress, L.K. (1990). Quality of life and rehabilitation differences among four ESRD therapy groups. *Scand. J. Urol. Nephrol.*, **131**, (suppl.), 7–22.

# 17

# Haematological disorders

*A. Fingret and P.M. Emerson*

## Introduction

In the context of employment, haematological problems arise either as the result of incidental findings during routine health screening procedures in industry or during the course of specific investigations of ill health by general practitioners or hospital consultants. Screening procedures in industry may be required statutorily because of exposure to toxic chemical substances or potentially harmful physical agents, e.g., lead, chemical solvents and, previously, ionizing radiation. Alternatively, many large industries have well-established policies for routine health screening of staff for various reasons.

Haematological disorders are common and it is beyond the scope of this chapter to encompass the full range. Some conditions, e.g., pernicious anaemia, are easily diagnosed, treatable, and curable, and these will not be described as they have little relevance to fitness for work. We have therefore concentrated on those conditions, mainly of a subacute or chronic nature where work performance, types of employment, or sickness absence are a problem, with special reference to up-to-date therapy and advances in treatment over the last two decades.

The conditions covered in this chapter include iron deficiency, polycythaemia, the significance of a high mean cell volume (MCV), the problem of the low platelet count, malignant haematological disorders, thalassaemia and the haemoglobinopathies, inherited coagulation disorders, and anticoagulant control.

Before proceeding to specific conditions a general word on the anaemic patient is relevant. Chronically anaemic patients may remain asymptomatic even with extremely low haemoglobin levels, particularly in the case of some congenital anaemias where a compensatory right shift in the oxygen dissociation curve allows patients with very low haemoglobin levels to have functional haemoglobins of several grams higher. For this reason it is absolutely essential to assess every patient individually with regard to employment; i.e., a low haemoglobin detected in an asymptomatic patient as part of a routine screening procedure obviously needs investigation and diagnosis but is not *per se* a contraindication for normal work.

## Iron deficiency[1]

Approximately 3 per cent of adult men and 14 per cent of post-menopausal women are anaemic and the prevalence remains relatively constant. Iron deficiency should be considered not as a diagnosis but rather as a symptom of an underlying disorder; certainly, treatment with iron is not sufficient and the cause should be sought assiduously. These causes are not listed as they are well known, but it is as well to remind readers that dietary lack, except in physiological states of increased need such as pregnancy, is unusual with the high quality foods now available, which are often fortified with iron. The most likely cause of iron deficiency in a previously healthy individual is occult bleeding from the gastrointestinal tract from such lesions as hiatus hernia, peptic ulceration, carcinoma of the colon, diverticulitis, and angiodysplasia. Aspirin and non-steroidal anti-inflammatory drugs may also cause gastrointestinal bleeding because of gastric irritation and their effect on platelet function.

Iron deficiency may be detected as part of a routine screen in an individual who feels perfectly fit but thorough investigation is still required. Patients who present to the doctor with symptoms of iron deficiency, which are non-specific, e.g., lethargy, fatigue or mild dyspnoea on effort, are often severely anaemic and it is not unusual for the haemoglobin to fall to below 9.0 g/dl and 7.0 g/dl in males and females respectively, before help is sought. Iron therapy can be started immediately whilst other investigations are in progress but should be continued long enough (at least three months) to replenish the depleted body stores after the haemoglobin has risen to normal (males: 13.0–18.0 g/dl; females: 11.5–16.0 g/dl).

It is difficult to assess how much iron deficiency affects work capacity but it should be remembered that iron is an essential cellular component of all tissues of the body in addition to haemopoiesis. There are often no symptoms at rest but these may occur during periods of demanding physical activity and more severely anaemic patients will almost certainly show reduced tolerance on exercise testing. In countries where iron deficiency is common it has been shown that work capacity and productivity are sub-maximal. Finally it should also be remembered that patients with α or β thalassaemia trait may have very low red cell indices (Mean Corpuscular Haemoglobin (MCH) and Mean Corpuscular Volume (MCV)) due to lack of the globin component of haemoglobin. Although these patients are usually iron-replete they can suffer from associated iron deficiency and this possibility should be considered in a previously healthy individual who becomes symptomatic.

## Polycythaemia[2]

Abnormally high haemoglobin levels give rise to problems which are potentially more hazardous than an equivalent fall in haemoglobin. The blood viscosity rises sharply when the haematocrit is above 0.50 and transient ischaemic attacks, visual disturbances, peripheral vascular occlusion, and other manifestations of ischaemia may occur at values above 0.55. Thus, the polycythaemic patient is more likely to have accidents at work or put his colleagues at risk than a moderately anaemic one. The upper limits of normal for adult males and females are haematocrits of 0.54 and 0.47 respectively, (Hb 18.0 g/dl and 16.0 g/dl).

Polycythaemia is classified as primary (polycythaemia rubra vera), or secondary, the latter being far more common. Polycythaemia rubra vera (PRV) is a clonal myeloproliferative disorder in which the total red-cell mass is increased and which requires therapy to keep the haematocrit and the platelet count, which is frequently raised, within the normal range. Treatment by intermittent venesection, radioactive phosphorus ($P^{32}$), or oral chemotherapy is essential as the median survival in untreated patients is less than 18 months. Patients can continue in full-time work and the condition runs a protracted course, the median survival being over 10 years. Time off work for attendance at hospital outpatients is variable but averages about once per month.

Secondary polycythaemia, in which there is also an absolute increase in the red-cell mass, is associated with conditions in which there is either a reduction in arterial oxygen, inappropriate secretion of erythropoietin, or rarely, an abnormal haemoglobin. Treatment consists of removing the underlying cause or venesection to reduce the haematocrit to a safe level which will depend on associated conditions such as cyanotic heart disease. Work limitation will depend on the severity of the associated condition. It should be stressed that patients presenting with either primary or secondary polycythaemia are at high risk from thromboembolic complications and no time should be lost in referral to an appropriate specialist. Occasionally a high haemoglobin is found in normal individuals who have returned from working abroad at high altitude; they require no special treatment as the haematocrit rapidly returns to normal.

Particular attention should be paid to the individual with what is now termed apparent or relative polycythaemia. Other terms used for this condition are Geisbock's syndrome, stress-, spurious-, or pseudopolycythaemia. These individuals have a high haemoglobin and haematocrit but while the red-cell mass is normal the total plasma volume is reduced more than 12.5 per cent below the predicted normal value. The condition is much more common in males, with a maximum prevalence in the 40–70 year age group. The cause is not known; contributory factors may be hypertension, smoking, diuretics, alcohol, and obesity but treatment or an improvement in lifestyle is not always followed by a fall in haematocrit. Suggestions that the condition is due to stress, inappropriate secretion of antidiuretic hormone, sleep hypoxia, or low aldosterone levels have not been confirmed. Arterial hypoxaemia is found in about one-fifth of patients but the extent of any possible vascular complications is still debatable. Venesection should be avoided unless there is persistently raised haematocrit.

# High mean cell volume and alcohol intake[3]

Since the introduction of modern automated equipment, the mean cell volume (MCV) is available as part of the routine blood profile but the normal range varies slightly with the equipment used. Generally speaking, however, a patient's red cells can be said to be macrocytic if the value exceeds 100 fl (femtolitre). As with iron deficiency and polycythaemia, abnormal values may be observed on a routine blood count and discretion as to when to investigate must be left with the physician, as it is not unusual to find a raised MCV in the presence of a normal haemoglobin. Having excluded the well-known causes, such as Vitamin $B_{12}$ and folate deficiency, the most common cause is excessive alcohol intake.

Alcohol abuse causes many haematological problems, ranging from the complications of liver disease, such as bleeding from varices, coagulation disturbances, hypersplenism and associated dietary folate deficiency, to a direct effect on the bone marrow itself. Alcohol is a tissue toxin and there is considerable evidence for a direct suppressive effect on all aspects of haemopoiesis. This is probably the cause of the macrocytosis in excessive drinkers who are otherwise healthy, as the MCV rapidly returns to normal on alcohol withdrawal. Physicians encountering a raised MCV as an isolated finding should take a detailed history of alcohol intake from the patient, especially if work performance is in doubt and appropriate help should be offered where needed. A persistently raised MCV suggests permanent liver damage or continued drinking (The problems of alcoholism are discussed in Chapters 13 and 21.)

In patients with no evidence of excessive alcohol intake or Vitamin $B_{12}$ or folate deficiency, macrocytic red cells may be due to myxoedema or myelodysplasia. The latter is a pre-leukaemic state and may last for many years before bone marrow failure ensues. Special investigations are required to confirm the diagnosis.

# Low platelet count

One of the problems regularly encountered by the haematologist is the patient, usually with refractory idiopathic thrombocytopenic purpura (ITP), who runs a persistently low platelet count. These patients are often young and may be concerned about its effect on their work. Generally speaking, patients with a count of more than $100 \times 10^9/l$ will be symptom-free and not bleed excessively following trauma; there may be haemorrhagic manifestations following trauma but otherwise few problems when the count is between 50 and $100 \times 10^9/l$ . The patient with a count persistently below this level and certainly below $25 \times 10^9/l$ may suffer from spontaneous bleeding, usually purpuric, the major risk to life being intracranial haemorrhage. This latter group is at risk and employment involving heavy manual work is best avoided and should be replaced by more sedentary occupations. It should be stressed, however, that some patients with counts in the 25–50 × 10$^9$/l range rarely bleed or even bruise easily and few restrictions on employment are necessary in such patients. There is a saying often quoted by haematologists, that the patient and not the platelet count should be treated.

Some patients with chronic ITP may be receiving steroid or immunosuppressive therapy, or have been subjected to splenectomy in the past. Splenectomized patients are prone to developing overwhelming and potentially fatal bacterial infections, especially by the pneumococcus and sudden collapse at work can occur. There should be no delay in referring the patient to hospital if this is suspected. A pneumococcal vaccine, which gives protection against most, but not all, strains is available and some clinicians recommend daily prophylactic penicillin in addition.

## Malignant haematological disorders[4,5]

### Incidence of disease and meaning of remission

Table 17.1 shows the latest available figures for the incidence of haematological malignant disease in the employable age group 16–64 years. These conditions are rare when compared with other forms of malignant disease and until 20 years ago their often rapidly fatal outcome precluded any consideration of return to work. The development of effective chemotherapeutic agents, together with improvements in supportive care, have led to increased remission rates and to

**Table 17.1** Annual incidence (per 100 000) of haematological malignant disease in the population of working age (16–64 years)[6]

| Type | Number |
| --- | --- |
| *All leukaemias* | 1217 |
| Acute myeloid leukaemia | 498 |
| Acute lymphoblastic leukaemia | 154 |
| Chronic myeloid leukaemia | 210 |
| Chronic lymphatic leukaemia | 253 |
| Other leukaemias | 102 |
| *All lymphomas* | 2938 |
| Hodgkin's disease | 880 |
| Non-Hodgkin's lymphoma | 2058 |
| *Multiple myeloma* | 599 |

the possibility of a 'cure' in some conditions. The definition of remission is of considerable importance concerning fitness to work. Generally speaking, a patient can be said to be in complete remission if no signs of active disease can be detected clinically in the laboratory, i.e., the patient feels well, has no organomegaly, a normal bone marrow and cerebrospinal fluid (CSF), and a blood count within the normal range except when depressed by chemotherapy.

During complete remission there is no reason why a patient should not return to almost any type of previous employment and many do but there is inevitably, especially with the acute leukaemias and some lymphomas, a period of absence from work during induction of remission. It is current clinical practice for a patient to be informed of the nature of his condition, the objectives of treatment, and given some idea of prognosis. Medical practitioners can be extremely helpful during this period by reassuring both the patient and his employer that the aim is to return the patient to normal life and to full-time employment as soon as possible.

## Aim of treatment and general effects of chemotherapy

The aim of treatment is to destroy as many abnormal cells as possible without permanently damaging the bone marrow or other tissue by the use of chemotherapeutic agents. Treatment is mainly by cytotoxic drugs but radiotherapy may be given as the treatment of choice or as an additional form of therapy. All chemotherapeutic agents have side-effects and are frequently used in combination, thus compounding these effects. The drugs are not specific for tumour cells and some damage to normal tissues is inevitable with adequate therapeutic dosage. Different drug combinations are used for the different conditions and a detailed description is outside the scope of this book. Broadly speaking, the more acute or high grade the malignancy the more likely the patient is to receive combination chemotherapy with up to four or more drugs.

## Acute myeloid leukaemia (AML)

In the age group 15–65 years, acute myeloid leukaemia (AML) and its variants are approximately twice as common as acute lymphoblastic leukaemia (ALL). The majority of patients in the United Kingdom are entered into one of the Medical Research Council's (MRC) trials of therapy. Treatment can be divided into three phases:

(1)  induction of remission;

(2)  consolidation of remission; and

(3)  a period of observation off treatment or bone marrow transplantation.

The patient is likely to be in hospital during the initial induction and intermittently during the consolidation period; these two phases together can last anything up to six months or longer but if the patient feels well enough he should be encouraged to return to part-time or even full-time work. From the patient's point of view the most distressing side-effects of chemotherapy are nausea and vomiting. The severity varies with the individual but can be prostrating in some cases. It is useful to give the patient, his family doctor, and the occupational physician a schedule of treatment so that times off work can be anticipated. Absence from work may also occur due to intercurrent infections as a result of immunosuppression, or the need for blood transfusion. Absence from work can be minimized by arranging blood transfusion and courses of chemotherapy over weekends.

With present therapeutic regimes patients in the relevant age group have a 75 per cent chance of attaining a full remission and a 25 per cent chance of being alive at the end of five years. Patients receiving an allogeneic marrow transplant from a compatible sibling have an estimated 50 per cent chance of survival at five years and this is currently the treatment of choice in remitting patients under the age of 40 years.

## Acute lymphoblastic leukaemia (ALL)

This is the most common leukaemia in childhood but constitutes only 20 per cent of adult acute leukaemia. In adults, the disease does not carry the excellent prognosis that it does in children where a 'cure' (i.e., five year survival after stopping treatment) can be expected in 75 per cent of cases. Approximately 12 per cent of patients have the Philadelphia chromosome on presentation which carries a poor prognosis. The complete remission rate for all adult cases is approximately 70 per cent and the median survival is between 2–3 years from diagnosis. Intensive induction and post-remission consolidation have produced better survival results but prolong the initial period of hospitalization. However, the majority of patients return to work early in the course of their disease. Maintenance therapy lasts for about two years and is almost entirely given on an outpatient basis. Bone marrow transplantation from a compatible sibling of high-risk patients in their first or second remission gives reported disease-free survival varying from 30–50 per cent at 2–4 years. However, marrow transplantation in ALL, particularly in first remission, is still controversial.

## Chronic lymphatic leukaemia (CLL)

This is a disease of the middle-aged and elderly and is often diagnosed incidentally during routine screening. These individuals feel fit and may not need therapy for many years and once it has been determined that the disease is not progressing, all that is required is a blood test at regular intervals. Progressive disease diagnosed by commencement of symptoms, anaemia or thrombocytopenia, and increase in size of lymph nodes or spleen, requires therapy. This will vary with the physician and may range from gentle oral therapy with *chlorambucil* and *prednisolone* to more aggressive combined chemotherapy. Whatever the treatment, the main problems are recurrent infections, usually respiratory, which require early antibiotic therapy and are often prolonged because of the associated immunosuppression.

It is important to recognize the relatively benign nature of the condition in many individuals, particularly in terms of employment, pension schemes, and life insurance. At one time, it was thought that younger patients had a more aggressive form of the disease but recent data have shown this not to be the case, the mean (50 per cent) survival for patients aged under 55 years at the time of diagnosis being 12 years. Death may occur from other medical conditions as in the general population. Attempts have been made to stage the disease and poor prognostic signs are anaemia (Hb less than 10 g/dl) and/or thrombocytopenia (platelet count less than $100 \times 10^9$l) at presentation, when the median survival is two years. The nature of the lymphocytic cell-surface immunoglobulin is also of prognostic significance.

### Chronic myeloid leukaemia (CML)

This may also be diagnosed on a routine screening procedure either as a result of a blood count or the detection of splenomegaly but once diagnosed therapy must be commenced immediately. CML has been designated a pre-leukaemic state by some authors, as progression to an accelerated phase and ultimately transformation into an acute leukaemia (blast-cell crisis) is the usual course of the disease. The condition is due to a mutation in a pluripotential stem cell and the blast-cell crisis may be either myeloid or lymphoblastic in nature. During the chronic phase the disease is usually treated by oral chemotherapy with either *busulphan*, *hydroxyurea* or by self-administered subcutaneous injection of *interferon* and the majority of patients continue in full-time work during this period which lasts on average under four years. Once patients enter the accelerated phase, thrombocytopenia and increasing splenomegaly present problems requiring regular supportive therapy and lost time from work is inevitable. In the absence of a compatible sibling for bone marrow transplantation the condition is incurable but occasional patients remain in the chronic phase for 10 years or longer. Once acute transformation has occurred the prognosis is poor. Patients are treated with a regime according to the type of transformation, the median survival for patients in lymphoblastic transformation being 12 months, compared with two months for those with myeloid markers.

### Hodgkin's disease (HD)

This has proved one of the more rewarding conditions to treat over the past 20 years. Eighty per cent of all patients can be expected to obtain a complete remission and of these approximately 65 per cent will be disease-free at 10 years. The condition is staged from I to IV prior to treatment, the higher numbers designating more widespread disease. Prognosis depends on histology, the extent of the disease at presentation, and the presence of non-specific symptoms such as weight loss and night sweats. Recurrent disease still remains a problem but the best series show a median survival rate greater than five years from the time of relapse. Radiotherapy is given to Stage I and some Stage II patients. The remainder receive chemotherapy which usually lasts for about six months to a year and the patient may be fit enough to work throughout treatment apart from a few days each month; others experience side-effects which limit activity but the high 'cure' rate of this condition means that patients need not be barred from most types of employment, nor be given heavy insurance loading. It is important that all physicians and employers are aware of the excellent prognosis of this condition compared with the uniform fatality before 1964, the year in which combination chemotherapy was introduced.

## Non-Hodgkin's lymphoma

The ability to give accurate statistics regarding remission rates and survival in this group of tumours has been bedevilled by the number of differing histological classifications and also by the lack of properly controlled clinical trials. The tumours consist of monoclonal proliferations of B cells, T cells, or histiocytes. They may occur at almost any site and are highly sensitive to irradiation and chemotherapy. The simplest classification for the purposes of this chapter is to divide them into low-grade, and high-grade lymphomas. The treatment and prognosis vary with each group and it is important to stress that there is now a possibility of cure of some cases within each group. As with Hodgkin's disease, the lymphomas are staged clinically from I to IV. Approximately 40 per cent of all cases of lymphoma are low-grade tumours. They have a long clinical course and occur in the older age-groups. Stage I and II tumours are usually treated by radiotherapy and Stage III and IV by chemotherapy, often with a single agent. Few patients are 'cured' in this group but very long remission rates (greater than 10 years) have occurred. The median time to relapse is approximately 4 years and survival is 7–10 years in most series. When relapse occurs it is often due to a transformation to a more aggressive form of the disease. High-grade tumours are more aggressive, affect younger patients, and early spread to the bone marrow, central nervous system, and other organs is common. These patients are always treated with multiple drug regimes wherever possible. The prognosis is poor but 'cures' are possible especially with the 'T' cell tumours. The treatment normally lasts from six months to a year and because of its intensive nature few patients feel fit to return to full-time employment during this period.

## Multiple myeloma

This condition affects mainly the elderly but there are over 500 cases per annum in those of working age. Response to chemotherapy has not been as satisfactory as in other forms of leukaemia and lymphoma and has improved very little in the past decade. Complete remissions are unusual and a greater than 75 per cent reduction in tumour burden is classed as a good response. The main clinical problems are bone pain, infection, and bone marrow suppression, either due to the disease or as a result of treatment. Poor prognostic indicators are a presenting pancytopenia and renal failure which cannot be reversed by rehydration. The severity of the condition varies greatly between individuals and some patients lead a relatively normal life for many months or even years and are capable of full-time work. Recent trials have been concerned mainly with comparing gentle oral therapy (*melphalan* and *prednisolone*) with more aggressive regimes using four or more drugs in combination and results have shown the latter to have a marginal advantage. Intractable bone pain can often be relieved by radiotherapy. The median survival in most large studies has been less than three years from diagnosis.

## General comments on malignant disease

It must be stressed that the haematological malignancies are unlike other forms of disseminated neoplasia in that the patient in complete remission is clinically disease-free and it is unusual for there to be a slowly progressive downhill course preceding relapse which is often of sudden onset. There is little literature about patients' attitudes to haematological malignant disease and their employment prospects. However, the majority feel capable of working and most return to their previous job within a year of diagnosis even though they are still receiving chemotherapy. After an initial period of intensive treatment the average time lost from work is less than four weeks a year. Negative attitudes of employers, who are uninformed about modern therapy, can be a problem and the attitude of the physician in encouraging patients to return to work is highly important; patients place great reliance on this advice, as optimistic outlooks encourage shattered morale and improve self-esteem. Practical advice on life insurance, pension prospects, and estates is also extremely helpful as individuals often feel greatly relieved if they have settled their affairs even though their condition carries a good prognosis. Close communication between all doctors involved in the patient's care (at work, hospitals, and family practice) is necessary and every effort should be made to organize chemotherapy and supportive treatment in such a way as to minimize interruption of the normal work routine wherever possible.

Another problem which concerns the occupational physician is whether and when to immunize or not. Certain patients on chemotherapy, or who are known to be immunosuppressed, should not be given live vaccines (polio, rubella, measles, mumps, and yellow fever, etc.) but immunization with other agents (triple, influenza, pneumovax, etc.) can be given although patients' ability to produce adequate antibody responses is variable. BCG vaccination has been given as part of the treatment for leukaemia but is no longer considered a useful ancillary agent. Finally, it should be mentioned that chemotherapy may result in sterility in both males and females depending on the type and amount of the various drugs used, and sperm banking and possibly ova storage, should be offered to younger patients.

## Thalassaemia and the haemoglobinopathies[7,8]

Of the many described variants of haemoglobin production and structure, only thalassaemia and sickle cell disease present problems which are likely to be encountered by prospective employers and occupational physicians.

### Thalassaemia major

In this condition there is insufficient production of adult haemoglobin because of the inability to manufacture the β chains of the haemoglobin A molecule. It is inherited as an autosomal recessive disorder, i.e., if both parents are carriers there is a 1 in 4 chance that the child will be affected. There are about 450 patients in the United Kingdom of whom 60 per cent are over the age of 16, most being the offspring of immigrants from Mediterranean and Asian countries. Antenatal diagnosis by means of trophoblast sampling early in pregnancy, followed by abortion of affected fetuses, has led to a substantial reduction in the number of patients under 10 years of age. Affected individuals present in the first year and require regular transfusions to maintain their haemoglobin at a level compatible with life; these repeated transfusions produce massive iron overload which ultimately affects vital organs producing cardiac, hepatic, and endocrine failure. The introduction of intensive iron chelation by the administration of *desferrioxamine* on five days of each week has extended the lifespan of patients and the majority now reach adult life. The need for regular transfusion at monthly or six-weekly intervals necessitates some absence from work but most centres arrange treatment over weekends so that time lost is minimal. Most British thalassaemia patients have not encountered major difficulties in obtaining employment, although most are employed below their potential because of previous loss of schooling.

### Thalassaemia trait

As mentioned on p. 324 affected individuals show a blood picture resembling iron deficiency. It is of considerable importance that these patients are not disadvantaged or advised wrongly about their work prospects, as the vast majority are symptom-free healthy individuals.

### Sickle-cell disease

Sickle-cell disease has arisen as a clinical problem in the United Kingdom in the past 30 years, mainly as a result of the large influx of immigrants of African ancestry. It is estimated that there are at least 4500 sufferers in the United Kingdom at the present time. Like thalassaemia major, it is inherited as an autosomal condition; heterozygotes are symptom-free but homozygous patients present with a severe and potentially crippling and life-threatening condition. Affected individuals have a point mutation resulting in the substitution of valine for glutamic acid on the β chain of haemoglobin A. The resulting haemoglobin S polymerizes under conditions of lower oxygen tension into rigid units which deform the red cell and produce the classical sickle or holly-leaf cell which can be seen microscopically. These abnormal cells give rise to the clinical effects, namely chronic anaemia (Hb 7.0–9.0 g/dl) due to haemolysis, painful episodic crises from stasis, and infarction in small vessels, aplastic crises due to intercurrent viral infections and sequestration crises when there is massive pooling of blood in the spleen in infants and more rarely in the liver of older patients. These three types of crisis should be treated as acute medical emergencies and the patient should be referred to hospital immediately if symptoms arise at work.

The incidence of sickle-cell trait in the United Kingdom is about 8 per cent among the Afro-Caribbean community and approximately 1:600 births in this population group will produce a homozygous individual. Antenatal screening should be routine and parents should be counselled about the possibility of producing an affected child. It is extremely important to differentiate between heterozygote carriers and patients with sickle-cell disease, as the former should be treated no differently from other members of the community with the exception that work in environments where there is a risk of low oxygen tension is best avoided.

Patients with sickle-cell disease should be given careful consideration when selecting a working environment. Because of the factors mentioned in the introduction they tolerate their anaemia remarkably well and a low haemoglobin level is not a contraindication to employment. Factors which may have an adverse effect on their condition are hypoxia, acidosis, extremes of temperature, dehydration, and changes in atmospheric pressure. There is no reason, however, why most forms of employment should not be undertaken, including outdoor relatively heavy work. Modern airlines have cabin pressures adjusted such that holiday travel is safe but sufferers should not be accepted as aircrew or divers. It is of considerable importance to note that a few patients with sickle-cell disease continue to manufacture a large amount of fetal haemoglobin (HbF) which protects against sickling; they can be regarded separately as they encounter far fewer problems.

There is little information about the employment prospects of patients with sickle-cell disease. Advances in supportive care rather than specific prevention of sickling, which is still a major therapeutic problem, have allowed many patients with sickle-cell disease to reach adult life and enter the job market. However, frequent absence from work due to intercurrent illness can prejudice the chance of long-term permanent employment and companies vary widely in their attitudes towards affected individuals.

## Glucose-6-phosphate dehydrogenase (G6PD) deficiency

This sex-linked condition affects approximately the same number of individuals and is present in the same ethnic groups as haemoglobin S and thalassaemia. Most sufferers are entirely symptom free and are unaware that they have the condition. Once diagnosed they should carry a list of drugs to be avoided as most problems arise as a result of haemolysis due to the ingestion of oxidative agents. The drugs considered unsafe are listed in the *British National Formulary*.[9] From the point of view of employment they should be advised not to work in chemical plants manufacturing naphthalene or trinitrotoluene. If there is a history of favism, agricultural work involving broad bean cultivation or processing should be avoided; otherwise there should be no problems with employment.

As in all these inherited conditions genetic counselling is essential, especially if the individual becomes pregnant.

## Coagulation disorders

### Haemophilia *A* and *B*[10] (see also Chapter 10, p. 189.)

There are approximately 5000 individuals with haemophilia A and 1000 with haemophilia B (Christmas disease) in the United Kingdom; these two disorders will be discussed together as their clinical presentation and treatment are similar. Both are sex-linked disorders and female homozygotes are extremely rare (estimate 1 per 50 million population) so, in practice, all patients are male. The condition varies in severity from mild cases who may not be diagnosed until adult life, to very severely affected individuals who require regular replacement therapy. The severity of the condition tends to run true in families and is assessed by measuring the blood coagulant activity of either Factor VIII or Factor IX. Haemophiliacs are classed as *severe* (Factor VIII coagulant < 1 unit/ml), *moderate* (1–5 units/ml), or *mild* (> 5 units/ml). The clinical presentation varies according to the level of activity, the most severely affected individuals suffering repeated haemorrhages into joints, deep tissues, and occasionally externally. These episodic bleeds can cause severe arthroses and contractures which, before the advent of modern treatment, led to crippling disability early in life. Mildly affected haemophiliacs, with Factor VIII coagulant levels of more than 5 units/ml, escape these deformities and tend to bleed only after accidental trauma, surgery, or dental extraction.

Modern therapy has greatly improved the prognosis with regard to mobility, motivation, education, employment, social activities and life-expectancy. Treatment consists of replacing the missing factor by intravenous injection as necessary, a procedure which takes about 15 minutes. There are designated Haemophilia Centres throughout the United Kingdom where programmes of replacement therapy are arranged to suit individuals. In home therapy patients are instructed to inject themselves with Factor VIII and this has been of major benefit in limiting the severity of bleeds and reducing travelling and waiting time at hospital. Other problems related to haemophilia are associated with chronic pain (there is a relatively high degree of drug dependency), unavoidable absence from school or college, and the psychological aspects of suffering from an inherited and potentially crippling condition. More recently, some haemophiliacs have also been inoculated with HIV through contaminated blood products (see Chapter 22).

The occupations which haemophiliacs can be expected to follow vary according to the severity of the condition. There are no limitations in obtaining driving licences unless debarred by associated medical conditions. Haemophiliacs are not accepted into the armed forces nor usually allowcd to fly passenger aircraft. In one instance a patient with a Factor VIII coagulant value of 2 units/ml, who had previously flown in Australia, was accepted as a commercial airline pilot in the United Kingdom but could not take up the position as insurance cover was refused (personal communication). Apart from these, no occupations are unsuitable for mildly affected individuals, but severely affected patients are best suited to sedentary jobs, such as office or clerical work, and heavy manual labour should be avoided. There is no fixed rule, however, as some haemophiliacs with extremely low coagulant activity seldom bleed, while some patients classed as moderately affected may suffer repeated haemorrhages.

About half of all haemophiliacs lose more than one month's schooling per year and are eventually officially classed as disabled, but on the positive side about half of all severely or moderately affected haemophiliacs follow a course of further education and about 20 per cent have a degree or diploma; many stay with the same employer for years. There is no doubt that self-treatment has improved employment prospects and as haemophiliacs have a remarkably accurate self-perception of early bleeding, a refrigerator should be available at their place of work for storage of emergency supplies of Factor VIII. Bleeds at work mainly result from accidental impact injuries rather than as a result of heavy work. The occupational physician can be of great assistance to haemophiliacs by assessing suitable employment and making arrangements for their self-treatment.

Unemployment among haemophiliacs is greater than the national average and there is marked geographical variation, unemployment being higher in the north of England and Scotland. Sufferers from haemophilia should not hesitate to tell prospective employers of their condition as most are sympathetic and helpful and will be guided by their occupational health advisers about the much improved prognosis through the recent advances in therapy.

Some haemophiliacs have experienced problems with life insurance and there is usually a 2 per cent loading. Information about insurance and pension schemes is best sought from the Haemophilia Society but the Disability Employment Adviser may be able to advise employers. In conclusion, although modern treatment has improved the general well-being of haemophiliacs it has not been shown to have improved their employment prospects but it has reduced absenteeism in employed haemophiliacs and probably increased the potential range of work. Better facilities for self-treatment at work are required and ignorance among employers about the condition is still encountered.

## Anticoagulant therapy

The exact number of patients on long-term anticoagulant therapy in the United Kingdom is unknown but the number is substantial: it has been estimated that up to 10 million coagulation control tests are performed per annum. At the John Radcliffe Hospital, tests are performed currently on approximately 1500 patients in a population of half a million. The major problems encountered are with dose control as response to therapy varies with changes in diet, alcohol intake, intercurrent illness, and medication. It is essential that the doctor responsible for controlling patients is informed of any alterations to therapy, as many drugs potentiate and some inhibit the action of the anticoagulants. A full list is available in the *British National Formulary*.[9] Patients are encouraged to continue in their present employment and no occupations are barred except those needing strenuous physical work. In practice, however, the patient's lifestyle may already have changed as a result of the underlying condition necessitating anticoagulant therapy.

## Selected references and further reading

1. Herbert, V. (1992). Iron disorders can mimic anything so always test for them. *Blood Rev.*, **6**, 125–32.
2. Landaw, S.A. (1990). Polycythaemia vera and other polycythaemic states. *Clin. Lab. Med.*, **10**, 857–71.
3. Pohorecky, L.A. (1991). Stress and alcohol interaction: an update of human research. *Alc. Clin. Exp. Res.*, **15**, 438–59.
4. Hoffbrand, A.V. and Lewis, S.M. (1989). *Postgraduate haematology*. Heinemann, Oxford.
5. Altmaier, E.M., Gingrich, R.D., and Fyfe, M.A. (1991). Two-year adjustment of bone marrow transplant. *Bone Marr. Transpl.*, **7**, 311–66.
6. *Cancer statistics registration*. Series MBI, No. 19. HMSO, London.
7. Weatherall, D.J. and Clegg, J.B. (1989). *The thalassaemia syndromes*. Blackwell, Oxford.
8. Serjeant, G. (1989). *Sickle-cell disease*. Oxford University Press.
9. *British National Formulary*. Published annually by British Medical Association and the Royal Pharmaceutical Society of Great Britain.
10. Bloom, A.L. (1991). Progress in the clinical management of haemophiliacs. *Thromb. Haemost.*, **66**, 166–77.

# 18

# Women at work

*L.H. Kapadia and G.V.P. Chamberlain*

## Introduction

Over 12 million (m) women are in employment in the United Kingdom, about 4 m in office work, 3 m in service jobs, and over 1 m in the health services and in education. There are now more women in paid employment outside the home than 40 years ago. Many work into pregnancy, 75 per cent of them into the last trimester. It might be expected that this would produce problems in the workplace, but they rarely happen.

## Pregnancy

### Specific hazards in pregnancy

Several specific hazards exist, physical, chemical, and biological.

Chemical hazards include:

- Metals, e.g., lead, mercury, copper
- Gases, e.g., carbon monoxide
- Passive smoking
- Insecticides
- Herbicides
- Pesticides
- Solvents, e.g., carbon tetrachloride
- Drugs during their manufacture
- Disinfecting agents, e.g., ethylene oxide

Physical hazards include:

- Ionizing radiation, e.g., X-rays
- Heat
- Vibration
- Humidity
- Noise
- Dust
- Lifting heavy loads

- Repetitive and fatiguing muscular work

Biological hazards include:

- Contact in crowded places, e.g., in travelling to work
- Contact with high-risk groups, e.g., schoolchildren with rubella
- Food preparation infections
- Water-borne infections
- Specific relevant infections such as brucellosis in lamb farming

Obviously these should be avoided in pregnancy, particularly in the first few weeks. Recent EU Directives have laid responsibility on the employer to provide protection for pregnant women against specific harmful industrial agents and processes, and even wider prohibitions apply to breast-feeding mothers.

It must be emphasized that most of the hazards listed above are only rarely relevant to working women but because the risks are greatest in very early pregnancy, advice may be needed before conception. Information needs to be given specifically, and should include plans to restrict exposure to these hazards for women who are planning to become pregnant.

### Non-specific problems in pregnancy

There are many general, non-specific problems which apply to all pregnant women. Fatigue occurs more rapidly in pregnancy and non-specific backache follows the alteration of the body's centre of gravity; the woman's bulk may make certain tasks difficult as she is forced further away from her work. Sickness in early pregnancy may lead to time off work while mental concentration may be affected by the metabolic changes of pregnancy. It is important to consider all aspects of an employee's work as soon as she becomes pregnant to see if they require modification.[1]

Most pregnant women can work the usual working hours, but provision of a time for rest after lunch may be desirable in later pregnancy. In other instances, shorter working hours or *flexitime* may be recommended to avoid tiring rush-hour travel. If work involves standing in a fixed position at a production line, or as a sales assistant in a retail outlet, alternative work, or part-time sedentary work should be considered as pregnancy progresses. Any employer keen to maintain the best productivity from employees will suggest less physical work for a pregnant member of staff. Repetitive lifting tasks should be avoided, as should work associated with climbing ladders that can often involve carrying merchandise or placing it in storage bins, which could precipitate premature labour.[2] The risks to safety should discourage any employer from keeping her in these types of work (Health and Safety at Work Act, Etc., 1974). Where transfer to another activity is not possible, the woman, under recent EU Directives, can be granted paid leave from work with protected employment rights.

Through modifications of such aspects of the pregnant employee's work, most women should be able to continue working until the last weeks of pregnancy if desired and if the physical demands are not excessive. Fatigue and repetitive or boring jobs have been considered to be associated with an increased risk of preterm labour and low birth-weight babies but sensible policies will minimize these risks. There is now an obligatory 2 week period of leave immediately before the expected date of confinement and a right to a total maternity leave of 14 weeks with payment equivalent to sickness benefit throughout.

## Legislation

The proposals for implementing the EEC Pregnant Workers Directive is still in the consultation stage at the time of going to press (January 1994) (Council Directive 92/85/EEC). In principle, it provides improved rights for pregnant workers. It was adopted in October 1992 for implementation no later than October 1994. The main requirements are that all pregnant women, regardless of the length of service or hours worked, must be given the right to a period of *at least 14 weeks* maternity leave—2 weeks of this leave around the time of birth will be compulsory and all contractual rights, except for a right to payment under the Contract of Employment, must be maintained during the full maternity leave period. It also states that implementing the Directive must not reduce existing rights in that country, if they are more favourable than those required by the Directive. If a redundancy situation arises the woman is entitled to be offered a suitable alternative vacancy where available. The woman then must, at least 21 days before she begins her leave, give her employer written notice of the fact that she is pregnant and the expected week of birth. She may have to prove this with a medical certificate if her employer requires it. She must also, at least 21 days before, give notice of the date that she intends to begin her maternity leave. This, however, has to commence after week 29 of pregnancy unless she is absent from work before this date because of reasons relating to pregnancy. She must give notice in writing that this is the case as her maternity leave will begin on the first day of absence. If the baby is born earlier than the expected date, maternity leave starts from the date of birth and the employer must be notified. If a woman wishes to return to work earlier than her maternity leave period, she must give her employer 7 days notice of that date. The right of the woman to return to work after maternity leave for those women who have worked 16 hours or more per week for two years and 8–16 hours per week for five years, must be given in writing confirming when she intends to return. This must be given at least 21-14 days prior to that date and no longer than 29 weeks after the date of childbirth. Employers with five or fewer employees are relieved of the requirements to take a woman back after maternity leave if it is not reasonably practicable to do so.

Many women leave work after 28 weeks of gestation (12 weeks before the expected date of delivery) which is the time when maternity benefits may first be claimed. However, many more are extending their working lives into late pregnancy quite safely but this requires greater understanding from their employers.

## Visual display units

Some of the fears which women may harbour in pregnancy cannot be substantiated scientifically. A typical example was the interest shown during the 1980s in visual display units (VDUs). Existing fears about X-rays and other electromagnetic radiation were extrapolated to VDUs from sporadic reports of spontaneous abortions, birth defects, and preterm labours among women VDU operators. These reports were mostly uncontrolled, small in numbers and anecdotal. It would be surprising if there was anything emitted by a VDU which would affect pregnancy or the fetus. The energy of X-rays emitted from VDUs is about 25 keV and is not detectable beyond the glass screen of the tube. Other non-ionizing radiations are at background levels, well below acknowledged international safety standards. No modern equipment emits more than 0.1 µSv/h of ionizing radiation; background natural emanation is about 0.3 µSv/h so no additional hazard exists there. Very low and extremely low frequency electric fields of the order of 1.8 kV/m and 10 millitesla are typically well below accepted levels. For example, these emissions equate one hour with a VDU to one minute with a food mixer.

A large and careful cohort study of the effect of VDUs on pregnant telephone operators has been performed in which the controls worked under similar conditions as the pregnant VDU operators, thus eliminating stress attributed problems or too long hours of work in an uncomfortable sedentary posture. The odds ratio for adverse pregnancy outcome in the VDU-exposed group compared to the controls was 0.99 (95 per cent CI 0.68–1.44) and there was no gradient with the amount of exposure. Women can be confidently advised that there is no evidence that work with a VDU will jeopardize pregnancy,[3] a conclusion also reached more recently by Roman (1992).[4]

## Diet

During pregnancy a woman should take a diet which is not necessarily bulky or very calorific but is nutritious. In some places of work, canteens provide enough variety for a pregnant woman to select appropriate food. However, in many instances employees buy their own lunches or snacks in nearby shops. Employers could help employees to improve their health by health promotion and good dietary advice for women in the reproductive age group who are at work. Specifically, the Department of Health has advised the taking of low doses of folate (0.4 mg folic acid daily) both when planning pregnancy and in the first 12 weeks of pregnancy, to reduce the risk of neural tube defects (NTDs). Such persons should also eat more folate-rich foods, e.g., bread (soft grain), sprouts, cornflakes and branflakes, and spinach.

## Cigarette smoking

Smoking has negative effects on pregnancy. In the male, fertility can be decreased; among women, those who are cigarette smokers may produce babies about 200 gm lighter than non-smokers at term. The menopause occurs earlier in women who smoke over 20 cigarettes a day; presumably ovulation stops sooner so reducing the duration of fertility. In pregnancy there is a risk of preterm labour and a higher perinatal death-rate.[6] In smokers, the congenital abnormality rate of conditions such as cleft palate and heart defects is higher[7,8] and the risk of a subarachnoid haemorrhage in the mother is six times that of a non-smoker;[9] while the prevalence of pre-eclampsia is lower in smokers and the severity of the condition is worse when it occurs. All in all, smoking is best discouraged in pregnancy or cut to the minimum and employers can help by prohibiting smoking at work which will also benefit non-smokers by reducing their exposure to 'sidestream smoke'.

### Alcohol and drugs

Health promotion at work should also draw attention to the dangers of excess alcohol and drugs in pregnancy. Excess alcohol may lead to the fetal alcohol syndrome in which the baby has a small head, mental retardation, and anomalies of the face, joints, and external genitalia. Some drugs, such as testosterone, anticonvulsants, and cytotoxics are also associated with congenital malformations.

### Travelling in pregnancy

Long-distance travelling is best left until after week 14 of pregnancy to avoid the risk of miscarriage. Most airlines refuse women on international routes over 34 weeks of pregnancy and over 36 weeks on domestic flights; they may need certification from a doctor about the length of gestation. This is mainly because airline owners are worried that premature delivery might occur in flight. Advice to air travellers is to stretch legs, drink plenty of fluids, and to take moderate exercise.

### Vaccinations

Vaccinations of killed or attenuated virus may be given in pregnancy. Live immunizations should be avoided as should rubella, mumps, and measles vaccines because of the risk of a pyrexia.

## Genetic counselling

Counselling may be requested for those who have a family history or a previously affected child with an inherited condition such as sickle-cell anaemia, cystic fibrosis, or other severe disorders.

Chromosomal abnormality risk increases with maternal age. The principal example of this is Down's syndrome where the incidence at birth is 1 per 3000 at 25 years, 1 per 300 at 35 years, 1 per 100 at 40 years, and 1 per 40 at 45 years. Chromosomal abnormalities can be detected in pregnancy by chorionic villus sampling (CVS) at 9–11 weeks of gestation or by amniocentesis at 13–16 weeks. Both are invasive tests with risks of miscarriage of 2 and 0.5 per cent, respectively. Several biochemical tests on maternal blood can be used and their results combined with maternal age to give more accurate risk predictions. These are known as the Barts and Leeds Tests and are done to assess whether the woman is in the high-risk category. If so, she may require sampling by amniocentesis.

## Pre-existing and coexisting illness

*Diabetes.* Pregnancy stabilization and control of insulin-dependent diabetes is important to reduce the risk of fetal abnormality. Good control of maternal blood sugar levels will ensure that the pregnancy is uneventful and the baby is a normal size. This will lower fetal loss from all causes, and so timing and dosage of insulin with meals is important. Regular meal breaks from work may be necessary at set times; this could interfere with some work timetables. Perinatal mortality used to be four times as high in diabetics as in the general population; this rate is related to the severity of the diabetes. The figure can be halved by good diabetic control.

*Heart disease* must be stabilized; the woman should be checked for any cardiotropic drugs which are known to interfere with organ formation in the fetus in the first trimester of pregnancy. There may be problems in pregnancy for a woman with a heart of a fixed volume, high left atrial pressure, and pulmonary vascular obstruction. In cyanotic heart disease the miscarriage rate is minimal, but extra rest is mandatory.

*Thromboembolism.* Pregnancy increases the prevalence of this condition fourfold. Patients on anticoagulation therapy who are at work need special advice and caution.

## Physical work

Women who have a long working week or whose work is physically tiring are thought to have a higher proportion of preterm births although there is little evidence for this. Heavy lifting, standing for long hours, and shiftwork have been associated with an increased risk of spontaneous abortion.[10] This has been challenged epidemiologically but is still perceived wisdom.

## Male reproductive factors

Evaluation of the male reproductive system is still subject to many variables. Well-established effects on male fertility are found with occupational exposure to the nematocide, 1,2-dibromo-3-choloropropane (DBCP) and to lead. More recently, employment as steel welders has been associated with reduced sperm quality presumably due to the hot environment of the work.[11]

Not only may fertility be affected but the contribution of the male gamete to successful pregnancy outcome has been questioned and paternal occupation in the glass, clay, stone, textiles, and mining industries has been associated with an increased risk of premature delivery while the wives of workers exposed to vinyl chloride have increased miscarriage rates.

## The enviroment

In the working environment conditions should be as safe as far as is reasonably practicable and when exclusionary policies are practised they often fail to acknowledge the male-mediated effects. Employers under COSHH and the Health and Safety at Work etc., Act, 1974 have to provide safe systems of work for their employees. In shiftworkers, tiredness may diminish sexual activity. Crossing time zones may disturb the menstrual cycle and may thus contribute to conception failure. If workplaces are hot enough to increase the core body temperature (such as in laundry, hairdressing, and kitchens) there is a slightly increased risk of miscarriage.

## Gynaecology

It is probable that women who are at work have a lower morbidity rate than those who are not employed (the healthy worker effect), but anyone employing many women is likely to encounter the consequences of the full range of gynaecological conditions.

In a survey among female employees of Marks and Spencer all consultations were categorized by complaint. In the last six months of 1992, 7769 women attended and 2481 or 32 per cent were for gynaecological complaints. Special clinics for cervical smears were held separately and many additional gynaecological problems were dealt with there. Approximately 60 per cent of the

**Table 18.1**   The most common gynaecologically related conditions found in the Marks and Spencer survey (see text)

| Reason for consultation | No. | Gynaecological attendances (%) |
| --- | --- | --- |
| Hormone replacement therapy | 345 | 13.9 |
| Menorrhagia and other abnormal vaginal bleeding | 306 | 12.3 |
| Cervical smears | 271 | 10.9 |
| Dysmenorrhoea | 230 | 9.3 |
| Problems associated with pregnancy | 199 | 8.0 |
| Abdominal pain of gynaecological origin | 157 | 6.3 |
| *Total* | 1508 | 60.7% |

gynaecological attendances were associated with six factors, see Table 18.1 (personal communication).

This reveals the nature of the gynaecological load that might be expected at an occupational health clinic. Occupational health staff must be trained to give appropriate advice and be prepared to refer on for specialist advice, without prejudice, those women who consult them or their employer.

## Infections of the genital tract

These might affect the vulva, vagina, uterus, fallopian tubes and ovaries or any combination. Usually the first two comprise lower genital tract infection and the last two pelvic inflammatory disease.

*Vulva*—pruritus vulva is a common presenting symptom.
The causes may be:

- Fungal—Candida (thrush)
- Viral—Herpes genitalis
- Parasitic—scabies, *pediculosis pubis,* or threadworms
- Sexually transmitted diseases, *Trichomonas vaginalis* or gonorrhoea
- Local skin atrophy

*Vagina*
Pathological causes may be:

- Infection

Inflammation from:

- Rubber allergy
- Douching, deodorants or chemicals
- Malignancy
- Foreign body: forgotten tampon
- Chronic skin conditions, psoriasis, eczema, *lichen planus* and *lichen sclerosis*

True pathogens of the lower genital tract include *Chlamydia, Trichomonas, Herpes simplex Type II, gonorrhoea, Treponema pallidum,* and *HIV*; most are sexually transmitted diseases. Opportunistic pathogens of the same area are *Candida, Gardnerella vaginalis,* and *mycoplasma.*

Vulvovaginitis and vaginal discharge are common presenting complaints; they can be managed easily and corrected by the patient's GP. Occasionally referral to a genito-urinary clinic is advisable when the sexual history shows recent casual contact. Others at risk include women after termination of pregnancy or where there is left iliac fossa pain and deep dyspareunia. Bacterial vaginitis from *Gardnerella* is probably the most common cause of vaginal discharge in the United Kingdom.

## Pelvic inflammatory disease (PID)

PID covers infections of the uterus, tubes, ovaries and parametrium. It is non-reportable; regional incidences vary with the incidence of sexually transmitted disease. It is an acute febrile illness with pelvic pain and local signs of genital infection. The diagnostic accuracy of the clinical picture is poor.

Primary ascending infection from the lower genital tract tends to occur most often after delivery or miscarriage. It may be iatrogenic at the time of termination of pregnancy, at salpingography, at dilatation and curettage (D & C) or following insertion of an intrauterine device. Seventy per cent of cases are due to ascent of endogenous vaginal and perianal flora. Of all women with PID, 70 per cent are under 25 years of age and 75 per cent are nulliparous.[12] The age-related risk of developing PID in sexually active women is:

| | |
|---|---|
| 15 years or less | 1 in 8 |
| 16–24 years | 1 in 10 |
| 25 years and over | 1 in 80 |

Infection rates are related to promiscuity.
The sequelae are:

*Chronic pelvic pain* in 20 per cent of patients; of these, 60 per cent will be infertile and suffer from dyspareunia.

*Heavy or irregular periods* because of pelvic inflammation.

*Infertility* which follows in 15 per cent to 20 per cent of cases, increasing to 60 per cent after three attacks of PID.

*Ectopic pregnancy* rates increase from 7- to 10-fold.

PID is treated with rest and avoidance of intercourse; long term antibiotics, such as *tetracycline* and *doxycycline,* should be taken. *Metronidazole* can be added. Two days to six weeks absence from work is usual.

# Menstrual disorders

Menstrual bleeding usually occurs every 28 days for 4 to 7 days. Periods commence at the age of 11, on average, and menstruation does not usually cause clots, pain or flooding. Many variations of menstruation may occur from absent or scanty periods to heavy, frequent, and irregular ones.

Scanty or absent periods often have a genetic or endocrine link and are occasionally associated with tumours. Psychological upsets and anorexia nervosa can also present in this way; here an occupational health physician or nurse may enable the woman to continue work and avoid lengthy absences. Counselling and advice for further referral help the employee to acknowledge the condition. Often a long period off work may be necessary especially if hospital admission is required for eating disorders.

## Menorrhagia

Menorrhagia is excessively heavy or prolonged periods which may cause problems at work especially if the woman becomes anaemic which is particularly common in vegans. Menorrhagia can occur in 18–25-year-old women when it may be linked to a fault in ovulation and fertility. Investigations are usually done as an outpatient but a minor gynaecological operation, D & C, is carried out as a day case to help diagnose the cause of the disordered bleeding. More often, it is the 35–40-year-old who has these problems, which may be linked with hormonal upsets and organic disease such as fibroids. Often, medication which may include hormones, antiprostaglandins or antifibrinolytic agents, will help to control symptoms. If, however, the woman is at the end of her reproductive life, a hysterectomy may be performed, which will require a 10 to 12 week period of convalescence before returning to work.

Laparoscopic, or minimally invasive, surgery has revolutionized gynaecological investigations for unexplained abdominal pain, infertility, sterilization and other problems such as ovarian cysts. Surgical time is short and occasionally a local anaesthetic can be used instead of a general anaesthetic. A small incision is made below the umbilicus and a small telescopic instrument, the laparoscope, is introduced into the abdominal cavity. A small incision may also be made in the pelvic area. The woman is in hospital either as a day case or occasionally overnight.

## Dysmenorrhoea

Dysmenorrhoea is painful menstruation. It presents as cramping low central abdominal pain in young women or teenagers just before the onset of a period. This is primary dysmenorrhoea which, at its worst, is a debilitating pain associated with nausea, diarrhoea, and flushes. Painful periods commencing after the age of 30 years tend to be due to pelvic disease; the pain is not fierce or spasmodic and builds up from a dull ache 2–3 days before a period lasting right the way through, often accompanied by backache. There may be other symptoms such as heavy periods or deep pain on intercourse.

Primary dysmenorrhoea may cause regular monthly absence from work in some young women. Investigations to exclude other causes of pain in this area may be required but often the diagnosis is obvious and treatment may be given in the form of the oral contraceptive pill or non-hormonal medication (antiprostaglandins).

In older women when the pain is secondary to fibroids, endometriosis or pelvic infection, treatment is that of the primary cause. This may require laparoscopic or ultrasound examinations to confirm the diagnosis and surger later.

**Table 18.2**    Women registered with gynaecological cancers reported in 1986 (latest year) and deaths (1990)

|  | Registrations (1986) | Deaths (1990) |
|---|---|---|
| Ovary | 4507 | 3995 |
| Endometrium | 3432 | 914 |
| Cervix | 4034 | 1781 |

# Cancer

Gynaecological cancer usually affects women over 40 years old. Figures for registration and deaths in England and Wales are shown in Table 18.2.

### Cancer of the ovary

This is one of the more prevalent fatal cancers of women aged 50–70, and in the United Kingdom, is the most common gynaecological malignancy. The disease is often asymptomatic in the early stages, presenting with poorly defined ill health or swelling of the lower abdomen. It is often first diagnosed by feeling a mass on examination; the tumour is confirmed at laparotomy. Ultrasound screening reveals pathology at an earlier stage and along with tumour markers in the blood, like CA 125, was considered as a potential screening system for ovarian cancer in the general population. However, it is felt that the way forward for ovarian cancer is to concentrate screening on the relatives of women with ovarian cancer as they have a four times greater risk of developing this cancer than the population at large.

Following treatment with surgery and chemotherapy, women are likely to be off work for some weeks and will require time off for further follow-up. Survival rates vary greatly, depending on the spread of the tumour at the time of first treatment. Unfortunately, the growth has often already spread widely when it is diagnosed and so this tumour is associated with a very poor prognosis, the worst of all gynaecological cancers.

### Cancer of the endometrium

In two-thirds of cases, endometrial cancer presents with post-menopausal bleeding but if it starts before the menopause there may be prolonged or irregular menstrual bleeding. The diagnosis is confirmed at curettage; surgical treatment is usually followed by radiotherapy. In a few cases, progestogens are given to reduce distant spread. This condition has a good prognosis and many women are back at work within 6 to 12 weeks of therapy. The range of survival rates is wide, but this tumour is usually slow to metastasize and is detected early; thus the prognosis is generally better than other cancers of the genital tract.

## Cancer of the cervix

This presents in the younger woman, usually between the ages of 35 and 50 years and is characterized by postcoital or intermenstrual vaginal bleeding. The diagnosis is made on vaginal examination or at colposcopy, and confirmed by biopsy. Depending on the stage of the disease, treatment may be by radical pelvic surgery, by radiotherapy, or by a combination of the two.

Of all the gynaecological cancers, cervical cancer has the best chance of being prevented. Cervical smear screening programmes often detect the condition at a pre-invasive stage when good chances of cure can be offered. The benefits to the working woman of providing this examination at the workplace are obvious. Good communication between the screening doctor, the general practitioner, and the individual about normal as well as abnormal results avoids misunderstanding. If screening is not available at the workplace, the working woman should be allowed time off to have this done at a clinic, or by her GP. However, cervical screening at work remains a valuable adjunct to the NHS facilities for those women who are reticent to come forward for screening and usually have the highest risk of cancer and for whom the workplace is the ideal venue for the examination.

In 1984, a survey of companies offering cervical cytology was carried out by writing to Company Medical Officers. Some 435 companies replied, a 29 per cent response rate. Of the responding companies, 42 per cent undertook cervical cytology screening programmes and, in 78 per cent of these, this was done at the place of work either by the company occupational health service or using the mobile units of the Women's National Cancer Control Campaign. Some 49 per cent of the companies undertaking cervical cytology screening offered the test to all female employees, irrespective of age, at three-yearly intervals; 20 per cent five-yearly, and 10 per cent annually. The cost-effectiveness of such a threefold increased load on the screening service has not been proven.

## Cancer of the vulva

This disease occurs in an older age group (usually over 60 years). The diagnosis is confirmed by biopsy and then usually treated with radical surgery. The woman may expect to be off work for several months. The prognosis is generally good as this cancer is a slow-growing tumour, with good survival rates for those diagnosed early.

## Breast cancer

See Chapter 19 pp. 367.

# Contraception

Effective family planning is an essential part of any health care programme while uncontrolled fertility usually adds to the deprivation cycle. Contraceptive enquiries are frequent topics for occupational health practitioners in companies with a large female workforce.

## Oral contraceptives

Steroidal contraception with synthetic oestrogens and progesterones is the most common method among young women in the United Kingdom. There are three frequently used types of oral contraceptive pill: combined low dose, progesterone only, and triphasic. The newer progesterones, *gestodene, desogestrel,* and *norgestimate* have fewer side effects than *mestranol* and *norethisterone*, and have less effect on lipid metabolism.

The interaction of both combined and progesterone-only oral contraceptives with drugs that induce hepatic activity, e.g., *griseofulvin, phenytoin,* and *phenobarbitone* must be considered. Short-term courses of enzyme-inducing drugs require additional contraceptive precautions for at least 7 days after stopping the course, whereas a long-term course of an enzyme-inducing drug requires a higher dose oral contraceptive pill. Some broad spectrum antibiotics, such as *ampicillin,* may interfere with oestrogen absorption and extra protection is suggested. This may present as menstrual problems at work.

Low-dose pills have few side-effects and can be used by women well into their 40s unless there are specific contraindications. Manipulation of the menstrual cycle occasionally will help during travel, in certain work situations and in athletics. It is ideal advice to stop the pill at least 4–6 weeks *before* elective major surgery and up to about four weeks *after* an operation.

Injectable steroids such as *Depo-Provera* can be given 3-monthly; these are effective, although they can cause weight gain and irregularity of menstruation so that a third of users get episodes of amenorrhoea. Despite 10 million users of this method every year world-wide, there has been no reported increase in cancer of the breast, endometrium or cervix; fertility usually returns to normal within 6 months of the last injection.

## Post-coital contraception

Post-coital contraception can be given within 72 hours of unprotected intercourse using either two 12 hourly doses of 50 μg oestrogen pill or the woman can be immediately fitted with a coil; the latter works if inserted within 5 days of unprotected intercourse by preventing implantation. *Mifepristone* is also an effective post-coital contraceptive, given as a 600 mg dose up to 60 days gestation. For medicolegal reasons the woman should be seen 3 weeks later to make sure the method has been successful.

## Intrauterine devices

The intrauterine contraceptive devices (IUDs) come in either an inert form or in copper. Those in copper are usually used for 5 years but the inert ones remain effective for much longer. Failure rates of 2–4 per cent in a year's exposure are reported. The coil is best put in just after menstruation, at a termination, 6 weeks post-delivery or within 5 days of unprotected sexual intercourse. Perforation of the uterus may occur in 1 in 1000 users and 2 per cent of users will develop pelvic inflammation within a year of insertion, the risk being greater to nulliparas and to the young. If pregnancy occurs with an IUD in place, the risk of spontaneous abortion is higher due to infection and therefore early removal of the coil is advisable if the threads are accessible. The risk of ectopic pregnancy compared with intrauterine pregnancy is 1 in 30 in IUD users and 1 in 300 in non-IUD users.

## Other methods of contraception

Chemical barriers to sperm, condoms, and diaphragms are well-established methods and have slightly higher failure rates than the pill or IUDs, although they are still effective if properly used.

## Problems arising from contraception

Most women of reproductive age will be using some form of contraception; in the UK the most common method used by married couples is still the sheath and this has no medical complications.

Health problems may occur from complications of oral contraception, especially during travel and crossing time barriers. The oral contraceptive pill should be taken slightly earlier rather than slightly later when this is the case. All methods have beneficial and adverse side effects but the former usually outweigh the latter. Some women develop irregular bleeding while others may have nausea, swelling of the ankles due to water retention and, more seriously, deep-vein thromboses. The latter occur more in older women who are overweight and smoke.

Common complications of IUDs are intermenstrual bleeding or heavy periods, while a smaller proportion of users report increased dysmenorrhoea. The treatment is often removal of the IUD, while some who have heavier menstruation are helped by prostaglandin inhibitors and antifibrinolytic agents. Abdominal pain as a consequence of contraceptive devices may present at work. It may be due to an extruding coil which would require removal and ectopic pregnancy or painful pelvic inflammation may occur in a woman with an IUD.

## Sterilization

Sterilization is becoming more popular among women in some parts of the UK; about 12 per cent of both females and males attending a family planning clinic elect for this. Female sterilization is usually carried out through a laparoscope and the fallopian tube is either banded or clipped. This procedure causes the woman to be away from work for a few days only. A small number of women report heavier periods after the operation. This may settle down or may need further treatment as discussed in the section on menstrual disorders.

## Miscarriage

The exact incidence of spontaneous miscarriage is not known. Probably up to 50 per cent of fertilized ova either do not implant or do not develop while between 10 per cent and 20 per cent of women who realize they are pregnant undergo a miscarriage characterized by vaginal bleeding and lower abdominal cramping pains. This can be serious, because a small number of women still die from miscarriage. Treatment is often in hospital, with evacuation of the uterus. A woman who has had a miscarriage will probably return to work one week after the evacuation unless physical or psychological complications occur.

## Legal abortion

In the United Kingdom, over 180 000 women have a therapeutic termination of pregnancy each year. If this is done early (before 10–12 weeks' gestation) it is a simple operation, performed through the cervix, which involves the woman being off work for three or four days only. The psychological effects, however, may last longer. After 10–12 weeks' gestation, difficulties in performing a termination increase in parallel with the delay; some women will require 2–3 weeks off for a prostaglandin termination performed up to 20 weeks' gestation.

*Mifepristone* (RU486) is used as an oral method of termination of pregnancy in women who are less than 9 weeks pregnant. It is not very widely used within the UK but it does not need hospital admission. It involves taking tablets and in most cases, the embryo dies and is reabsorbed. There may be a lower emotional trauma rate than with surgical termination. There is only an occasional need (5 per cent) to evacuate the uterus for retained products.

## Prolapse and stress incontinence

After 40 years of age, many women who have had children may develop some weakness of the ligaments supporting the pelvic organs and develop a genital prolapse. Symptoms may be non-specific, such as backache or a low dragging pain in the lower pelvis; more specifically, there can be an associated involuntary loss of a little urine on sneezing or coughing (stress incontinence). The diagnosis is made by examination and assessment of the degree of laxity. A few women who are unfit, or those in the younger age group wishing for further pregnancies, may elect to try a vaginal pessary in an effort to compensate for the weakness. Such pessaries need changing at intervals and vaginal hygiene has to be strict. Occupational health staff may be of assistance in helping women to adjust to this and in advising on hygiene procedures; they may recommend that employees with prolapses should avoid jobs which involve heavy lifting or standing in one position for long periods.

More commonly, reparative surgery is performed to reduce and support the prolapse. A vaginal hysterectomy is sometimes required, but alternatively an anterior and posterior wall buttress operation will support the organs. These operations will involve the woman being off work for 6–12 weeks depending on the extent of surgery performed. On return to work she should be advised that, for about 3 months, she should avoid duties involving repetitive lifting, or standing in a fixed position without an opportunity to sit down periodically.

## Backache

Backache in women is not usually gynaecological but from ligamentous or muscular strain of the lower spine associated with activity at home or at work. The diagnosis must be considered with care and causes elucidated. See Chapter 9.

## Infertility

Infertility affects 10–15 per cent of couples in this country; in 40 per cent of those investigated a female cause is found, in a further 15 per cent there is a male cause, and among the rest, no cause is discovered. The female factors include blocked fallopian tubes and non-ovulation; in the male, there may be poor sperm production or an inability to maintain an erection. In others, sperm antibodies may be found which diminish sperm action after ejaculation.

Infertility does not produce physical symptoms but the emotional stress is considerable, particularly at the time of the monthly bleed, when the woman is often depressed and disappointed that no pregnancy has occurred. Infertility does not intrude on a woman's work physically, but the mental stress and the time off for the repeated and unpleasant investigations needed may affect work performance and come to the attention of the employer.

## The menopause

The menopause is the time when menstruation ceases, and the climacteric is the transitional period during which the woman's reproductive capacity ceases. The average age of the menopause has slowly increased since the mid 19th century so that in the United Kingdom it is now 50 years; this is concomitant with women's life expectancy increasing from 45 to 82 years of age. There are approximately 10 million post-menopausal women in the United Kingdom, many of them still at work. Often those who were part-time employees while their family was growing up return to full-time work at this age.

Symptoms of the menopause frequently begin before the cessation of menses. Interlinked groups of symptoms are:

*Vasomotor*: hot flushes and night sweats lead to insomnia and tiredness so affecting work during the day.

*Emotional*: lack of concentration, irritability, depression, and lability of mood can follow, and these also may affect work performance.

*Sexual symptoms*: decreased libido and dyspareunia may cause anxiety but do not relate to work directly.

*Urinary symptoms*: cause frequency and urgency which may be a problem in people who have to do long shifts, and those who are unable to have easy access to lavatories.

*Musculoskeletal*: laxity of ligaments and decreased muscular strength may predispose to aches and pains which affect any lifting or handling procedures.

The menopause can occur before the age of 40 following oophorectomy or from early ovarian failure, possibly due to auto-immune disease, to viral infections (e.g. mumps) or to cytotoxic drugs. These women have a greater predisposition to osteoporosis and hormone replacement therapy (HRT) should be considered where possible. Women who have had bilateral oophorectomy at the time of hysterectomy also require HRT. Symptoms of the menopause may be confused with those of other medical disorders such as hypothyroidism which should be excluded.

Psychological symptoms in perimenopausal women may be related to sleep disturbance while difficulty in making decisions and loss of confidence may be features of the menopause itself. These women are probably unsuited for shiftwork.

Although 70–85 per cent of women experience some climacteric symptoms, only 10 per cent seek advice. HRT relieves 85–100 per cent of the patient's symptoms. However, compliance is poor after one year.

As well as treating the acute symptoms of hormonal withdrawal, oestrogen replacement protects against osteoporosis and reduces the risk of coronary heart disease. HRT has a beneficial effect on the rate of fatal and non-fatal myocardial infarction in post-menopausal women halving the relative risk, and probably producing a similar benefit in cardiovascular disease. In addition, oestrogens maintain skin collagen and therefore offer protection against varicose ulceration. Oestrogens are more beneficial than calcium chloride, thiazide diuretics or vitamin D, in conserving bone and preventing fractures. In women who have not had a hysterectomy, it is important that cyclical progesterone therapy is given for the latter 7 days of every month to prevent endometrial hyperplasia. This, however, will mean she will continue to have a monthly bleed and this may prove unwelcome. The new hormonal preparations which do not cause monthly bleeding will, it is hoped, improve compliance.

Contraindications to HRT are breast cancer and other oestrogen-dependent tumours, and severe liver disease. Oestrogen replacement can be given as oral therapy, implants, vaginal pessaries, or transdermal therapy. For those women who feel that the continuing repeated menstrual bleed is no longer acceptable, low-dose hormone replacement may be prescribed where no obvious endometrial proliferation occurs.

The progestogenic component can cause symptoms similar to the premenstrual syndrome such as irritability, mood swings, and weight gain and there is often a high drop-out rate from treatment where this occurs. It also reduces some of the protective effects of oestrogen on coronary heart disease by countering the lowering of high density lipoprotein (HDL) and cholesterol levels.

## Selected references and further reading

1. Chamberlain, G. (1984). Women at work in pregnancy. In *Pregnant women at work,* (ed. G. Chamberlain), pp. 3–13. Royal Society of Medicine and Macmillan, London.
2. Mamelle, N., and Laumon, B. (1984). Occupational fatigue and preterm birth. In *Pregnant women at work,* (ed. G. Chamberlain), pp. 105–15. Royal Society of Medicine and Macmillan, London.
3. Schnoor, T.M.I. *et al.* (1991). Video display terminals and risk of spontaneous abortion. *New Engl. J. Med.*, **324,** 727–33.
4. Roman, E. (1992). Spontaneous abortion and working with VDUs. *Brit. J. Indust. Med.*, **49,** 507–17.
5. Blackwell, R. and Chang, A. (1988). Video display terminals and pregnancy—A review. *Brit. J. Obstet. Gyn.*, **95,** 446–53.
6. Naeye, R.L. (1978). Effects of maternal cigarette smoking on fetus and placenta. *Brit. J. Obstet. Gyn.*, **85,** 732–7.
7. Buncher, C.R. (1969). Cigarette smoking and duration of pregnancy. *Amer. J. Obest. Gyn.*, **103,** 942–6.
8. Evans, D.R., Newcombe, R.G., and Campbell, H. (1979). Maternal smoking habits and congenital malformations. *Brit. Med. J.*, **2,** 171–3.

9. Royal College of Physicians (1992). *Smoking and the young.* Royal College of Physicians, London.
10. Armstrong, B.G., Nolin, A.D., and McDonald, A.D. (1989). Work in pregnancy and birth weight for gestational age. *Brit. J. Ind. Med.*, **46,** 196–9.
11. Blond, J.P. (1990). Semen quality and sex hormones amongst steel and stainless steel welders. *Brit. J. Indust. Med.*, **47,** 508–14.
12. Stirrat, G.S. (1987). Pelvic infections. In *Aids to obstetrics and gynaecology,* (2nd edn), Churchill Livingstone, Edinburgh.

# 19

# Surgery

*D.P. Manning and I. McColl*

## Introduction

There is no general agreement amongst surgeons about the time interval between operation, ambulation, hospital discharge, and return to employment, but the trend towards early activity continues. During World War II an army order decreed that all patients must be kept in bed for 21 days after inguinal herniorrhaphy,[1] but by the 1950s early ambulation had become popular. Advances in laparoscopic and electrocautery surgery, the removal of kidney stones by lithotripsy, together with day case surgery, are now contributing to rapid recovery and early return to work. Hernia repairs, appendicectomy, and cholecystectomy can all be performed through an endoscope thereby reducing the size of incisions and the amount of post-operative pain. The Royal College of Surgeons lists hernioplasty and laparoscopy amongst operations suitable for day case surgery and states that up to 50 per cent of elective surgery could be performed on a day case basis.[2] In suitable patients, laparoscopic cholecystectomy can also be done as a day case. Some surgeons have predicted that within the next five years 80–90 per cent of abdominal surgery will be carried out laparoscopically.

The most recent statistics on the numbers of surgical operations quoted below refer to surgical practice in England during the year 1989–90.[3] There were 3.276 million ordinary hospital operations and 1.032 million day case operations. During the next decade the number of day case procedures is likely to move steadily towards 50 per cent of surgical admissions and an increasing number of operations will be performed through an endoscope. All these advances in treatment methods will gradually reduce the time taken to recover from surgery and facilitate earlier return to work.

## Abdominal and hernia operations

Every year more than a quarter of a million patients require advice about the degrees of activity and exertion which may safely be undertaken during convalescence following surgery and many of them need guidance on the length of absence from work and on the type of work compatible with their surgical operations.

Factors which influence return to work after abdominal and hernia surgery are discussed below

## Wound strength

Since 1945, the Shouldice Clinic in Toronto has advocated early post-operative activity, and in 1972 Iles described the procedure followed for 75 000 abdominal herniorrhaphies.[4] Repairs were carried out under local anaesthesia and patients were discharged from hospital 72 hours later and advised to resume immediately any activities they could carry out in reasonable comfort. By the fourth week, the most strenuous activity was permitted, including piano-moving. The Shouldice technique consists of a double-breasted repair of the fascia transversalis, followed by a Bassini-type procedure using a continuous suture. Glassow[5] reported in 1984 that survivors to 10 years whose hernia had been repaired by a consultant using this technique had a 99 per cent expectation that the hernia will remain sound. Use of non-absorbable sutures is essential for early ambulation and also for early return to work.

A study of wound healing revealed that wound strength was 70 per cent of normal immediately after operation, provided that non-absorbable sutures were used, whereas scar tissue strength improved slowly and after 8 weeks was only 41 per cent of normal.[6] Three further studies in the literature confirm that return to any kind of employment one month after an operation for unilateral inguinal hernia does not increase the risk of a recurrence. Laparoscopic repair of inguinal hernias was introduced in 1990 and involves stapling mesh over the internal surface of the inguinal region. As this produces far less damage of tissue with no suturing or tension, post-operative pain is minimal and the patient returns to work within a week. The results of long-term follow-up are awaited to see if laparoscopic repair will rival the recurrence rate of less than 1 per cent of the Shouldice repair. (Advice to patients is discussed on p. 359.)

## Size and location of scar

A small scar from a gridiron incision for appendicectomy can be expected to reach maximum strength quickly due to the crossing layers of the abdominal wall. A paramedian incision, in which the rectus abdominis muscle is sandwiched between two layers of connective tissue, may also be expected to heal soundly with more strength than midline abdominal scars. Transverse or oblique incisions involve fewer nerve segments, even though muscle is divided, and are therefore less painful. A midline incision through the linea alba leaves a weak scar, but current surgical practice is to use a continuous nylon suture four times the length of the wound, with 2 cm bites, and this technique reduces the incidence of incisional hernia to the same order as that for paramedian incisions. Laparoscopy wounds do not significantly weaken the abdominal wall and rarely cause herniation except at the umbilicus where hernia may occur in 1–2 per cent unless sutured with suture material which lasts for three months.

## Wound dehiscence

Partial or complete disruption of the deeper layers of a wound can occur in the early post-operative period and may be symptomless. Unless the wound is immediately re-sutured an incisional hernia will develop and seriously prejudice the permanent strength of the abdominal wall (see p. 361).

## Wound infection/haematoma

Superficial wound infection should not weaken the wound, but infection of the deep fascia and lower layers of the wound will delay healing and may lead to permanent weakness and recurrence. A haematoma of the deep layers of a wound also delays healing.

## Persistent pain or paraesthesia

Pain and tenderness in the scar or paraesthesia or hypoaesthesia usually resolve rapidly following most surgical operations. Transverse abdominal incisions which divide few sensory nerves are the least painful in the post-operative period, whereas vertical incisions dividing numerous nerve branches are more painful. Operations for inguinal hernia sometimes divide or trap the scrotal branch of the ilioinguinal nerve and cause pain or hypoaesthesia which may delay a return to full activity. Some occupations involve leaning across benches or against machine guards, and tenderness of abdominal scars may delay a return to work.

### Occupation

In many occupations the intra-abdominal pressure arising from exertion and the forces applied to the scar by muscular contraction are unlikely to exceed the forces generated by normal physiological functions such as defecation and coughing. In occupations which involve manual handling of loads or other forms of muscular effort, the force applied to the scar will be considerable.

### Advice to patients

The most important factor determining the interval between surgical treatment and return to work is motivation. Some patients who have a keen interest in their work or career, or who cannot afford to lose money, will return to work very soon after an operation, sometimes on the next day. Others are more cautious and may appreciate professional advice; some will require persuasion. In practice, most patients will delay their return to work until it suits them, but pre-operative advice is important in determining not only length of stay, but also time off work. For instance, if a patient is told that the operation will require 3 days inpatient treatment he or she will be champing at the bit if kept any longer. Conversely, if told beforehand that the expected length of stay in hospital is 10 days, the patient will be disgruntled if discharged after 3 days. The same principle applies to time off work, and **much unnecessary absence from work could be avoided by counselling patients appropriately before their operation about expected time off work.**

The following guidelines are proposed. It should be borne in mind throughout that, except where complications are mentioned, they refer to patients who have made a normal recovery. Surgeons may sometimes deviate from these guidelines because of strong personal preferences or variations in surgical technique.

## Unilateral inguinal herniorrhaphy and epigastric hernia operations

More than 76 000 inguinal hernias are repaired annually.[3]

The two long-term studies by Bourke *et al.*[7] and Taylor and Dewar[8] recommended a return to full activity and normal work within 28 and 21 days respectively. A leading article in the *Lancet* in 1985[9] stated that 'we should therefore recommend return to work within two weeks for sedentary workers and after four weeks for those in more strenuous occupations', but 'any physical activity that causes pain should be avoided'. Since most surgeons now use a nylon darn or a Bassini-type operation for repair of inguinal herniae, these recommendations are reasonable and evidence from the Shouldice Clinic[4] is most convincing that any occupation may be resumed safely after four weeks. Patients should be advised not to drive for two weeks following inguinal herniorrhaphy, as they may be slower to operate the brake due to wound discomfort.

## Bilateral inguinal hernia operations

A prospective study of bilateral inguinal hernia repair concluded that simultaneous repair of bilateral hernias can be carried out with no greater morbidity than a unilateral repair and the return to normal activity is as rapid: hernias should be repaired simultaneously rather than sequentially.[10] Most patients after laparoscopic hernia repair return to work within a week.

### Reassurance

It is traditional for some doctors to recommend a period off work of up to three months, and of light work for 3–6 months, following operations for inguinal hernia. However, there is no evidence of clinical benefit from such a prolonged period of inactivity, and patients should be reassured that they are not increasing the risk of recurrence, or of other complications arising, if they return to normal work after a shorter interval. Patients who have residual discomfort in the scar due to peripheral nerve involvement will need an explanation and reassurance that the discomfort can be ignored.

**Femoral hernia operations/uncomplicated appendicectomy with gridiron incision**

More than 51 000 appendices are removed and 6000 femoral hernias repaired annually.[3]

The majority of patients should be able to resume sedentary work after two weeks, and heavy occupations after three weeks.

**Umbilical hernia operations**

The period of restriction tends to be longer and may be extended to three months for a large umbilical hernia.

**Hernia scars weakened by infection or haematoma**

The scar may be permanently weakened and healing will certainly be delayed. Those employed in heavy occupations or indulging in strenuous leisure pursuits should be advised to avoid heavy exertion if they wish to reduce the risk of developing a hernia, but for those who must return to heavy work there appears to be no advantage in reducing activity more than three months from the time of operation.

**Operations for recurrent inguinal hernia**

A second repair of an inguinal hernia is less likely to produce a sound scar than the primary repair. Patients will also be more reluctant to risk a further recurrence due to heavy exertion. There is no reason why the patient should remain inactive during the post-operative period, but he should be advised against heavy exertion for a period of three months.

Recurrent hernias are best treated laparoscopically and the return to work is usually after two weeks.

**Operations for incisional hernia**

Incisional hernias vary in size. Return to a sedentary occupation should be possible within two weeks following repair of the smallest hernias, and to more strenuous occupations after six weeks. Repair of a large incisional hernia is unlikely to achieve sufficient strength to withstand heavy manual exertion and there will remain a high probability of further breakdown of the scar. Heavy exertion should, ideally, be avoided permanently and return to manual work delayed for three months. Use of a suitable corset, however, can give some protection for those who must undertake heavy exertion.

## Cholecystectomy and cholecystitis

More than 32 000 gall bladders are removed annually in England.[3]

Endoscopic cholecystectomy is rapidly replacing the traditional operation through a Kocher's incision, both for elective removal of gallstones and for acute cholecystitis.[11] Recovery is rapid and the patient is able to return to normal activity within a few days of surgery. The traditional transabdominal approach leaves a painful wound which restricts activity for about six weeks and most patients would remain absent from work during this time; those in heavy manual occupations may not be able to resume work for three months from the time of operation.

Acute cholecystitis usually resolves in several weeks and a period of convalescence of two weeks may be required before the patient returns to work. Endoscopic cholecystectomy in the acute phase is being carried out in many centres and appears to shorten the period of recovery. There are reports of patients returning to work within 21 days after operation.

## Operations on the stomach and duodenum

There are about 13 000 open operations yearly on the stomach and duodenum.[3]

Operation wounds usually become pain-free within a month, enabling patients to resume employment, with progression to heavy manual work within three months. Following partial gastrectomy small frequent meals are necessary and patients must take regular meal-breaks. Shiftworkers should remain on regular days for a few weeks or longer if any digestive symptoms occur. This is not an absolute requirement for all patients as there are those who obtain more rest during daylight hours.

## Post-gastrectomy syndromes

Post-operative abdominal and vasomotor symptoms are seen in the majority of patients following gastric surgery, but they usually diminish with time. Early symptoms occurring shortly after a meal may persist in 5–12 per cent of patients, who must be able to eat small meals separate from drinks, and this may require concessions by management when the patient returns to work. Patients should also avoid sugar. Late symptoms occurring about two hours after a meal are treated by taking food, and here too, when the patient returns to work he or she must be able to obtain food when required. Following gastric surgery it is common for patients to lose weight and to suffer from nutritional disturbances which may limit their capacity for physically strenuous work. Placement in alternative, less active work is sometimes desirable.

## Resection of the colon and other major abdominal operations

At least 36 000 resections and other major abdominal operations are performed each year.[3]

The recommendations are similar to those for conventional cholecystectomy, viz., a return to sedentary occupations in six weeks, with a maximum of three months avoidance of heavy exertion in manual occupations. Alteration of bowel function, causing more frequent bowel actions, sometimes requires immediate access to a toilet which should be taken into consideration. This applies especially to low rectal anastomoses and operations in which the ileocaecal valve has been removed and to extensive intestinal resection for Crohn's disease and other pathology which also frequently results in malabsorption and loss of weight. Nevertheless, working capacity may be retained in half of the patients. Permanent colostomy is discussed in Chapter 13 (p. 254).

## Pancreatitis

The course is so variable that each patient needs individual assessment.

### Patients waiting for operations

Patients waiting for surgery may be receiving treatment and may be unfit for work due to the symptoms of the illness. Those waiting for hernia repair or for cholecystectomy, however, will usually be capable of attending work. In the early stages, during the development of an inguinal hernia, patients may experience aching discomfort due to stretching of tissue as the hernia enlarges, and symptoms are increased by exertion. During this time the patient may be able to attend work if he can avoid manual exertion and excessive walking. As the hernia enlarges, symptoms may disappear and a return to any kind of work is possible, although it is usual to avoid heavy work while waiting for operation. The patient should be warned, however, that if pain occurs in the hernia or abdomen, he should immediately lie down and reduce the hernia. If this is not possible or if the pain continues, medical advice must be obtained without delay. A truss is an acceptable aid to some patients waiting for repair of an inguinal hernia.

## Anal region and pilonidal sinus

### Incidence of operations

There are more than 53 000 operations per year including 7500 for pilonidal sinus and 27 000 for haemorrhoids.

### Haemorrhoids

Perianal haematoma has been described as the five-day painful self-curing lesion of Milligan, and most patients present after a week and need no treatment. Discomfort is increased by walking and sitting on hard surfaces. Absence from work is usually not justified, but alternative employment may be necessary for a few days.

*Prolapsing internal haemorrhoids* may cause disability. Symptoms usually can be relieved by immediate reduction, but if strangulation and/or thrombosis occur the patient will be unable to attend work. A diet with increased roughage will reduce the incidence of symptoms.

Patients who suffer from recurrent prolapse of piles often assume that the condition will be aggravated by sitting on hard or warm surfaces. They should be reassured that their fears are groundless.

### Operative treatment

Most prolapsing internal haemorrhoids are treated in outpatients using rubber band ligation, or injection. However, some patients require admission for day case surgery including dilatation under general anaesthesia. These treatments cause little post-operative discomfort and the patient can return to any form of employment next day. Those requiring general anaesthesia may be unable to work for two or three days and should be advised not to drive for 48 hours. Following haemorrhoidectomy, the patient should be able to return to work without a restriction on activity or exertion after two or three weeks. A high roughage diet and administration of stool softeners will expedite recovery.

### Ischiorectal abscess and perianal abscess

Following surgery, symptoms should rapidly disappear and return to work will be determined by availability of dressing facilities. If there is an occupational health unit at the place of work, the patient could be referred there by letter for wound dressing. Otherwise a return to work should be postponed until the patient can cope with wound treatment. In occupations involving prolonged sitting, the patient should be advised to sit on a soft foam pad.

### Fissure-in-ano and fistula-in-ano

Following anal dilatation or lateral partial internal sphincterotomy, the patient will be able to return to work within two or three days. Occasionally there may be temporary impaired control of faeces or flatus which would delay the return to work.

Most fistulae are low and patients can return to work in a week or two after operation. Earlier return may be possible if dressing facilities are available at work. Higher fistulae will need a much longer period of absence from work.

### Pilonidal sinus

There is no ideal treatment. About half of all cases present with an abscess which is treated by incision, curettage, and drainage. Complete healing occurs within a month but 40 per cent of patients will require further treatment of a sinus. Sinuses treated by phenol injection or by laying-open will probably heal within one to two months. Excision with primary closure may be followed by healing within two weeks whereas healing takes two to three months after excision and laying-open.[12] It is possible for well-motivated patients to return to work quite soon after laying-open and dressing facilities at work would assist. Patients treated by primary closure return to work earlier, sometimes within three weeks of operation; six to seven weeks is more usual. Pressure over the coccyx should be avoided by sitting on a soft foam pad.

# Arterial system

## Incidence of cardiovascular operations

At least 25 500 open heart operations are performed annually including 11 400 coronary artery bypass grafts.

## Heart valve surgery

Between 65 and 80 per cent of patients resume work after heart valve surgery. The avoidance of lengthy sick leave by operation at an early stage in the disease has been shown to improve the quality of life and the rate of return to work.

## Coronary artery angioplasty and bypass surgery

The dilatation of narrowed coronary arteries by an inflatable balloon catheter (angioplasty) is now an established method of treatment for coronary artery disease. Compared to the bypass operation, angioplasty has the advantage of a shorter hospital stay, earlier return to work, and lower psychological stress.

A randomized intervention trial comparing coronary angioplasty (percutaneous transluminal coronary angioplasty or PTCA) with coronary artery bypass grafting (CABG) (1993)[13] found that one month after treatment the PTCA patients had higher mean exercise times, were more physically active and had less coronary related unemployment than CABG patients. Recovery after CABG takes longer than after PTCA but the latter patients required more supplementary revascularization procedures, had more repeat diagnostic arteriography, and more myocardial infarctions than CABG patients. After one year the mean exercise times of both groups had increased by three minutes. Mortality in the two groups was not significantly different. Patients will be followed-up for three years.

Following coronary artery bypass surgery for more extensive artery disease, between 47 and 79 per cent resume work in two months to one year after operation. In most studies more than 65 per cent eventually resume work. Up to 97 per cent returned to work in low exertion jobs in one series but only 47 per cent in high exertion jobs.[14]

Permanent unemployment after operation is more likely for patients having lengthy sick leave prior to operation and for those with persistent angina.

There is some evidence that: (a) vocational counselling by an occupational physician; and (b) rehabilitation including exercise between 2 and 6 months from the time of operation, both benefit the patients and may improve the prospect of resuming work. (See also Chapter 14.)

## Cardiac transplantation

The numbers of successful heart transplant operations is steadily increasing and many patients are able to resume work. In one series of 250 patients 45 per cent were employed and most had returned to their previous occupation.[15]

Following any heart surgery patients may be anxious that physical activity and exertion could be harmful. Clear advice from the surgeons about suitable exercise and the type of employment which may safely be undertaken will help to reassure patients and encourage early return to full employment.

## Aortic aneurysm

It is possible for patients in sedentary occupations to continue in employment while waiting for surgery, providing they are well, blood pressure is controlled, and they avoid driving. Those employed on manual tasks which might raise blood pressure should not work.

## Aortic grafts and aorto-iliac grafts

Patients should avoid all physical exertion for four weeks and be able to return to sedentary work after six weeks and any other work after three months.

The results of aorto-iliac grafts are excellent and should enable the patient to return to any form of employment. However, there may be a restriction on activity due to the underlying arterial disease. Cessation of smoking, control of weight, and blood pressure, and a healthy low-fat diet are thought to improve the prospects for a full recovery.

## Femoro-popliteal grafts

Patients with ischaemic limbs may be saved from amputation by a femoro-popliteal graft. The results of surgery are less successful than for aorto-iliac grafts, but patients may be able to resume sedentary work in four weeks, and more active occupations in 12 weeks, depending on the symptoms and the degree of atherosclerosis affecting other organs. They should not return to occupations involving crouching and repetitive knee flexing.

### Carotid stenosis

Ability to work is liable to be determined by the underlying arterial disease and residual symptoms. Recovery from surgical operations on the internal carotid artery should be complete in four or five weeks.

### Further care after cardiovascular surgery

Drug therapy to prevent potential complications following cardiovascular surgery is often required. This may include anticoagulant therapy to prevent emboli, antibiotics to prevent the infection of grafts, and immunosuppressive drugs following transplantation procedures. Such therapy is not incompatible with most types of work though the employee may need to take short absences from work to attend special clinics for the monitoring and adjustment of dosage.

Driving is not contraindicated in these patients provided that cardiovascular function is acceptable. Although strenuous exertion may need to be avoided on immediate return to work, these patients will all benefit from moderate exercise and they should not be unduly restricted. Those on immunosuppressive drugs should not be employed in areas where exposure to infection is likely.

## Breast

During 1989–90 there were about 11 000 breast excisions and 61 000 other breast operations.[3]

### Biopsy and surgery for innocent cysts and swellings

Lumpectomy together with chemotherapy and radiotherapy have drastically reduced the number of total breast excisions.

Aspiration of cysts need not lead to absence from work, but operations involving an incision may require an absence of a few days.

### Simple mastectomy

Following simple mastectomy, the principal obstacle to resuming normal activity and work is motivation. It is usually in the patient's best interest to return to work as soon as the wound is healed. Breast reconstruction or fitting a prosthesis immediately after the operation will assist the patient to adjust to the disfigurement.

Evidence for the beneficial effect of psychological support is growing. Weekly group therapy with self-hypnosis for pain relief and psychological support by a well-trained nurse, have been shown to assist social recovery and return to work.[16]

Following simple mastectomy, it is common for a serous discharge to drain from the wound for up to one week or more. Patients should be warned about this, provided with suitable dressings and reassured that it has no serious import.

### Radical mastectomy

Radical mastectomy is not often undertaken now, but the operation sometimes leads to oedema of the arm and shoulder stiffness which may interfere with employment. Patients will usually require a period of absence extending to at least two months.

### Radiotherapy

Radiotherapy and adjuvant therapy with either endocrine or cytotoxic drugs, are likely to delay a return to full-time or part-time work owing to systemic disturbance.

## Genito-urinary tract

More than 120 000 major open operations are performed together with 50 000 endoscopic operations on the prostate and 5000 lithotripsy procedures.[3]

### Shock-wave lithotripsy

Major surgery to remove kidney stones is being superseded by ultrasonic shock-wave destruction of stones. Patients are treated as day cases or may be admitted for one or two days. Fragments of stones are usually passed completely within three months but additional surgical procedures are required in about 8 per cent of patients.[17] The majority return to normal work within two weeks. The traditional surgical operation usually leads to an absence of about eight weeks.

### Nephrectomy

Patients frequently complain of discomfort in the scar which is aggravated by bending and twisting movements. A return to clerical-type work should be possible within six weeks, but avoidance of repetitive stooping and heavy lifting for a further period of six weeks would be reasonable in some manual occupations.

Patients having lost one kidney are anxious about possible injury to the remaining kidney. In practice the risk of injury to a kidney at work is remote.

Patients can be reassured that loss of a kidney does not prevent manual work in any occupation (Chapter 16).

Laparoscopic nephrectomy is being carried out in some centres and results in much less morbidity.

### Prostatectomy

Following transurethral prostatectomy patients usually leave hospital within a week and will require at least a similar period of convalescence before resuming work. The chief consideration regarding return to work is adequate control of micturition and ready access to a toilet. The type of work is of less importance.

### Testicular torsion

The patient will be able to return to any kind of work when scar tenderness settles, usually within two weeks.

### Hydrocoele

Aspiration treatment should not lead to absence from work. Following operation the scar will be tender, which will reduce activity for one or two weeks.

### Orchidectomy

Orchidectomy should only require a reduction in activities, such as walking, until tenderness has diminished to an acceptable level—possibly a week or so. Treatment of the underlying disease, e. g., by cytotoxic drugs or radiotherapy, may delay return to work.

### Vasectomy

One study showed that 46 per cent of patients do not lose time from work following vasectomy, and the percentage could be much higher if the operation is performed on a Friday.[18] Those who were absent lost an average of 5.12 days. It is possible that patients with more active manual occupations find it necessary to take time off work. The occurrence of a haematoma or of infection may require an absence of 10 days.

## Head and neck

During 1989–90 there were 10 000 thyroid operations and at least 306 000 other operations excluding eye and dental operations, on the head and neck.[3]

## Thyroidectomy

Patients usually make a rapid recovery from thyroidectomy, but convalescence may be prolonged if the patient previously had hyperthyroidism, especially if there have been symptoms of cardiac involvement. Most patients will be capable of normal work after two weeks, with a further restriction on heavy physical exertion for two months in all.

## Operations on the salivary glands

Removal of stones from the ducts of salivary glands causes few operative problems, and patients should be capable of any type of work within two weeks.

## Operations for malignant tumours

Depending on the site of the malignancy there is likely to be disfigurement and disability. Radical surgery for tumours of the sinuses and mandible are especially disfiguring and early fitting of a prosthesis is highly beneficial. Reconstructive surgery by skin and muscle flap grafts are major advances in cosmetic rehabilitation. Radical neck dissection to remove tumour and lymphatic tissue may cause persistent shoulder pain and many patients in manual occupations are forced to give up work, especially if the accessory nerve is divided. Patients in non-manual occupations should be able to return to work.

Excision of laryngeal tumours causes partial or complete loss of voice which may damage promotion prospects in some occupations. Re-acquisition of speech has been shown to be an important factor for employment. Laryngectomy is usually performed on patients in their late 50s or older; nevertheless 24 of 62 patients returned to competitive employment in one series.[19]

The surgical formation of a fistula between the oesophagus and the trachea together with the insertion of a stomal valve (speech button) enable the patient to force a greater volume of air into the oesophagus and up to 90 per cent of patients achieve fluent speech. Dedicated and well-trained staff are required to provide a speech button maintenance service.[20]

## Craniotomy and operations on the circle of Willis

There are about 11 000 intracranial operations per annum, including 1400 on brain aneurysms and arteries.[3]

## Subarachnoid haemorrhage and operations to clip a berry aneurysm

Disability following surgical treatment varies considerably. There may be residual neurological disability from the haemorrhage or from the surgery. This varies from minor symptoms from which the patients may recover in a few weeks to more serious disability, but most patients will require lengthy rehabilitation. A minimum absence of two months is to be expected.

Successful operations to clip the aneurysm will eliminate the need for any restriction on physical activity, but for a period of some two years the safety of the patient should be considered as there is an increased risk of an epileptic seizure. Employers should be advised that the patient could fall without warning and should not, therefore, work at heights, work with unguarded moving machinery, or drive vehicles during this period.

On returning to work, patients with a post-operative skull defect who are liable to strike their heads against structures may require protection in the form of a padded cap or safety helmet.

### Operations on the middle and inner ear

Operations to control infection of the middle ear or to close perforations of the tympanic membrane are normally followed by a resumption of work in about two weeks but dressing facilities may be required and patients will not be able to wear ear protection in a noisy environment until healing is complete; avoidance of a hearing hazard is essential. Operations on the inner ear may be followed by disability lasting from weeks to several months. Patients have to avoid noise and hazardous situations in which loss of balance might lead to injury. For example, patients should not climb, drive, or work near moving parts of machines if unsteady. Hearing protection is necessary when resuming work in a noisy environment. Ear muffs or plugs can be worn when there is no longer any risk of introducing or aggravating infection but advice from the surgeon is essential.

# Ingrowing toenails

### Treatment of ingrowing toenails

There are over 23 000 admissions per annum for nail operations.[3]

Ingrowing toenails lead to a great deal of needless absence from work; absence for more than 24 hours is quite unnecessary for the majority of these patients. Symptoms are relieved almost immediately by excising a triangle of nail where it is irritating the nail fold; avulsion of the nail causes tenderness of the nail bed and absence from work of at least one week. Recurrent ingrowing toenails requiring additional treatment, such as cryotherapy or excision of a strip of nail and ablation of a small piece of the nail bed with phenol, justify an absence of a few days until tenderness has cleared and the wound is healing. Complete removal of the nail bed requires an absence of at least two weeks and probably longer for patients whose work involves much walking.

# Thorax

More than 29 000 surgical procedures per annum involve opening the chest. They include 11 000 coronary bypass grafts and 3000 excisions of lung.[3]

## Thoracotomy scars

Incisions for pulmonary operations usually follow the dermatome, but injury to the sensory branches of intercostal nerves sometimes leaves residual tenderness and paraesthesia which may interfere with employment. An explanation of the cause of symptoms should help to convince the patient that there is no need to restrict activity or avoid heavy exertion.

## Partial and total pneumonectomy

In addition to symptoms from scar tissue, exercise tolerance may be limited, particularly following total pneumonectomy. Pneumonectomy is commonly undertaken in middle life or in older persons whose pulmonary reserve has already been compromised by smoking. Dyspnoea at rest or on very slight exertion will prevent travel to work or any physical activity. Nevertheless, a long-term study in the Netherlands revealed that of 37 male pneumonectomy patients 14 resumed full-time work and 9 part-time work.[21] Patients have a better prospect of re-employment following partial pneumonectomy. The minimum period of absence is likely to be two months, extending to six months for the most disabled.

## Hiatus hernia and reflux oesophagitis

Although as many as 1 in 14 of the population may have heartburn from reflux oesophagitis only 5 per cent of patients referred to hospital need surgery.

Patients waiting for operation should be able to attend work providing that there is no requirement to stoop to waist level or lower; symptoms are aggravated by reflux of acid while stooping. In those who fail to respond to medical treatment surgery will usually eliminate the symptoms from reflux. The surgery may involve an abdominal incision or a thoracotomy. A minimum absence of six weeks is to be anticipated for sedentary workers and up to three months for manual workers (see also Chapter 13) Laparoscopic fundoplication has greatly reduced morbidity and patients can leave hospital after two days and return to work in a week or two.

## Operations on the oesophagus

Operations on the oesophagus will usually require a transthoracic approach, and the factors described on p. 372 may apply. Post-operative disability depends on the extent of the operation and will be maximal following resection of a carcinoma. This usually entails a combined abdominal and thoracic approach, and may involve radiotherapy. Very few patients will return to work. After a laparoscopic Heller's operation for achalasia the patient can leave hospital in two days and return to work in a week or two.

## Spontaneous pneumothorax

Following spontaneous pneumothorax the patient is advised to avoid exertion for at least two weeks to allow full expansion of the lung. A further period of restriction is sensible to permit sound healing of the defect. An absence of six weeks would be reasonable for manual workers. Recurrent pneumothorax will require a longer period of protection from heavy physical activity, for up to 12 months, and operative intervention may be indicated. Factors discussed on p. 301 may apply following operation. There are particular restrictions on divers and hyperbaric workers (see Appendix 4).

## Varicose veins and venous thrombosis

Over 47 000 varicose vein operations are performed annually.[3]

### Varicose veins

There is no general agreement about the symptomatology of varicose veins, but patients frequently complain of aching legs. They should be reassured that walking and general activity is beneficial to the circulation; muscular movement in the leg helps to empty the veins. Conversely, standing still or sitting still may increase symptoms, but there are few occupations in which a person stands still; any movement of the feet is beneficial. Elastic stockings may be preferable or supplementary to operative treatment. Thus, there is no need for patients to lose time from work while waiting for hospital assessment or treatment.

Patients who are liable to strike their legs against objects at work should wear a protective covering to prevent haemorrhage from rupture of a varicose vein. They should also be instructed that bleeding from a ruptured varicose vein is easily stopped by raising the leg and the application of gentle pressure over a clean dressing.

### Injection of varicose veins

Following injection of a sclerosing agent, the patient is usually advised to walk at least 5 kilometres a day, hence there is no reason to lose time from work. Nevertheless, a study in 1972 revealed that the average number of days absence from work following injection was 6.4.[22]

### Operations on varicose veins

Scars sometimes remain tender for several weeks, but most patients should be able to return to work within 14 days, and 90 per cent within three weeks. The average number of days lost from work in the study mentioned above was 31.3.[22] Stripping of varicose veins is much less popular now. Simple ligation of perforators and avulsion of small veins is now preferred.

### Superficial thrombophlebitis

A small area of thrombophlebitis may be treated while the patient attends work, but if there is evidence of spread the patient should rest at home while undergoing treatment. It would be unusual to lose more than two weeks from work unless ligation of the vein is required; in such circumstances an absence of one month may be necessary, with the possibility of some restriction on walking until tenderness resolves.

### Deep vein thrombosis (phlebothrombosis) and white leg

Thrombosis of the deep veins has far more serious implications. Initially, the patient will require observation and anticoagulant treatment for a minimum of four weeks before returning to work in order to permit stabilization of the prothrombin level, but the period of disability is liable to be greater. Persistent swelling of the leg, even with an elastic support, is likely to limit the amount of walking, although patients do need to exercise the leg as much as possible. Those employed in occupations requiring continuous walking may need alternative work. Similarly, prolonged standing is not practicable. Patients receiving continuous anticoagulation treatment should be instructed on methods of stopping bleeding should they receive an open wound at work.

### Ulceration of the lower leg

Although this is mainly a problem with the elderly, some employed persons may suffer from a leg ulcer. The first essential is to prevent trauma to the leg in those with venous insufficiency as a minor blow may precipitate an ulcer. Treatment of an ulcer in an occupational health department is quite feasible if staff are provided with dressings and advice on the recommended method of treatment. The patient should be encouraged to continue wearing an elastic stocking in order to help prevent a recurrence.

## Pulmonary embolism

The size of an embolism will be the chief determinant of disability. Small infarcts heal with no long-term disability. Large infarcts may limit exercise tolerance and possibly lead to persistent pleural pains and prolonged absence from work.

## Axillary vein thrombosis

Axillary vein thrombosis is rare, but may cause prolonged disability due to swelling of the limb, with associated clumsiness of movement. Patients will usually be reluctant to use the arm, fearing that exercise may cause a relapse. Following the initial period of treatment, normal use of the arm should be encouraged, while avoiding situations which would apply pressure to the axilla.

## Selected references and further reading

1. Farquharson, E.L. (1955). Early ambulation with special reference to herniorrhaphy as an outpatient procedure. *Lancet*, **2,** 517–9.
2. Royal College of Surgeons (March 1992). *Report of the working party on guidelines for day case surgery,* (rev. edn). Royal College of Surgeons, London.
3. DOH (Department of Health). *Hospital episode statistics,* Vol. 1. Finished consultant episodes by diagnosis, operation and specialty. England: Financial year 1989–90. (ISBN 1 85839 100 8.) DOH, London.
4. Iles, J.D.H. (1972). Convalescence after herniorrhaphy. *JAMA,* **219,** 385–8.
5. Glassow, F. (1984). Inguinal hernia repair using local anaesthesia. *Ann. Roy. Coll. Surg. Eng.,* **66,** 382–7.
6. Lichtenstein, I.L., Herzikoff, S., Shore, J.M., Jiron, M.W., Stuart, S., and Mizuno, L. (1970). The dynamics of wound healing. *Surg. Gyn. Obstet.,* **130,** 685–90.
7. Bourke, J.B., Lear, P.A., and Taylor, M. (1981). Effect of early return to work after elective repair of inguinal hernia: clinical and financial consequences at one year and three years. *Lancet,* **2,** 623–5.
8. Taylor, E.W., and Dewar, E.P. (1983). Early return to work after repair of a unilateral inguinal hernia. *Brit. J. Surg.,* **70,** 599–600.
9. Editorial (1985). British hernias. *Lancet,* **1,** 1080–1.
10. Serpell, J.W., Johnson, C.D., and Jarrett, P.E. (1990). A prospective study of bilateral inguinal hernia repair. *Ann. Roy. Coll. Surg. Engl.,* **72,** 299–303.
11. Wilson, R.G., Macintyre, I.M.C., Nixon, S.J., Saunders, J.H., Varma, J.S., and King, P.M. (1992). Laparoscopic cholecystectomy as a safe and effective treatment for severe acute cholecystitis. *Brit. Med. J.,* **305,** 394–6.
12. Allen-Mersh, T.G. (1990). Pilonidal sinus: finding the right track for treatment. *Brit. J. Surg.,* **77,** 123–30.

13.  Coronary angioplasty versus coronary artery bypass surgery: The randomised intervention treatment of angina (RITA) trial (1993). *Lancet,* **341,** 573–80.
14.  Sim Munro, W. (1990). Work before and after coronary artery bypass grafting. *J. Soc. Occup. Med.,* **40,** 59–64.
15.  Paris, W. *et al.* (1992). Social rehabilitation and return to work after cardiac transplantation—a multicentre survey. *Transplantation,* **53,** 433–8.
16.  Editorial (1991). Psychological factors in breast cancer. *Brit. Med. J.,* **302,** 1219–20.
17.  Rajagopal, V. and Bailey, M.J. (1991). Mobile extracorporeal shockwave lithotripsy. *Brit. J. Urol.,* **67,** 6–8.
18.  Randall, P.E., and Marcuson, R.W. (1985). Absence from work following vasectomy. *J. Soc. Occup. Med.,* **35,** 77–8.
19.  Goldberg, R.T. (1975). Vocational and social adjustment after laryngectomy. *Scand. J. Rehab. Med.,* **7,** 1–8.
20.  Editorial (1992). Voice after laryngectomy. *Brit. Med. J.,* **304,** 2–3.
21.  Laros, C.D. (1979). *The patient after total pneumonectomy. A long-term study. Selected papers,* Vol. 19. The Royal Netherlands Tuberculosis Association, The Hague.
22.  Piachaud, D. and Weddell, J.M. (1972). The economics of treating varicose veins. *Int. J. Epidemiol.,* **1,** 287–94.

# 20

# Psychiatric disorders

*J.L. Kearns and D. Prothero*

## Introduction

This chapter provides a brief account of the major characteristics and patterns of psychiatric illness, and their implications in the selection for, retention in, and departure from work. It emphasizes the importance of excellent communication between those concerned in their varied roles, and the potential counter-productivity of excessive confidentiality.

Given appropriate support, many psychiatrically ill people can successfully be accommodated in industry. For this to occur, those caring for the patient need to recognize that the patient's interests may conflict with the demands of a commercial environment, and to consider how this potential conflict can be resolved in each individual case. This depends on both a clinical prediction of the likely future performance of the patient, and an understanding of the working environment. Occupational health staff have an essential role to play in the resolution of that conflict.

Frank psychiatric disease may commence with a phase of prodromal signs and symptoms, such as early morning waking in the period before an anxiety/depressive state develops. Health professionals in general may be aware that these abnormalities represent only the 'tip of the iceberg' of mental distress. In the development of psychiatric disease, the occupational physician or nurse may recognise an earlier long phase of behavioural change, which may also have been noted by the patient's manager or work colleagues.

Assessment of the patient against the following criteria will help the physician to reach a diagnosis, and determine appropriate clinical therapy and the wider aspects of management at work. They suggest the functional disabilities which may flow from the abnormality and which must be taken into account in determining the future employment of the patient; if necessary, after rehabilitation in the former position, and after considering redeployment should that be necessary and feasible.

1. *Behaviour*: appearance, posture, social behaviour, disorders of motor behaviour, excitement, restlessness, and immobility.

2. *Speech*: flights of ideas, pressure of speech expressing thoughts arising in abundance, thought block, illogicality, disordered thinking.

3. *Mood*: depression, elation, loss of affect in blunting or incongruity of emotion.

4. *Depersonalization* and feelings of unreality.

5. *Obsessional phenomena*: compulsive rituals.

6. *Delusions*: false beliefs, misinterpretation of things that exist, feelings of persecution.

7. *Illusions*, hallucinations, misperceptions with or without an originating stimulus, e.g., hearing voices.

8. *Orientation*, in time, place, person.

9. *Attention* or concentration.

10. *Memory*.

11. *Insight*.

Beware of misinterpreting the transient effects of alcohol or drug abuse, the dazed state after head injury, the recovery period after a fit, or an overdose of drugs.

## Classification and prevalence of psychiatric disorders

The prevalence of psychiatric morbidity in the workplace is not known, and is difficult to assess precisely. The most common problems presenting in the workplace are anxiety and depression, whose symptoms are those which also describe normal feelings. Illness is only present when those symptoms are severe, persistent, and disabling. A number of epidemiological studies show that about 100–250 per 1000 adults have a psychological disorder in any one year. This is mostly depression and anxiety but in 1–3 per cent is psychosis, mostly schizophrenia and affective psychosis. A number of epidemiological studies carried out in industry suggest that depression and anxiety are also common in people at work. The majority of those affected are in the 15–64 age range, which is that of the working population.[1]

It is helpful to understand various distinctions which are used in psychiatric classification.

*Personality disorders* involve deeply ingrained maladaptive behaviour patterns which continue throughout most of adult life, more evident at one time than at another.

They may present at work as unsatisfactory behaviour or performance. A major task for occupational health staff is to explain that such a problem will not improve. It can be a major disadvantage to 'medicalize' a personality disorder, and to imply that treatment may modify the behaviour in some way. It is much easier to cope with the complex issues if the disorder is managed in an entirely management milieu, to determine whether the performance of the individual exhibiting these personality traits is beneficial to the employer or is, at least, acceptable.

*Psychiatric illnesses* usually have a defined beginning and are characterized by the patient behaving in a manner which deviates from his normal pattern. There is a distinction between organic and functional illness.

*Organic mental illness* is the consequence of known physical disease affecting the brain. This can be structural pathology of the brain, such as a tumour or a toxic, infectious, metabolic or systemic disturbance affecting the brain, e.g., dementia.

*Functional illness* is a psychiatric illness with no apparent physical cause, e.g., anxiety state.

There is a further distinction between *neurotic* and *psychotic* illness.

*Psychoses* are mental disorders in which mental function is impaired to a degree that interferes with insight, the ability to meet ordinary demands of life, and to maintain adapted contact with reality. The psychotic patient often misperceives the world about him, as for example when hallucinating—'hearing voices'.

*Neuroses* are mental disorders in which the patient does not confuse his morbid subjective experiences and fantasies with external reality. He is, if you like, living in the real world, but has difficulty in coping because of severe and disabling symptoms.

Depression and anxiety can be presenting symptoms of both psychotic and neurotic illnesses, and may be associated with other diseases.

## Neurotic illness

### Anxiety states

Patients with anxiety states show various physical and mental manifestations of anxiety, not attributable to real danger, occurring either in attacks ('panic attacks') or as a persisting state.

These symptoms are frequently physical. Examples are palpitations, breathlessness, chest pain, sweating, faintness, trembling, difficulty in swallowing, dizziness, and frequency of micturition. Mental symptoms include tension, irritability, fear of collapse or of physical or mental illness, and impaired concentration. Behaviour at work may be affected; it may be interrupted by anxiety or panic attacks. The patient may be too preoccupied with his own symptoms to concentrate on the job in hand, or he may defer it repeatedly.

*Anxiety and depression* often go together and may develop into a cycle of anxiety: worry → poor sleep → poor performance → malaise → depression → more anxiety → worse depression, and so on.

*Prevalence.* Anxiety states are the most common form of neurotic illness. They can be found at any age, but often start in the young adult, and are more common in women. The prevalence has been variously estimated at between 2 and 6 per cent of the population.[2]

### Phobic anxiety state

This form of anxiety state includes an intense fear of certain objects or specific situations which would not normally have that effect. Work problems may arise from avoidance of feared situations, e.g., open spaces, closed spaces, tunnels, public transport, etc., and may result in absence from work, or reluctance to do certain work.

Behavioural treatments are often very effective in phobic anxiety states and patients may be maintained in regular work if consideration is given as to how symptoms occurring at the workplace may be overcome. Behavioural therapy is becoming widely used in the NHS, but sometimes the waiting time for treatment impedes its availability.

### Neurotic depression

Depression is a common temporary mood in normal people, but illness is only judged to be present when the depression is severe, persistent (i.e., lasting weeks), and disabling. The more severe symptoms found in affective psychosis, including biological changes in appetite and sleep, are not normally present in neurotic depression.

Symptoms of depression include low spirits, loss of interest, energy and drive, poor enjoyment of life, and possibly suicidal thoughts. Thinking is coloured by pessimism. Depression may sometimes present with physical symptoms, notably back pain or facial pain. There may be a clear precipitating situation, such as bereavement or a failure to obtain promotion, but the complaint of depression is often of disproportionate degree in that it is an excessive response to the provoking situation.

*Prevalence.* The complaint of depression is more frequent than the diagnosis of depressive illness, which has a point prevalence of 3 per cent for men and 7 per cent for women.

### Hypochondriasis

This is a neurotic illness in which the patient has excessive concern with his physical health or less commonly, his mental health. He may be cancerophobic, or worried about the functioning of some part of his body. These symptoms tend to be of long standing and do not respond to medical reassurance. They can be associated with anxiety or depression, and the complaints become exacerbated if the patient becomes depressed and return to their usual level if the depression is treated. Many such patients manage to continue working successfully, although they may incur repeated absences for a day or two when seeking medical consultation.

## Psychotic illness

### *Schizophrenic psychosis*

Schizophrenic psychoses are characterized by disturbance of the following mental functions:

1. *Disorders of thinking,* e.g., feeling that thoughts are being withdrawn from or inserted into the mind, or that one's thoughts are being broadcast.

2. *Disorders of emotion,* e.g., incongruous emotional response to situations, or emotional flatness.

3. *Disorders of motor function,* e.g., excitability, stupor.

4. *Disorders of perception*—delusions (false beliefs)—hallucinations, i.e., perception through the special senses such as hearing, for which there is no originating stimulus.

In practice, schizophrenic illness is divided into acute and chronic forms. The above symptoms may not all be present and may be present in varying degrees in different patients. The most frequent symptoms of acute schizophrenia are summarized in Table 20.1.[3]

The prognosis of the acute attack depends on prompt and thorough treatment.

- Approximately 25 per cent recover completely
- 25 per cent recover, but have a recurrence of illness at some time in the future
- 25 per cent improve, but are left with residual symptoms

**Table 20.1** The most frequent symptoms of acute schizophrenia[3]

| Symptom | Frequency (%) |
| --- | --- |
| Lack of insight | 97 |
| Auditory hallucinations | 74 |
| Ideas of reference | 70 |
| Suspiciousness | 66 |
| Flatness of affect | 66 |
| Voices speaking to the patient | 65 |
| Delusional mood | 64 |
| Delusions of persecution | 64 |
| Thought alienation | 52 |
| Thoughts spoken aloud | 50 |

- 25 per cent do not recover and are disabled by chronic schizophrenia which affects them socially and in their occupation

*Prevalence.* The lifetime risk of developing schizophrenia is approximately 0.85 per cent.

*Treatment.* Pharmacological treatment is through neuroleptic drugs such as *chlorpromazine, haloperidol,* and *trifluoperazine.* Side-effects such as tremor, inco-ordination, drowsiness, and postural hypotension may be significant at work. Depot neuroleptic drugs are slowly absorbed, long-acting drugs administered by intramuscular injection by the community psychiatric nurse or the occupational health nurse at the place of work. All these drugs help to prevent relapse.

Psychological treatment includes counselling and rehabilitation to a more normal way of life, including a structured work pattern which is within the capability of the individual. It is important to understand that the content and objective of such counselling is the reconciliation between the demands of a job and the capability of the individual. It cannot be carried out in an exclusively therapeutic mode. For instance, it is necessary to address the problem posed to management by the behaviour of the individual.

An awareness and an expectation that there are standards of performance to be met are essential, even at the risk that they may appear to be disciplinary strictures.

The presenting symptoms of the disorder seriously reduce the opportunities for rehabilitation and redeployment. Supervisory middle and senior management tasks are likely to be beyond the capability of the schizophrenic. Suitable tasks may only be available in lower levels of clerical and manual operations. The statistics quoted show that a proportion of schizophrenic patients are left with a greater or lesser degree of disability after an acute illness. The potential for un-satisfactory performance is therefore undeniable.

However, many schizophrenics will be capable of making a useful contribu-tion at work.[4] The symptoms of chronic schizophrenia include social withdrawal and lack of drive, but lay impressions of chronic schizophrenia leading to total unemployability are false. Some sufferers are able to encapsulate their strange beliefs and experiences and to perform normally and effectively in the other parts of their lives. It is important that superiors and colleagues understand the condition. The person suffers from a genuine illness and is not being lazy, awkward, or devious. Such persons need time on their own with minimal social stimuli to cope with their state of high arousal. Hallucinations are very real ex-periences with feelings similar to any normal person's when hearing, good, bad or frightening news by telephone. If strange ideas are expressed, it is unproduc-tive to argue and they are best ignored.

If allowance is made for the patient's recognized psychological disability, he may achieve satisfactory work despite the continuing background of strange ideas.

A major contribution to the individual's welfare is to allow leave for depot medication which may be required every three or four weeks. It may be possible to administer depot medication at work. Work should be arranged to allow for a

**Table 20.2** Factors predicting the outcome of schizophrenia[5]

| Good prognosis | Poor prognosis |
| --- | --- |
| Sudden onset | Insidious onset |
| Short episode | Long episode |
| No previous psychiatric history | Previous psychiatric history |
| Prominent affective symptoms | Negative symptoms |
| Older age at onset | Younger age at onset |
| Married | Single, separated, widowed, divorced |
| Good psychosexual adjustment | Poor psychosexual adjustment |
| Good previous personality | Abnormal previous personality |
| Good work record | Poor work record |
| Good social relationships | Social isolation |
| Good compliance | Poor compliance |

measured social withdrawal by reducing pressure to perform or the expectation to meet high standards or urgent deadlines. After an acute episode, a trial period can clarify both work ability and the level of pressure which can be tolerated.

The community psychiatric nurse is the key professional in the satisfactory maintenance of persons with chronic schizophrenia. Close liaison between occupational health services and those caring for the patient in the community is essential; case conferences should be arranged to cope with crises and for review.

Marked withdrawal, persisting depression, agitation, or threats of self harm, are indications for urgent assessment.

It is possible to predict which patients are likely to become more severely or less severely handicapped by schizophrenia. The indicators of future likely behaviour are set out in Table 20.2.[5]

## Affective psychosis

### Manic depressive psychoses

Affective psychoses are mental disorders, usually recurrent, in which there is a severe disturbance of mood, e.g., depression or elation. This disturbance may be unipolar, as in recurrent depression, or bipolar where the patient suffers at different times from depressed and hypomanic episodes. These episodes may be mild or severe and recurrent depression is the more usual form. There is a genetic predisposition, although attacks may be precipitated by emotional or physical stress.

True mania, in which the patient is so overactive and excited as to be uncontrollable, is nowadays rare. Hypomania consists of a state of elation or excitement out of keeping with the person's circumstances. The patient is overactive, garrulous, and may be grandiose or self-important. There is pressure of speech, flight of ideas, and increased energy with sleeplessness. The patient is irritable to others and the illness is more noticeable to others than to the patient himself, who will indeed say that he has never felt so well. This denial of illness and consequent refusal of medication and advice makes management difficult. There is a danger that the patient may physically exhaust himself through over-activity. Excessive spending is common and in such an attack a patient may ruin himself and his family financially if appropriate measures to preserve his financial interests are not taken. The refusal to accept help coupled with the danger to the patient's health and his irritability towards others, often results in the need for treatment on a compulsory basis under the Mental Health Act 1983.

In a depressive bout, the patient shows low mood which may or may not have a precipitating reason. There is diurnal variation of mood, the mood being worse in the morning. There is loss of appetite and consequently loss of weight, loss of energy and libido, loss of interest and concentration, and a sleep pattern characterized by early morning wakening. The patient may express low self-esteem and feelings of hopelessness and there is a risk of suicidal behaviour.

*Prevalence.* Annual incidence is approximately 12 per 100 000 for men and 18.3 per 100 000 for women. The lifetime morbidity risk is 0.6 to 1 per cent.


## Dementia

Dementia is a generalized impairment of intellect, memory, and personality occurring in the absence of clouding of consciousness. Because this mainly affects older age groups, it usually strikes after retirement, but some groups of workers may continue to work into their old age. Dementia is a progressive illness, but it is important to distinguish this diagnosis from the depressed patient, who may also show forgetfulness and increasing incapacity to cope with his work. The main causes of dementia are cerebral arteriosclerosis and Alzheimer's disease, but there are rarer causes which may commence below the age of 65. These include dementia due to the toxic affects of chronic alcoholism and poisoning by heavy metals, such as mercury, lead, arsenic, and thallium. The onset of dementia is insidious. One of the first signs is a loss of short-term memory, while distant memory remains intact. Subsequently, there is general intellectual decline, paralleled by a decline of social behaviour and self-care.

The brain is an organ with no power of regeneration, so treatment can only arrest the dementing process but cannot restore functional loss due to the death of brain cells. The exacerbation of the confusion which can occur in general illness improves when the latter is treated.

Dementia in a worker may be concealed by the misguidedly 'generous' acts of colleagues who may cover up his mistakes in order to prevent his dismissal. Because loss of judgement is one of the symptoms of dementia, this illness occurring in someone at senior management level can have serious consequences if appropriate action is not taken.

**Table 20.3** Percentage change in population distribution by age

| Age | Age variation (%) |
| --- | --- |
| 65–69 | –0.4 |
| 70–74 | +10.9 |
| 75–79 | +3.5 |
| 80–84 | +11.3 |
| 85+ | +59.7 |

*Prevalence.* The incidence of dementia in society is increasing as a consequence of its ageing population and is more common in women. Demographic changes in the United Kingdom indicate that the proportion of elderly people is increasing rapidly. The Office of Population Censuses and Surveys (OPCS)[6] suggested in 1989 that between then and the year 2011 the proportions of age groups will alter as shown in Table 20.3. Ineichan's 'rule of thumb' suggests that the prevalence of dementia in the 65–74 age group is 1 per cent, rising to 10 per cent in those over 75 years of age.[7]

**Acute confusional state**

This is an illness in which the patient becomes confused and disorientated and there is clouding of consciousness and frequently, visual hallucinations. It is secondary to physical illness within the brain or general systemic illness affecting the brain. The latter includes toxic, infectious, and metabolic illnesses. A key diagnostic feature is fluctuating clouding of consciousness. At times, the patient appears drowsy and has an impaired awareness of self and surroundings. The patient may at times appear to be semi-comatose, but at other times there is disorientation of time, place and person, as well as hallucinations. The patient may become labile, fearful, and agitated, particularly in delirium tremens, a form of acute confusional state found in the chronic alcoholic, where the patient may hallucinate, seeing animals, such as rats or spiders, and becoming afraid of them. The underlying physical cause may arise from the toxic effects of alcohol, drugs of abuse or prescribed drugs, industrial chemicals, head injury, epilepsy, and other infectious vascular or metabolic diseases affecting brain function. The causes of acute confusional states are similar to the causes of coma, so that unless the underlying physical cause of the acute confusional state is energetically investigated and treated medically, it is possible for such patients to slip progressively into coma and subsequent death.

*Prevalence.* Although these illnesses are fairly common in hospital inpatients, their incidence at the workplace is not known, but is probably rare and is more likely to occur in patients with known established medical conditions which may be intracranial, such as epilepsy, or extracranial, such as diabetes and chronic cardiac failure.

In most cases the patient can be successfully managed if there is good communication between occupational health staff, the employee's own doctor, and the manager of the department.

## Mental handicap

Patients with mild mental handicap form an important component of the working population and present few problems. Their intelligence quotient (IQ), ranges from 50 to 70. Problems arise when the mental handicap is associated with additional disabilities or social handicaps. These include speech disorders or lack of social skills. The limited intelligence of these people makes them slow in learning new skills at work, but many such individuals become reliable and conscientious workers. Some are aware of their limitations and deliberately compensate for them by working harder.

*Prevalence.* Mild mental handicap is estimated at 20–30 per 1000 of the population.

# Special work problems

### Suicidal risk

Suicidal risk must be assessed in the depressed patient as a guide to the degree of urgency for further referral. It is a myth that the person talking of suicide will not attempt it. Questioning the patient about suicidal thoughts or intentions will not provoke suicidal behaviour and may be of relief to the patient.

The patient should be asked whether he has made a previous suicide attempt in his life and should be asked whether at the present time he has suicidal thoughts and whether he has any suicidal intentions.

The state of a severely depressed patient can be evaluated from his answers to the two questions shown in Table 20.4.

Successful suicide attempts are more likely to occur if the patient is over 55 years of age and isolated, particularly if he has drink, drug, or physical problems. However, suicide attempts may occur at any age and often take the form of a gamble with death, i.e., leaving one's future to be decided by fate.

Sometimes, patients at risk pose a major additional problem to the employer despite his most generous intention. For instance, the severity of depression may be prolonged and after several months, may seem likely to be prolonged indefinitely. Occupational health staff then have the task of facing the possibility that news of the termination of service may be an additional burden possibly leading to the suicide of the employee.

**Table 20.4** Assessment of suicidal risk in a severely depressed patient

| | | | |
|---|---|---|---|
| Do you have suicidal thoughts | Yes | Yes | No |
| Do you have suicidal intentions | No | Yes | No |
| COMMENTS: | These are the most common answers from a severely depressed person. While caution is needed, such replies should not provoke serious concern. | This patient is saying he or she is actively suicidal and must be treated as such. | Most, if not all, severely depressed patients have suicidal thoughts. These answers suggest that the patient is denying or blocking any thoughts of suicide so that the risk of suicidal action is present despite the patient's denial. |

Clearly this situation has to be handled with extreme delicacy, since the management objective has to be the replacement of the individual who is no longer performing his role, and is likely to remain so disabled. It is therefore up to the occupational health department to act as broker between those caring for the patient and those responsible for his financial security and pension in managing the departure of the individual from the organization with as little further distress as possible. The possibility that this compassionate confrontation of irreconcilable objectives may not be a success has to be faced, and occupational health staff must prepare those they advise to bear the consequences of necessary decisions.

### The psychiatric patient at work

Prejudice towards psychiatric illness is as common in the workplace as in society as a whole, but many psychiatrically ill people can successfully be accommodated in industry. Education and advice by occupational health staff can help to achieve the necessary balance between rejection of the sick worker on one hand and too high an expectation of him on the other.

The psychiatric patient/employee in a production, construction or service industry may pose a threat to the safety of himself and others. He may make errors dangerous to large numbers of people, or extremely costly to the employer. Legitimate management anxiety about the performance of the individual is increased by ignorance and fear of mental disease.

It is a great help to the occupational health department if people are not referred directly to it without prior consultation with the relevant manager, so that all the stages in the management of the problem are planned in advance, before the patient is seen by the occupational physician.

Health workers playing the primary therapeutic role must try to understand the basis for the anxieties of the employer and the patient's co-workers, so that the commercial constraints upon rehabilitation and redeployment at the workplace are taken into account while they advise the patient upon his return about leading as normal and active a life as possible.

### The prospective employee

The employer's policy regarding the employment of the mentally disabled is crucial. It is vitally important to involve those who have been caring for a psychiatric patient in the assessment of his work capability before any appointment is made.

These factors must be taken into account in assessing the patient's condition and prospects. The patient must be fit enough at the outset for an environment which demands satisfactory performance. Selection requires close co-operation between those caring for the patient and the personnel and occupational health departments of those enlightened employers who are willing to give the disadvantaged a chance of work when it is practical to do so. Health professionals who have not worked in a production or service industry may assume too easily that any work can be used as therapy. It is surprising that the patient with a psychiatric disorder is often recommended or encouraged to take up 'work with people' in personnel or health care roles, where psychological professional demands are more likely to be negative than positive factors. It is not sensible to expect a nurse, doctor or health worker to use the circumstances of the work as therapy, or to avoid decisions about the future, knowing that at the end of a long training period, the individual may be quite unable to do the job. However, each case must be assessed on its merits.

In the process of rehabilitation from mental illness, the patient must have progressed sufficiently in a therapeutic environment before being returned to the rigours of a commercial and competitive environment to complete his recovery.

Close co-operation is necessary between occupational health staff and those treating the patient to determine whether the patient may remain at work despite the possible side-effects of treatment. If there are grounds for confidence that the patient will in the near future be able to resume full working responsibilities with a low likelihood of recurrence, they should be declared. General support may be obtained from the local office of MIND, the National Association for Mental Health (for their address see Appendix 9). There are provincial centres throughout England and Wales. Further help in re-training may be available from Remploy through the Disability Employment Adviser of the local Employment Services Office. Facilities for re-training which were formerly available in the large mental hospitals are disappearing as those institutions close. The Social Services Departments of Local Authorities in the United Kingdom may provide residential care as an interim measure to support those most socially disadvantaged patients who have suffered a mental health crisis and which has caused them to lose their jobs.

## Management of an acute emergency

The care of the mentally disturbed patient demands tact, sympathy with, and understanding of the patient, and the reassurance of onlookers. The patient may be unco-operative, disturbed and/or violent and may cause concern for his safety. If there is difficulty in dealing with the case because of violence, or lack of co-operation by the patient, the Authorized Social Worker at the Local Authority Social Services Department should be contacted and given a brief account of the patient's condition and previous history if known.

### Within a production/service department

If the patient is still at his workplace, the arrival of the nurse may be reassuring both to the patient and onlookers. When the nurse arrives, she should greet the patient first, and then ask a competent person for an account of what has happened. She should then talk to the patient in privacy, others being asked to withdraw, if the patient is not violent. Minimum restraint of the patient should be exercised. A uniformed security guard, a burly foreman or similar figure who may, possibly, be seen to be threatening should stay in the background. If possible, the patient should be taken to the treatment room. If not, the situation must be dealt with where it has arisen.

*In the treatment room*

In no case of mental disturbance should the patient be left alone, until handed over to a responsible relative, medical colleague, or Authorized Social Worker. If it is necessary to make phone calls, or to write notes, do so with the patient in view, or close by with an escort (a manager, forelady, personnel officer, etc.). Be prepared for long delays; it may be hours before the Authorized Social Worker and/or doctor arrives. The patient may be allowed freedom appropriate to his state, but should not be allowed to 'escape' from care. Threat of possible restraint may provoke violence by the patient, who might otherwise be persuaded gently to stay where he or she is. Remember that the patient may be in some confusion, so he should be treated gently, but with sympathetic firmness if necessary. When the patient has been sent home or to hospital, write full notes of what has happened, and send a copy to the general practitioner and the hospital.

It is useful, at this stage, to reassure the patient's co-workers, and to prepare them to receive their colleague back without prejudice about 'madness'.

## The absent employee

An absence control policy is an essential factor in the management of psychiatric problems. As soon as a psychiatric diagnosis is suspected, correspondence should begin between the occupational health department and those caring for the patient, so that the transition between the patient role and the employee role can be as smooth as possible as a result of careful planning. Line management must be informed and involved.

Occupational health staff will have the task of determining, in correspondence with those treating the patient, whether return to work is practicable.

It is essential for the patient's welfare that he should be brought to terms with the reality of the situation. If those who control the therapeutic and the working environment can work together, the management of the case will be more effective and potentially more compassionate than it would be if clinical and line management is split into two phases each managed with different objectives.

Some diagnoses allow the hope that the patient will eventually return to full capability. Others may virtually disqualify the patient/employee from ever returning to his normal post. The manager will welcome early information on the likely date of return to work and likely capability at that time.

The major role of occupational health staff is to attempt to predict the likely progress of the condition. The timescale is set by commercial imperatives, and a period of three months for the assessment of progress might be considered generous. Although the patient may eventually make a full recovery the question to be answered by occupational health staff is whether or not he will have recovered sufficient capability to perform all the functions expected within three months and to be reasonably likely to render an efficient service thereafter without further problems. It may be necessary to make some very broad predictions about how long the patient may be expected to cope before he has a relapse.

# The employee returning to work

## Drug treatment and its management at work

Many patients return to work still taking their psychotropic medication and the effects of this at work are discussed below (see also Chapter 3).

## Specific treatment for various conditions

### Antipsychotic drugs (British National Formulary: *BNF 4.2.2*)

This group includes the phenothiazines such as *chlorpromazine*; the butyrophenones, such as *haloperidol*; and similar drugs such as *pimozide* and *fluspirilene*, which are mainly used to treat schizophrenia and other psychiatric illnesses. For maintenance therapy, long-acting injections are used to ensure better patient compliance.

### Antimanic drugs (BNF 4.2.3)

*Lithium carbonate* is used both in the treatment and prophylaxis of mania, manic depressive psychosis, and recurrent depression. *Carbamazepine* is used for the prophylaxis of manic depressive psychosis unresponsive to lithium. Patients on lithium should carry a card explaining the side effects; need for lithium levels, etc.

### Antidepressant drugs (BNF 4.3)

Drugs used for the treatment of depressive illness fall into 3 groups:

1. Tricyclic and related antidepressant drugs.
2. Monoamine oxidase inhibitors.
3. Serotonin uptake inhibitors.

Patients taking monoamine oxidase inhibitors should carry a card giving instructions about suitable diet and warning of interaction with other medicines while the drug is taken or for 14 days after it is stopped.

### Hypnotics and anxiolytics (BNF 4.1)

These drugs are sometimes used for the short-term relief of insomnia or severe anxiety respectively and are usually prescribed in patients with an anxiety state.

## Response to treatment

### Antipsychotic drugs

Follow up studies of acute schizophrenia suggest that the outcome of treatment of the acute attack may produce a varied response. Prompt treatment is essential. Prognostic factors are listed in Table 20.2.

Compliance with prescribed medication is important in preventing relapse into further illness.

### Antimanic drugs

Patients respond well to treatment of the individual attack, although many patients with hypomania will quickly become depressed during the period of treatment before they recover. *Lithium* is markedly successful in some patients with manic depressive psychosis in preventing relapse, but less so in others. The patients need to be encouraged to comply with the treatment regime and associated blood investigations.

### Antidepressant drugs

Although many patients complain that depression is the worst of all illnesses in the suffering it engenders, it does usually respond fully to treatment. Most antidepressants take between 10–14 days before they begin to relieve symptoms, and patients need to be encouraged to continue medication for *one month* at least. After recovering the patient should not discontinue the medication abruptly, as this may produce relapse. Antidepressants should be discontinued by gradual weaning off the drug under medical supervision.

### Hypnotics and anxiolytics

These drugs do not affect the underlying psychiatric condition. They are prescribed only for the short-term relief of symptoms, which will recur when the medication is discontinued, unless other action has been taken to combat the cause of the sleeplessness or anxiety.

## The effect of treatment on work performance

### Antipsychotic drugs

Many of these drugs impair psychomotor performance and the degree to which they do so depends on the amount of sedation they produce. Psychotic patients show impairment of psychomotor function even without drugs, and in some this will be improved by treatment. Therefore, both the effects of the illness and of the medication need to be considered when advising patients about the possible risks associated with driving or particular work tasks where alertness is important. Photosensitization and contact sensitization can occur; patients taking *chlorpromazine* need protection from the sun if working outdoors.

*Antimanic drugs*

*Lithium* probably has little effect on performance, although impairment of some laboratory tests of psychomotor function has been described.

*Antidepressant drugs*

Many antidepressants produce sedation, especially at the onset of treatment, and this is potentiated by alcohol. Psychomotor impairment is related to the sedation effect. As tolerance develops to the sedative effects of antidepressants, it seems sensible to advise patients not to drive or undertake work which could be affected during the first few days of treatment with the more sedative antidepressants.

Side-effects of these drugs which may affect performance include tremor, blurring of near vision, and postural hypotension. The latter is more likely to occur with the older tricyclic antidepressants and with monoamine oxidase inhibitors. Antidepressants may affect central temperature regulation, and anticholinergic side-effects may interfere with sweating, so patients on these drugs should not be exposed to extremes of temperature.

*Hypnotics and anxiolytics*

These are central nervous system (CNS) depressants and consequently impair psychomotor function, slow down responsiveness, and impair motor skills and co-ordination. Most hypnotics produce residual effects the following morning. The effects on psychomotor function are potentiated by alcohol. Barbiturates should not be prescribed for this purpose to patients who drive or operate machinery. The benzodiazepine drugs differ in their effect upon performance but all these drugs can affect performance in susceptible patients. In particular, they affect the performance of memory-based tests; the prescription of anxiolytics during the day could affect the performance of a wide range of activities.

*Occupational exposure to CNS depressants*

Employees who work with solvents or in atmospheres where a potential build up of gases or fumes can depress the CNS are at risk if they are also taking any of the medications listed above. Safe occupational exposure limits assume an employee is not on medication, and the CNS depressant action of the gas or solvent may summate with the CNS depressant action of the medication.

The role of occupational health staff in supervising psychiatric patients is fundamentally dependent on liaison with the general practitioner. Some patients may be managed successfully by their own doctor without referral to a consultant. Those patients who do require more complex assessment and therapy will virtually always be in the care of their local practice prior to their return to work.

'Rehabilitation should begin as the patient departs from work in the ambulance!' Employees are in the care of their managers. Line and personnel managers will be aware of absence patterns. Care of the sick employee should lead to correspondence between occupational health staff and the general practitioner as the illness unfolds and resolves.

It is for the GP to explain the side-effects of treatment to the patient, and the interest of occupational health staff may supplement the supervision. It should be possible to negotiate the return to work, perhaps gradually, of the employee/patient. Once back at work, benign and discreet care can be continued by occupational health staff and the patient may have recourse to the Occupational Health Department if there is need for it.

Yet again, the integration of occupational nursing and medicine into the organization can smooth the transition of a patient, often hesitant and lacking in confidence, from a state of residual mental turmoil to the stability necessary to function effectively at work, and as a normal individual in the community.

It is important for both the manager and the patient that the issue of a planned return to work is discussed at an early stage, as this can allay fears of immediate dismissal. Contact between the practitioner in charge of the case and occupational health staff is important, and will make it more likely that practical recommendations made with regard to retraining or restructuring of the employee's work can be implemented. In planning return to work all those concerned should consider if changes in the work, counselling, re-training or a job more suitable for the individual could lessen the risk of relapse and improve performance.

In phobic states, or during the anxious phase of recovery, the journey to and from work is a greater obstacle than the work itself. Transport by a willing co-worker may be arranged, since it is usually impractical to expect an employer to arrange to transport one of his employees to and from work. This is an excellent example of the way in which occupational health staff can mobilize work colleagues to help others in their temporary misfortune.

After return to work it may be necessary to review progress discreetly with managers and co-workers to determine whether the performance at work is acceptable. If it is not, clinical management may need to be adjusted. Should such adjustment be unsuccessful, redeployment or termination of service will have to be considered. This review period has to be measured in weeks rather than months to enable the department in a production/service industry to survive in a hostile economic climate.

### Ill-health retirement

The major contribution of the occupational health staff will be to assist a manager to deal compassionately with a disorder which disqualifies the individual from continuing in his current post.

The right balance between encouragement and coming to terms with the likely outcome of the crisis depends fundamentally upon a sound relationship between those treating the patient and those with responsibility to the employer for the maintenance of effective work performance.

## Conclusions and recommendations

Occupational health staff should become integrated into the personnel department activities, such as organizational/management development and performance appraisal, and contribute some advice to laymen in the recognition of stress, which is dealt with at greater length in Chapter 21. It is a test of the efficiency, competence, and trust of the occupational health department that those found wanting at performance review can be discussed informally without transgressing ethical constraints. Such an approach allows occupational health staff to contribute to the development of a healthy organization.

The competent management of a particular case provides an opportunity for them to promote general education about mental health to combat prejudice.

The occupational health staff must interpret the individual clinical picture, predict the likely performance of the patient, without risk to people, activity, product or service. Only they can support the patient in his or her recovery to being an effective employee in a demanding environment.

## Selected references and further reading

1.  Jenkins, R. (1992). Prevalence of mental illness in the workplace. In *Prevention of ill health of workers.* HMSO, London.
2.  Weissman, M.M. and Merikangas, K.R. (1986). The epidemiology of anxiety and panic disorders. *J. Clin. Psychiat.,* **47,** (suppl.), 11–17.
3.  WHO (World Health Organization) (1973). *Report of the international pilot study of schizophrenia,* Vol. 1. WHO, Geneva.
4.  Harding, C.M., Zubin, J., and Strauss, J.S. (1987). Chronicity in schizophrenia; fact, partial fact or artifact? *Hosp. Commun. Psychiat.,* **38,** 477–86.
5.  Gelder, M., Gath, D., and Mayou, R. (1989). *Oxford textbook of psychiatry,* (2nd edn), p. 113. Oxford University Press.
6.  OPCS (Office of Population Censuses and Surveys) (1991). *Sub national population projections—1989.* HMSO, London.
7.  Ineichan, B. (1987). Measuring the rising tide: How many dementia cases will there be by 2001? *J. Psychiat.,* **150,** 193–200.
8.  Gelder, M., Gath, D., and Mayou, R. (1989). *Oxford textbook of psychiatry,* (2nd edn). Oxford University Press.
9.  WHO (World Health Organization) (1992). *The ICD 10 classification of mental and behavioral disorders: Clinical descriptions and diagnostic guidelines.* WHO, Geneva.
10. Sims, A. and Snaith, P. (1988). *Anxiety in clinical practice.* Wiley, Chichester.
11. Kelly, D. and France, R. (1987). *A practical handbook for the treatment of depression.* Parthenon, Carnforth, Lancs.
12. Seemen, M.V., Litman, S.K., Plummer, E., Thornton, J.F., and Jeffries, J.J. (1982). *Living and working with schizophrenia.* Jenson Pharmaceutical Ltd, Oxford.
13. Mental Health Act (1983). HMSO, London.

# 21

# Stress, alcohol, and drug abuse

*G. Smith and M.S. Lipsedge*

## Introduction

A CBI survey in 1993 estimated the cost of stress to industry at £1.3 billion per year.[1] It also indicated that 30–40 per cent of absence from work is due to some form of mental or emotional disorder and that 71 million days are lost per annum due to mental illness, much of which is stress-related, out of a total 147 million days of sickness absence in general.

## Causes

Stress might be defined as an excess of environmental demands over the individual's capacity to meet them.[2] It is a multi-factorial phenomenon with interactions between physical, personal, social, and environmental elements. In the work situation, stress may develop when there is a poor fit between the worker and the job, when the worker cannot control his work conditions and if he lacks social support. Work stresses include both overload and underload, unpleasant working conditions, repetitive work, and shiftwork. Other potentially disruptive situations include transitions in the place of work such as technological changes, reorganization, and relocation. Conflicting demands and loyalties are further sources of stress. There might be conflicts between one's role as an employee and as a parent or spouse.

Dissatisfaction can be due to problems in the work environment (poor physical conditions such as noise and over-crowding), role ambiguity, role conflict, under-promotion, over-promotion, lack of financial security, poor relationship with employer or employees and little participation in corporate decision-making. The workload may be excessive or too complex with unrealistic production-targets. Some employees feel threatened by information technology. Factors related to the work environment include unpredictability or a change in responsibilities without consultation or explanation, inducing a sense of impotence.

When the fit between work and worker is poor, various pathological mechanisms come into play. They might be cognitive with impaired concentration, indecision, and loss of creativity, but they can also be emotional with feelings of anxiety, depression, apathy, and demoralization. They might also be behavioural with risk-taking, aggressive feelings and behaviour, and substance abuse, or they might be physiological with the development of cardiovascular or gastrointestinal disease (typically hypertension or irritable bowel syndrome).

A particularly high-risk situation at work is a mismatch between the individual and the environment in terms of ability and demands, with the development of a pervasive feeling of lack of personal control. This may induce one of the stress-related reactions of self-destructive, resentful, passive/aggressive behaviour. It has been suggested that chronic feelings of anger and frustration can lead to a state of depression on the basis of learned helplessness, when repeated exposure to an unsatisfactory outcome leads to the belief that events are beyond one's control and that one is powerless to change the situation.

A lack of influence over organizational decisions affecting employees leads to stress, as can lack of consultation and appreciation by superiors. Thus, operators in a clothing factory working on machine-controlled production processes have higher catecholamine levels than workers on manually operated machines, which allow more control over the workpace and greater utilization of skills. This suggests that if an individual can influence his situation he can modify the stressors.[3]

High-risk groups of employees include those with chronic low self-esteem; lack of assertiveness; a constitutional tendency to a high level of anxiety; and a propensity for Type A behaviour. As a result of the interaction between high-risk situations and vulnerable personality, employees will react emotionally, and/or cognitively and/or physiologically and in the absence of protective 'buffering' the individual is at risk of developing one of the stress diseases and low morale. Peer group support and participation in decision-making can lead to cohesiveness and improvement in morale. Clarification of role responsibilities and formulation of realistic goals can also help. The effects of occupational stressors can be further modified by teaching coping skills and by social support.

A personal review (Dr M. Samuel, personal communication) of 42 consecutive referrals for specialist psychiatric opinion from the occupational health adviser to a large public utility permitted an analysis of the causes of failure to cope with work. The 42 employees included semi-skilled and unskilled manual and clerical workers and middle-managers, roughly equally divided between men and women and with an age range of 21–64 years, average 46. These employees had been on continuous sick leave for over four weeks. They were mainly certificated by their family practitioners as suffering from depression and/or anxiety. Only six were found to be suffering from formal psychiatric disorder: bipolar affective disorder, severe 'endogenous' depression, schizophrenia, chronic paranoid state, and early dementia. There was also one case of anorexia nervosa. An employee with severe endogenous depression showed features of the 'impostor complex'—an inaccurate perception of herself as having been over-promoted and incapable of performing her duties, at which in fact she excelled when euthymic.

The majority however were suffering from 'stress'. In 22 cases the source of the tension could be located in the workplace while in the remainder (14 cases), domestic crises, bereavement, marital tension or psychiatric disorder in the spouse had led to the absenteeism.

There was an interesting phenomenon in which stress at work presented as physical symptoms disproportionate to organic disability. Two employees who had had myocardial infarctions presented with 'cardiac neurosis'. In fact, their reduced exercise tolerance was a form of agoraphobia, induced by fear of visiting notoriously violent housing estates in the course of their duties. One employee with 'sphincter phobia' could not cope with a more demanding schedule because of his irrational fear of having to urinate frequently while at work.

In this series, the most common sources of dissatisfaction at work were: relocation and missing former colleagues and/or having to cope with increased travel time (6 cases). Other employees felt that their training was inadequate or that they had been allocated insufficient staff or resources. One specifically identified increased productivity targets as the trigger for his sickness absence. Failure to achieve promotion, or demotion following reorganization accounted for three cases. Eighteen employees lacked appropriate assertiveness skills and 6 could not delegate effectively while 7 complained of poor relationships with supervisors and colleagues. Those lacking in assertiveness skills sometimes behaved in the workplace in a resentful, passive/aggressive manner or with inappropriate forcefulness. Six cases were of post-traumatic stress disorder. Whilst 4 of these were induced by accidents at work (exposure to explosions, burns, etc.), 2 were due to trauma in the domestic setting (one employee had been raped and the other had been the victim of two burglaries).

## Outcome

Overall the majority of these employees were able to resume their duties after a course of cognitive behavioural therapy undertaken by clinical psychologists with an interest in occupational stress. Twelve had to take medical retirement.

A personal review of over 100 claimants of sickness benefit on the grounds of psychiatric disorder showed a similar paucity of major psychiatric illness. The majority of these claimants, who had similarly received the anxiety/depression label, were 'refugees' from various types of work stress. These included difficulties in handling colleagues, lack of assertiveness, failure to delegate, poor time management, lack of resources, relocation, inadequate training, and unrealistic targets. Many of these problems could be avoided, or at least minimized with appropriate training and psychological intervention with cognitive-behavioural therapy.

Prevention of stress in the workplace centres mainly on the removal of its causes, which have already been described, and the better matching of people to jobs. The treatment of stress in the workplace may vary from the provision of counselling and employee assistance programmes to the provision of exercise facilities and anxiety management training, utilizing a variety of techniques, any of which may be effective in individual cases but none of which are useful in all cases. The multi-factorial causes of stress demand a flexible and varied approach to its treatment but, to be really effective, the major emphasis should be on prevention through the eradication of the 'stressful work situation'.

## Alcohol and drug abuse

Alcohol and drugs, whether illicit or prescribed, are of concern to an employer and to a company medical officer when the use of these substances interferes with work performance or with relationships with colleagues.

Alcohol and drug abuse are an important cost to industry in terms of loss of production, reduced speed of work, mistakes in procedures, damaged equipment, and compensation claims for accidents and injuries. Accident proneness, frequent sickness absence, poor work performance, and erratic behaviour should all raise the possibility that the employee may be affected by drugs or alcohol. Alcohol has been implicated in a variety of industrial accidents including drowning, falling from a height, burns, and road traffic accidents. Also, it is well recognized that substance abuse leads to lost time and impaired productivity.

It is thought that about 4 per cent of the population in England and Wales and over twice that proportion in Scotland, are problem drinkers in the sense that their alcohol consumption has adverse effects on their health, occupation or social and domestic life. Occupational physicians should be concerned with both overt drinking which has an obvious and immediate effect on the handling of dangerous machinery, and longer-term alcohol abuse which leads to absenteeism and inefficiency, with colleagues possibly colluding with and covering up for the alcohol-dependent employee.

A list of features suggesting a problem with alcohol includes absenteeism, frequent accidents, obvious physical changes (such as tremulousness, conjunctival injection, and the odour of alcohol), changes in personality and erratic behaviour at work. Colleagues and supervisors might be aware of inappropriate talkativeness, and a tendency to be argumentative. It is known that alcohol and drug-using employees have a high absenteeism rate.[4,5] In addition, they have more accidents and injuries, cause more breakages, demoralize the sober work force, and may even steal from them to support drug use.

Certain occupations are associated with a substantially higher rate of problem drinking. Male liver cirrhosis mortality is the best available indicator of the relative prevalence rates of alcoholism. High rates of this condition are found in licensees, members of the catering and hotel trade, seamen, the armed services, sales representatives, brewers and distillers, journalists, and medical practitioners. Factors contributing to this wide occupational spread include the availability of alcohol at work (which might even be provided free or at a reduced price), social pressure to drink, and self-selection by people with established drink problems for entry into jobs where alcohol is easily or cheaply available. Freedom from supervision is a factor in independent professions such as medicine and journalism. Other groups, such as servicemen and seamen who are separated from normal social relationships and have limited opportunities for recreation, may resort to drinking excessively.

## Alcohol and industrial accidents

The risk of causing a driving accident increases 3-, 10-, and 40-fold if the blood alcohol exceeds 80, 100, and 150 mg/100 ml, respectively. In fact, many skills and cognitive processes begin to decline with a blood alcohol level of 50 mg/100 ml, a level which can be produced by just two units of alcohol consumed within an hour. In the US Armed Forces a blood alcohol level of 50 mg/100 ml or above indicates unfitness for duty and such a level merits disciplinary action. At this level, memory transfer from immediate recall to long-term storage may be disturbed. Companies operating North Sea oil and gas rigs ban alcohol completely and refuse access to the worksite to anyone reporting for duty under the influence of alcohol.

It has been shown that driving at levels below the prescribed blood alcohol level (80 mg/100 ml), introduced in the Road Traffic Act 1967, is not free of hazards. Even 'safe' levels of alcohol may be associated with significant impairment of driving ability. Drivers who have consumed fairly low doses of alcohol and have blood levels between 30 and 60 mg/100 ml, are likely to show impaired ability to negotiate a test course with artificial hazards.

Laboratory and simulated studies, as well as the performance of typical driving tasks on a closed-course circuit, indicate the detrimental effect of alcohol even with moderate levels of intoxication. Furthermore, by measuring driving performance in a controlled obstacle course which closely parallels actual driving situations, it has been shown that the combination of alcohol and cannabis (see below), even at low levels of the drugs has a potentially hazardous effect on the driving task. The impairment created by the combination of these two drugs is much greater than that created by either drug alone.

A strong association has been demonstrated between a raised gamma GT (glutamyl transferase) and road accidents in drivers aged over 30, indicating that a large proportion of these accidents may be caused by problem drinkers. A high prevalence of raised liver enzyme activity has also been demonstrated in those over the age of 30 who apply for licences as drivers of large goods and passenger carrying vehicles.

## Cannabis

Cannabis use is now widespread in the United Kingdom. Large-scale market research by Gallup in 1989 in the 15–25 age group found that 12 per cent of males and 9 per cent of females reported cannabis use at some time. Seizures of cannabis by Customs increased sevenfold in the period 1978–88. Cannabis is attractive as a workplace drug of abuse because of its compact packaging and rapid onset of action.

Five years ago a series of 162 offshore oil and gas rig workers in the North Sea were subjected to urine analysis for cannabinoids immediately prior to deployment offshore. Positive results were found in over 9 per cent.[6]

Ten experienced pilots each smoked a cigarette containing 19 mg of tetrahydro-cannabinol. Twenty-four hours later their performance on a simulated landing task showed trends towards impairment in all variables. Despite these deficits the pilots reported no awareness of impaired performance, or of difficulty in precisely aligning and landing the aircraft down the centre of the runway.[7]

Cannabis interferes with motor vehicle operation which is comparable to the operation of many industrial machines, the degree and nature of the impairment being similar to that seen with alcohol. Cannabis-intoxicated drivers are over-represented in fatal accidents and it is potentially as dangerous as alcohol in this context, and especially when the two drugs are taken together.

Cannabis users have been found to have twice the normal frequency of road traffic accidents in the 6–12 months before they are convicted for cannabis use. In a study of 710 fatally injured drivers in the United States, over half had used alcohol, 8 per cent were taking benzodiazepines, while 38 per cent had also used cannabis.[8]

In fact cannabis users have nearly as many accidents under the influence of cannabis alone as they do under the influence of alcohol with or without cannabis. On a driving simulator, cannabis has a much stronger effect than alcohol on the estimation of time and distance, and has correspondingly more potent effects on braking time. In controlled laboratory studies, cannabis adversely affects perception, co-ordination, braking time, and other motor skills. Again, cannabis is especially potent in its effects on these skills when combined with alcohol.

There is an extensive literature on human performance under the influence of cannabis and effects on memory, attention span, and perception have been demonstrated. This has implications not only for piloting aircraft but also for operating complicated, heavy equipment, driving railway trains or operating signals.

Accidents in the United States involving rail road crews performing complex tasks have been associated with cannabis detected in the urine of a signalman on one occasion and of a driver on another. A pilot in a fatal commercial air crash was found to have smoked cannabis 24 hours before the crash and there is concern that the use of this drug can lead to impaired piloting performance after such a length of time.

It is known that cannabis can have an adverse effect on any complex learnt psychomotor task involving memory, skill, concentration, sense of time and orientation in three-dimensional space, and on the performance of multiple complex tasks. Cannabis impairs judgement, performance, and immediate recall, while alcohol tends to affect the transfer process from short- to long-term memory stores. With cannabis, cerebellar dysfunction (slurred speech and ataxia) does not occur, but there is impairment of glare recovery, peripheral vision, and sense of time. Visual illusions and the intrusion of inappropriate memories can also occur.

There can be temporal disorganisation with disruption of the correct sequencing of events in time, and work requiring a high level of cognitive integration is adversely affected. A single 'joint' of cannabis can cause significant impairment of skills that is measurable for more than 10 hours. This cognitive impairment lasts for long after the euphoria has disappeared. Psychophysiological activities impaired by cannabis include tracking ability, complex reaction time, hand steadiness, complicated signal interpretation, and attention span. There are, therefore, deficiencies in perception, memory, and cognition. Cannabis has a particularly deleterious effect on pilots who have to orientate themselves in three-dimensional space. A single cannabis 'joint' grossly interferes with the execution of a relatively simple landing pattern in a flight simulator.

In the intoxicated state cannabis, like alcohol, impairs short-term memory in proportion to the dose. However, unlike alcohol, moderate cannabis use is associated with selective short-term memory deficits that persist following a period of several weeks of abstinence.

## Prescribed medication

Both sedative psychoactive medication and alcohol reduce the overall level of alertness of the central nervous system. Certain antidepressants, anti-anxiety agents, and hypnotics have side-effects which reduce skilled performance, concentration, memory, information-processing ability, and motor activity, as demonstrated in both volunteers and patient populations. All these effects increase the risk of driving accidents. It is for this reason that airline pilots are prohibited from flying while under the influence of prescribed psychotropic medication. It is also known that the use of both prescribed and illicit drugs is associated with an increased involvement in road traffic accidents.[9] (See also Chapter 3.)

The relative contribution of mental illness and psychotropic drug use have not been analysed in many of the epidemiological studies. It is therefore possible that some patients with mental disturbance would have been even more hazardous as drivers if they had not been taking their medication. On the other hand, after taking their drugs in normal therapeutic doses, such patients might still remain unsafe drivers. Laboratory studies on the effects of psychotropic drugs on driving-related skills of chronically treated patients are rare. However, it has been demonstrated that patients receiving diazepam do in fact perform worse, showing impaired visual perception and impaired anticipation of dangerous events when driving.

The official report of a 1974 railway accident in Scotland (March 1974, Glasgow Central Station) concluded that the use of diazepam by the train driver was a contributory cause and Scandinavian researchers have found that serum concentrations of benzodiazepines are significantly greater in drivers involved in road traffic accidents than in control groups. Laboratory assessments of psychotropic drugs on sensory and motor skills, steering, brake reaction time, divided attention, and vigilance have shown specific impairment following the administration of minor tranquillizers and tricyclic antidepressants, as well as on the morning after taking benzodiazepine hypnotics. Data from the Netherlands have shown that hypnotics, minor tranquillizers, and tricyclic antidepressants cause driving deficits in real-life conditions on the open road including lateral deviation of the position of a car driven along a motorway. Even fairly low doses of psychoactive drugs have a detrimental effect on the performance of car-driving tests and related measures of psychomotor ability.[10]

These detrimental effects have been demonstrated with the hypnotic *nitrazepam* in a dose as low as 5 mg, *flurazepam* 30 mg, *amitriptyline* 50 mg, *mianserin* 10 mg, *lorazepam* 1 mg, *diazepam* 5 mg, and *chlordiazepoxide* 10 mg. The hypnotics were assessed for their residual activity the morning after night-time sedation, while the effects of the antidepressants and anxiolytics were measured during the day. The amnesic effects of some benzodiazepines is such that drivers fail to remember routines and cannot read maps competently.

The sleep disturbance caused by jet-lag might lead pilots or other people whose work requires vigilance, motor skill, and a high level of decision-making, to take a hypnotic. A benzodiazepine with a short half-life might appear to be an attractive option because of the reduction of day-time sedation, but amnesia may persist after the sedation has disappeared. For sedatives/hypnotics, the available data show that their use could more than double the road accident risk factor.

Although both *amitriptyline* and *dothiepin* impair performance on laboratory analogues of car-driving and related skills, the 5 hydroxytryptamine re-uptake inhibitor, *fluoxetine*, in a dose of 40 mg showed a lack of cognitive and psychomotor effects when administered in an acute dose to volunteers.

Since *fluoxetine* has a long half-life however, it is possible that if administered to patients over a therapeutic period, there might be some impairment of skill performance and car-handling ability.

## Company drugs and alcohol policies

Although substance abuse can be a generic term to include alcohol and solvent misuse as well as drugs, the term is commonly reserved only for drugs, and that convention will be followed here. Obviously alcohol misuse cannot be ignored, indeed it is almost certainly the larger of the two problems, but by separating the two entities it is easier to draw up parallel policies which show the areas of commonality as well as the differences. Solvent abuse is different again and it is also difficult to know how much of a workplace problem it represents as it tends to be a problem predominantly of the young. Nonetheless, the management and rehabilitation of staff found to have solvent abuse problems has much in common with the alcohol and drugs situation.

The principle underlying the workplace management of alcohol and drug abuse is that both are health matters and the onus is on the employee to co-operate with treatment and achieve abstinence. There is evidence that the costs of dismissing an employee who has a drink problem, which include those relating to formal discipline and grievance procedures and legal liability, are greater than of rehabilitation, even allowing for impaired productivity, absenteeism, and accidents.

Employers must also realize that it is a criminal offence for the occupier of any premises knowingly to allow the use, possession or production of any controlled substance (Misuse of Drugs Act 1971). This includes cannabis, so an employer would be committing a criminal offence if he permitted smoking of cannabis on the premises. Also, it is counter-productive to provide a bar with alcohol available at subsidized rates or where alcohol is freely available for entertaining visiting clients.

If a manager suspects a problem on the basis of absenteeism or poor performance the employee should be referred to the occupational health service either directly or through the personnel department. Quite often, the problem only comes to light after a criminal offence has been committed or a serious breach of company rules has occurred. In such cases, it is usually better to proceed with the disciplinary action, if appropriate, and then implement the rehabilitation process. Unfortunately, in some organizations, particularly those with high safety sensitivity, e.g., the offshore gas/oil industry and railways, the disciplinary process can mean summary dismissal. It is for that reason that staff are encouraged to self-declare problems, and in the case of railways, managers are briefed on the identification of problem drinkers/drug abusers so that positive action to help can be initiated.

When staff request assistance or are encouraged to seek professional help, the employee should be allowed time off work for treatment and follow-up appointments. If he has a relapse, further treatment should be offered providing the employee has co-operated up to that point. The management of dependency problems is best achieved as a 'partnership' or 'contract' between the employee, the manager, and the occupational health department. Failure of the employee to follow the treatment programme, maintain abstinence, and achieve regular attendance can lead to termination of the programme for that individual, followed by dismissal.

In setting up a company alcohol and drugs policy it is essential that wide consultation is held at the draft stage, particularly with staff associations/trades unions. The acceptance and co-operation of these organizations is crucial to the success of any alcohol and drugs policy and the better they are briefed, and therefore have understood it, the more successful it will be.

In those cases where employers wish to screen for alcohol or drug addiction in a pre-employment medical examination, the informed consent of the job applicant has to be obtained. For these purposes the physician has to explain the nature of the blood and/or urine tests and has to obtain the prospective employee's consent to disclosure of the test results to the prospective employer. Positive specimens at a screening examination must be confirmed by a further laboratory analysis before being reported as such.

It may be advisable for employers to include a term in the contract of employment which requires abstinence from alcohol for 12 hours before starting a shift.

### Drug-screening programmes

The comprehensive Company Substance of Abuse Screening Programme comprises a triad of measures all of which interrelate in the workplace management of the problem. The three main components are:

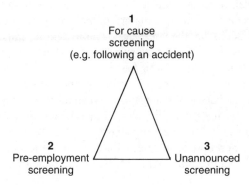

Whilst acknowledging that some components of the triad, particularly pre-employment screening, are easier to implement than others, it is emphasized that it is only with all three that management can consider that it has given itself the maximum opportunity of reducing drug abuse, within its workforce, to the lowest achievable level. Taking each in turn the following points can be made.

### 1. Pre-employment screening

This is the easiest of the three to introduce because, at the selection stage, there is no contractual relationship between the job applicant and the prospective employer. It also provides the opportunity for the organization to make a 'statement' on the whole question of substance abuse, making it clear to prospective new entrants that drug usage is incompatible with employment in that particular firm. It is therefore important that the screening policy is as open as possible, including the provision of information leaflets which clearly spell out the position.

It is not unknown for drug users to maintain abstinence long enough to pass the drug screening test and then resume their habit once they have been taken on. Also, it is important to be alert to the applicant who, having failed the screening test at one place may re-apply to the same firm but in another part of the country. On the second occasion, the applicant 'passes' the drug screening test as he has had a sufficient period of abstinence. The only effective way of avoiding this situation is to maintain good records of the pre-employment candidates screened. Also, those who have failed should be time-barred for some specified period (e.g. three years), during which they may not re-apply to join the company. However, it is important to be aware of the known practice of some job applicants who deliberately abstain so they may pass the drug screening test. Clearly they will almost certainly continue their habit once employed which provides the strongest reason for introducing and maintaining the other two components of the comprehensive screening programme referred to above.

## 2. For cause screening

In the workplace itself managers and supervisors often refer to this as 'post-incident' screening which is, in fact, a major component of for cause screening. However, it is considered that the latter term is more flexible and therefore more useful, particularly as it avoids any argument as to whether a particular event constitutes an 'incident' or not.

In defining for cause screening, it is probably best described as the drug screening of staff at the behest of management when there is a situation in which the manager/supervisor feels that drug abuse might be a relevant consideration, or from which he wishes to exclude drug abuse.

Also it is entirely appropriate to screen for alcohol at the same time, as it is almost certainly a far more common underlying reason than drugs for workplace accidents/incidents.

## 3. Unannounced (random) screening

This third component of the screening triad is possibly the most difficult to introduce in terms of both acceptability to staff and the scope of its application. Not only is it necessary to decide whether to screen the entire workforce or merely those in safety-sensitive jobs, but also the frequency at which screening should be done. Although logistics influence the former, particularly if the workforce is both large and geographically diffuse, it is the frequency of screening which can create most problems. If screening is too infrequent then it loses its deterrent effect as the factor of uncertainty will be blunted by a low expectation of being screened. On the other hand, at too great a frequency there is a risk of it becoming irksome and intrusive and causing staff resentment rather than acceptance of what should be perceived as a necessary part of the total drug abuse management programme. The most effective system for any group selected for unannounced screening is an annual screen for everyone plus the possibility of second screening tests within the same year for, say, a further 10 or 20 per cent of that same population. If the number of designated personnel within that selected group is relatively small then such a system is manageable but again, the size and geographical dispersion of the workforce are significant factors in considering the feasibility and cost.

### Screening on other occasions

In addition to the three basic components regarded as essential to a comprehensive screening programme, other opportunities to screen may also be taken, for example, if staff are either promoted or transferred into different jobs within the company, and in conjunction with standard, periodic medical assessments. Whilst it may be assumed that, because screening on such occasions is predictable and therefore provides forewarning none will be detected, practical experience proves otherwise. The adoption of such a system also provides management with a further opportunity to demonstrate its refusal to tolerate drug abuse.

## The role of the occupational physician

In considering the role of the occupational physician in drug screening, organizations which adopt policies against drug and alcohol abuse often expect active involvement of the occupational physician in their programmes. Not only are occupational health departments the most appropriate place for undertaking urine sample collections but the maintenance of confidentiality and the proper interpretation of the results of the analyses are also very definitely medical responsibilities. With respect to the actual urine samples, these have to be collected under conditions such that neither adulteration nor substitution of the sample can occur, the entire process from voiding the sample through the laboratory analysis process to the receipt of the result in the occupational health department being known as a 'chain-of-custody'.

The occupational physician also has to maintain strict impartiality in implementing his part of the company alcohol and drugs policy, maintaining confidentiality being especially important both for individuals at the personal level as well as ensuring the maintenance of programme credibility and acceptance.

Finally, but certainly not least, the reasons why the occupational physician's role in drug screening is so crucial, is the medical review officer process. This task is vitally important as it provides the confidential interpretation of both the analytical findings from the laboratory and the clinical information which the sample collection officer has obtained from the donor. This information may include recent medically prescribed drugs as well as over-the-counter medication being taken by the donor. The importance of this information cannot be overestimated, as it will become part of the structured dialogue which must take place between the medical review officer and the toxicologist responsible for the analysis of the donor's urine sample. The purpose of this discussion is to ensure that proper account is taken of any medication or food (e.g., culinary use of poppy seeds) which may have been taken during the preceding 7–10 days before the drug screen test so that false positive reporting does not occur.

Employers who are considering the introduction of a drug screening policy on, for example, job applicants or employees, require expert advice on the selection of the drugs to be screened for, and their metabolites, as well as the collection of the biological specimens, their identification, storage, preservation and transport, and the validity and reliability of the subsequent chemical analyses. They also require advice on the reporting of the laboratory-generated results and the interpretation and use of those results. Although blood, breath, hair, saliva, and urine are biological specimens which can be used for drug testing, it is urine which is most usually tested, both in the military and civilian settings.

Commercial laboratories can screen for opiates, barbiturates, amphetamines, cannabis, and cocaine metabolites. Heroin is broken down to morphine and is reported as such while part of ingested codeine is converted to morphine, so an individual taking codeine as an analgesic might have a positive urine for morphine as well as codeine. Any immunoassay test which produces a positive result must be confirmed by gas chromatography/mass spectrometry if the result is to be defensible in the event of legal challenge.

A urine test for cocaine metabolites can be positive for up to 72 hours and in a daily user of cannabis, urine can be positive for at least two weeks because the drug is deposited in fat stores. However, the results of urine tests *alone* cannot be used to determine whether or not the donor was actually impaired by drugs or their metabolites or was unfit to undertake any given task. Furthermore, a positive urine drugs test result cannot be used by itself to establish what dose of a drug was administered or when.

Given the steadily increasing number of organizations setting up drug screening programmes it is important that occupational physicians have a full understanding of their role within them, this being achieved by careful attention in setting up the programme so that actions and responsibilities are both clearly defined and communicated. Guidelines on this have already been produced by the Faculty of Occupational Medicine.[11]

## The mechanics of alcohol and substance abuse screening

Acts of Parliament, i.e., the Road Traffic Acts and the new Transport and Works Act 1992, which applies to the railway, allow for screening to be done on samples of breath, blood, and urine in the case of alcohol, and on blood and urine in the case of drugs. In the workplace, it is considered that the most effect-ive method for alcohol screening is an analysis of breath and for drugs an analy-sis of urine. Avoidance of any procedure involving blood is recommended as it is both time consuming as well as carrying the risk of needle-stick injury and its associated problems.

In undertaking the sample collection work, it is essential to maintain 'chain of custody' security. This is an auditable process whereby the sample donated by each identified donor is uniquely identified and remains secure at all times. A common method of achieving this is to use barcode labels which are unique to the particular donor, the code itself accompanying the sample throughout the entire process. This requires an extremely high level of consistency of operation and attention to detail, with carefully written procedures and a clearly defined audit trail so the progress of the sample can be followed at every stage. To em-phasize the importance of the integrity of the chain-of-custody procedure it is recognized as the most productive area for demonstrating procedural and/or security errors, thereby challenging the entire drug screening procedure.

The laboratory analytical procedure is either a one- or two-step process de-pending on whether the first step is positive. The initial screening procedure, which is now largely automated permitting a high throughput of samples, is an immunoassay system, set up to identify whatever range of analytes the pro-gramme requires. If the immunoassay tests for the various analytes all prove negative then nothing further will be done and the laboratory will report the screen to the medical review officer as negative. The sample is then usually re-tained for a period of up to two weeks before being destroyed. Samples testing positive on immunoassay have to undergo a second entirely separate confirmation test using gas chromatography/mass spectrometry. This is the definitive method of identification and if the analytes initially discovered on im-munoassay are proved to be present then the sample will be reported as positive to the medical review officer. It is at this stage that discussion takes place so that the interaction of any previously disclosed medication can be taken into account. In a number of cases, laboratory 'positives' are reported to management as nega-tive because a satisfactory explanation for that result has been agreed between the medical review officer and the toxicologist.

## The problem drinker: early recognition and intervention

A health screening programme identifying all individuals with a raised serum gamma GT as a means of identifying employees with a drinking problem, can potentially reduce the absenteeism rate for all alcohol-related conditions by 50 per cent, if it is combined with counselling about reduction of alcohol intake and serial gamma GT estimations at three monthly intervals to monitor progress.

Covering up for the problem drinker by colleagues leads to delay in recogni-tion. Alerting factors include absenteeism, especially on Monday mornings, and also certain observable features including redness of eyes and tremulousness, irritability, indecisiveness, procrastination, errors, and poor productivity.

One of the most important aspects of a company's alcohol and drugs policy is to get the employee to do something about his drinking. This requires demonstrating to the problem drinker the link between his presenting work problems and his alcohol intake as well as deterioration in his general health and his social and domestic life. It is valuable to teach the patient the concept of units (1 unit = 1 glass of wine or sherry; 1 measure of spirits; $\frac{1}{2}$ pint of beer), to maintain a drinking diary and to identify emotional or social triggers for heavy drinking. To avoid futile debate about whether a particular employee is 'an alcoholic', it is more constructive to describe the presenting problem in terms of the damage, whether social, occupational or medical, which that particular individual's drinking is causing. Referral to a counselling agency and also to organizations, such as Alcoholics Anonymous, can also be extremely helpful. Some physicians recommend a supervised *disulfiram (Antabuse)* programme. This chemical deterrent might have a place provided its limitations are recognized. It should, however, be regarded as a short-term measure to provide a respite from drinking while counselling with both the individual and the partner begins to take effect. It is certainly not to be regarded as a substitute for counselling and education.

## Drug and alcohol rehabilitation programmes

When establishing any programme of alcohol and substance abuse screening it is essential that the company or organization also sets up a formal rehabilitation programme both for those who self-declare a dependency problem and request assistance with it; as well as for those found positive on screening who are then directed towards the rehabilitation procedure as part of the corporate disciplinary process. Obviously, the nature and scope of the rehabilitation programme will depend very much on the management style of the company and also the nature of its activity. However, irrespective of whether rehabilitation is offered as a totally in-house service or resourced mainly by outside agencies, it is essential that the responsibility for the programme itself is managed from within the company rather than passed in its entirety to an external provider. The principal reason for this is the need to maintain appropriate managerial control of the rehabilitation programme such that those members of staff within it are properly followed-up to ensure compliance within the terms of the programme. In this respect, it is essential that management is kept informed of progress, or lack of it as the case may be, particularly as, in the latter situation, it may be necessary to terminate employment.

It is therefore considered that the corporate occupational health service is the most appropriate organization through which to manage a company dependency rehabilitation programme, thereby building up an appropriate relationship between:

(1)  the member of staff concerned;

(2)  the management;

(3)  any external agency that might be involved; and

(4)  the occupational health department itself.

There should, in principle, be no difference between the programme for staff with alcohol dependence and for staff with drug dependence; both are varieties of chemical dependence.

However, employers and perhaps also trade unions seem to be much more 'comfortable' with the reformed problem drinker than the reformed drug user. It would seem that drug dependency is commonly perceived as a life-long, irretrievable addiction, whereas alcohol dependency is not. However, it is up to the company occupational health service to convince line managers that dependency problems must be treated in a uniform way and the outcome of each judged upon its merits, particularly when there has been scrupulous compliance with the rehabilitation programme and total commitment to recovery on the part of the particular employee.

## Acknowledgement

We are most grateful to Dr Margaret Samuel for help in the compilation of this chapter.

## Selected references and further reading

1.  CBI (Confederation of British Industry) (September 1993). *Working for your health: Practical steps to improve the health of your business*. CBI, London.
2.  Fingret, A. (1985). Stress at work. *The Practitioner*, **229**, 547–55.
3.  Spillane, R. (1984). Stress at work. *Int. J. Hlth. Serv.*, **14**, 589–604.
4.  Hore, B.D. and Plant, M.A. (ed.) (1981). *Alcohol problems in employment*. Croom Helm, London.
5.  Banta, W.F. and Tennant, F. (1989). *Complete handbook for combatting substance abuse in the workplace*. Lexington, MA.
6.  Calder, I.M. and Ramsey, J. (1987). A survey of cannabis use in offshore rig workers. *Brit. J. Addict.*, **82**, 159–61.
7.  Yesavage, J.A., Leirer, V.O., Denar, M., and Hollister, L.E. (1985). Carry-over effects of marijuana intoxication on aircraft pilot performance. *Amer. J. Psychiat.*, **142**, 1325–9.
8.  Glauz, W.D. and Blackburn, R.R. (1975). *Drug use among drivers*. Technical contract report to the National Highway Traffic Safety Administration. Department of Transportation, Washington, DC.
9   Skegg, D.C.G., Richards, S.M., and Doll, R. (1979). Minor tranquillisers and road accidents. *Brit. Med. J.*, **1**, 917–19.

10. Hindmarch, I. (1986). The effects of psychoactive drugs on car handling and related psychomotor ability. In *Drugs and driving*, (ed. J.F.O' Hanlon and J.J. de Gier), pp. 71–9. Taylor & Francis, London.
11. Faculty of Occupational Medicine (1994). *Guidelines on testing for drugs of abuse in the workplace*. Faculty of Occupational Medicine, London.

# 22

# Acquired immune deficiency syndrome (AIDS)

*A. Cockcroft and N.M. Foley*

## Introduction

Fear, anxiety, and ignorance still surround HIV infection and AIDS. In this chapter the spectrum of HIV disease is reviewed and the recent epidemic summarized. The main problem in the workplace is the concern of non-infected workers; this should be tackled by a clear policy and an effective education programme. The virus is only transmissible by certain limited means and occupational transmission is rare, even in the health care setting where the risk can be reduced by implementing guidelines for safe practice. In most workplaces employees with the acquired immune deficiency syndrome (AIDS) can continue at work as long as they are physically and mentally able, and the considerations for their work are the same as for any progressive debilitating illness. There are special considerations in the health care setting, where new guidelines advise that HIV-infected workers should not participate in certain invasive procedures. The management of HIV-infected health care workers requires a sensitive, informed approach. Confidentiality is of particular importance in the occupational issues surrounding HIV infection.

A major problem for workers infected with human immunodeficiency virus (HIV) is the general public's perception of AIDS. No other health problem has had such wide publicity or engendered so much fear and anxiety. There is still considerable ignorance about the risks of contracting infection with HIV. It is widely perceived as being contagious—transmissible by casual and accidental contact in everyday life—despite good evidence to the contrary. Additionally, in the Western world HIV infection is most prevalent amongst male homosexuals and injecting drug users; the behaviour of these groups is seen by some as deviant or morally reprehensible. Prejudice and misconceptions often influence the way that people with HIV infection are treated by others.

In reality, HIV infection is not confined to certain so-called high-risk groups. Although the prevalence of infection in 'low-risk groups' remains low, the rate of increase in the heterosexual population now exceeds that in the traditional risk groups. The virus is only transmissible by certain limited means and in the vast majority of jobs there is no risk of workers becoming infected or of transmitting the infection to others. In the health care and laboratory setting there is a risk of occupational transmission of the virus, but even here the risk is very low and can be virtually eliminated by proper precautions.

However, occupational health professionals must recognize and play a part in reducing the fear, ignorance, and prejudice which still surround HIV disease. If employees discover or suspect that a colleague is HIV-infected, or even suspect that he is at greater risk of infection, considerable problems and disruption can occur. Stigmatization and ostracism of such individuals can increase the burden on their physical and mental well-being where infection does exist. Such problems can be prevented by pre-emptive action in the workplace. This should include education about HIV infection for all employees and support for any that are infected with HIV. The employer must decide how to tackle HIV infection in an employee and review existing policies and procedures relating to ill health to ensure that they are robust enough to cope with HIV disease should it arise.

The HIV epidemic is a problem for everyone. Workplace initiatives can have an important influence. They can help the community to accept the need for the changes in attitude and behaviour that are necessary to control the spread of infection and to provide adequate care for those who are already infected or who will become so.

## Clinical aspects affecting work capacity: spectrum of disease

HIV infection results in a spectrum of disease, over a variable but prolonged time.[1] (see Fig. 22 1.)

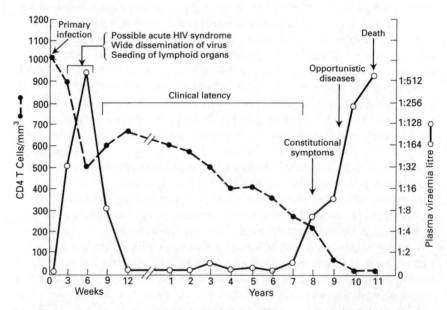

**Fig. 22.1**   Viraemia, CD4 lymphocyte count, and clinical disease in HIV infection (reprinted by permission of the *New England Journal of Medicine*, 1993, pp. 328–9).

Individuals with HIV infection often remain asymptomatic for many years and, even with symptoms, are often fit enough to continue at work. Most people with HIV infection can and should be in employment. During the asymptomatic phase they usually have an unaltered work capacity, although anxiety and depression can lead to difficulties, especially soon after the diagnosis has been confirmed. During the asymptomatic phase many people are unaware that they are infected.

In a proportion of those infected with HIV an initial acute retroviral illness occurs about two to eight weeks after infection. It is self-limiting and may go unrecognized, often being attributed to 'flu' or glandular fever. Antibodies to HIV, which are not protective, appear in the blood after about 12 weeks, while at the same time the titre of virus in the blood falls from the high level that may occur soon after infection (see Fig. 22.1). After a variable period of years, symptoms begin to appear and there is a rise in the level of viraemia and a fall in the CD4 (T helper cell) lymphocyte count, indicating damage to the immune system. The latest US definition of AIDS includes HIV infection with a low CD4 count, even in the absence of other AIDS-defining features. In the United Kingdom, a low CD4 count alone is not AIDS-defining.

Clinical syndromes related to AIDS[1] include persistent generalized lymphadenopathy (PGL), which can occur relatively early after infection and may be associated with fatigue which limits the capacity for full-time work, especially if it is physically taxing. Later symptoms include fever, night sweats, significant and rapid weight loss, malaise, and skin rashes. As AIDS progresses there may be repeated episodes of opportunistic infections, such as *pneumocystis carinii* pneumonia, *cytomegalovirus* infections, systemic fungal infections, and infection with mycobacteria. Infection with *mycobacterium tuberculosis* is an increasingly frequent feature of AIDS in the United States and in developing countries. While tuberculosis is not yet a prominent feature in the UK AIDS epidemic, it may become so in the future.

Malignancies, such as Kaposi's sarcoma and lymphoma, can affect almost any part of the body. Neurological involvement in AIDS includes dementia, specific neurological deficits and psychotic syndromes. AIDS dementia has been reduced by antiviral treatment but minor degrees of mental impairment are common in the late stages of HIV disease. Once AIDS has developed, there is usually serious debility, even between acute episodes of infection, so that most people are unable to continue in full-time work.

The prognosis of AIDS is very poor, with nearly all cases dead within five years, and most dead within two years of diagnosis of AIDS. Better treatment and prophylaxis of opportunistic infections has improved the prognosis a little and has led to an improved quality of remaining life. Anti-retroviral therapy is progressing from the use of *zidovudine* alone to the use of combinations of agents. A number of trials of combination therapy are currently in progress, with the hope that such treatment will prolong survival and/or improve the quality of life by reducing the frequency of opportunistic infections.

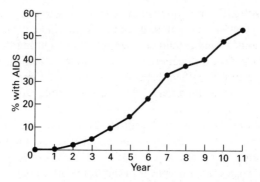

**Fig. 22.2**   The development rate of AIDS among a cohort of San Francisco men with HIV infection followed up for 11 years (from Professor P. Griffiths, drawn from data published by Multi-Center AIDS Cohort Studies Group).

Prediction of the rate of disease progression in individuals is difficult. Among a cohort of HIV-infected individuals in San Francisco, more than half had developed AIDS after 11 years and there is so far no evidence of a slowing of the rate at which AIDS develops (Fig. 22.2). There is evidence that the presence of co-factors, such as *cytomegalovirus* infection, can increase the risk of progressing to AIDS. So far, there is no good evidence that any treatment of asymptomatic individuals can slow the rate of progression. Advice to HIV-positive persons to lead as healthy a lifestyle as possible, and to avoid unhealthy behaviour, such as smoking and excessive drinking, seems reasonable. Since stress can affect the immune system, it also seems wise to avoid stressful situations as far as possible, including those at work.

A major morbidity of HIV-infected people is psychological. Anxiety and depression are common, especially if individuals have not received adequate counselling before and after HIV testing. Psychological problems are often severe enough to affect the capacity for work, at least in the short-term. Most HIV-infected individuals learn to cope with the diagnosis with the help of counselling but problems in coping with work will be worsened if they receive a negative and unsympathetic response from employers and colleagues to whom they reveal their diagnosis.

## Prevalence: the developing epidemic

HIV infection in the United Kingdom has been mainly spread by sexual intercourse, especially between men. However, there are increasing numbers of AIDS cases contracted through heterosexual intercourse and injecting drug use. In the United Kingdom, AIDS cases to the end of April 1993 are shown in Table 22.1. The number of cases has continued to rise, as shown in Table 22.2 and

**Table 22.1** Cumulative AIDS cases in the United Kingdom from January 1982 to end March 1993

| Route of transmission | Male | Female | Totals |
|---|---|---|---|
| *Sexual intercourse* | | | |
| – Between men | 5527 | | 5527 |
| – Between men and women | | | |
|   'High risk partner'* | 24 | 53 | 77 |
|   Other partner abroad | 356 | 213 | 569 |
|   Other partner UK | 37 | 31 | 68 |
|   Under investigation | 9 | 1 | 10 |
| *Injecting drug use (IDU)* | 243 | 101 | 344 |
| – IDU & sex between men | 120 | | 120 |
| *Blood* | | | |
| – Blood factor | 353 | 6 | 359 |
| – Blood/tissue transfer | | | |
|   abroad | 13 | 31 | 44 |
|   UK | 19 | 19 | 38 |
| *Mother to infant* | 38 | 45 | 83 |
| *Other/undetermined* | 88 | 14 | 102 |
| *Total* | 6827 | 514 | 7341 |

* 'High-risk partner' is a partner who is an injecting drug user or a man who has sex with other men.

From: AIDS and HIV infection in the United Kingdom: monthly report. *Communicable Disease Report*, 1993, **3**, p. 77, table 1.

Fig 22.3. Figures for HIV positive people are less reliable, based only on confidential reporting by physicians, but are clearly much higher than the number of AIDS cases. Table 22.3 gives the numbers of HIV-infected persons in the United Kingdom to the end of March 1993.

**Table 22.2**    Incidence of AIDS cases in the UK (by quarter) to June 1993

| Year | Quarter | | | | Total | Deaths by Dec. 1992(%) |
|------|---|---|---|---|-------|------------------|
|      | 1 | 2 | 3 | 4 |       |                  |
| 1982 | 1   | 0   | 0   | 2   | 3    | 100 |
| 1983 | 2   | 6   | 10  | 8   | 26   | 92  |
| 1984 | 12  | 9   | 28  | 28  | 77   | 96  |
| 1985 | 34  | 32  | 45  | 47  | 158  | 92  |
| 1986 | 48  | 59  | 96  | 95  | 298  | 93  |
| 1987 | 147 | 143 | 197 | 154 | 641  | 92  |
| 1988 | 202 | 167 | 194 | 193 | 756  | 89  |
| 1989 | 207 | 178 | 272 | 185 | 842  | 80  |
| 1990 | 321 | 278 | 366 | 304 | 1269 | 66  |
| 1991 | 352 | 303 | 317 | 390 | 1362 | 46  |
| 1992 | 335 | 360 | 413 | 380 | 1488 | 25  |
| 1993 | 418 | 361 |     |     |      |     |

From AIDS and HIV infection in the United Kingdom: Monthly report. *Communicable Disease Report*, 1993, **3**, 154, table 4.

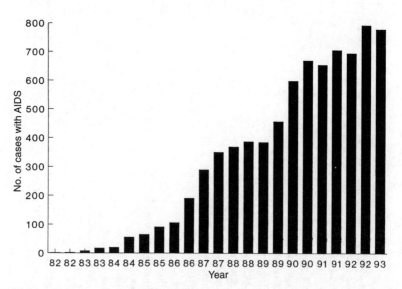

**Fig. 22.3**   Incidence of reported UK AIDS cases in 6-monthly periods from January 1982 to June 1993 (from *Communicable Disease Report*, 1993, **3**, 154, table 4.)

**Table 22.3**  HIV infections in the UK (by exposure category and date of report) to week 13 of 1993.

| Route of transmission | No. of cases Weeks 14/91–13/92 | | | No. of cases Weeks 14/92–13/93 | | | Total cases Weeks 45/84–13/93 | | |
|---|---|---|---|---|---|---|---|---|---|
| | M | F | NS | M | F | NS | M | F | NS |
| *Sexual intercourse* | | | | | | | | | |
| – Between men | 1503 | | | 1466 | | | 11 809 | | |
| – Between men and women | | | | | | | | | |
| 'High risk partner'* | 14 | 51 | | 8 | 41 | | 61 | 302 | |
| Other partner abroad | 235 | 213 | | 236 | 240 | | 973 | 836 | 4 |
| Other partner UK | 23 | 27 | | 20 | 36 | | 100 | 139 | |
| Under investigation | 24 | 21 | | 35 | 50 | | 109 | 138 | |
| *Injecting drug use* (IDU) | 170 | 67 | | 132 | 54 | | 1635 | 744 | 8 |
| IDU & sex between men | 31 | | | 23 | | | 257 | | |
| *Blood* | | | | | | | | | |
| – Blood factor | 7 | | | 9 | | | 1203 | 11 | |
| – Blood /tissue transfer abroad/UK | 11 | 16 | | 11 | 3 | | 88 | 87 | 1 |
| *Mother to infant* | 22 | 17 | | 16 | 15 | | 85 | 78 | |
| *Other/undetermined* | 53 | 19 | 1 | 85 | 20 | 6 | 683 | 133 | 40 |
| *Total* | 2093 | 431 | 1 | 2041 | 461 | 6 | 17 003 | 2468 | 53 |

* 'High-risk partner' is a partner who is an injecting drug user or a man who has sex with other men.

NS, sex not stated on report.

From AIDS and HIV infection in the United Kingdom: monthly report. *Communicable Disease Report*, **3**, p. 78, table 2 (1993).

## Modes of transmission: general

By far the most common mode of transmission of HIV is via sexual contact, both between men and between men and women. Sexual contact between men has been particularly prominent as a means of transmitting HIV in the Western world but in many countries heterosexual contact is more important. The majority of cases of HIV infection world-wide are acquired by heterosexual contact. Transmission can occur via transfusion of infected blood or blood products (such as factor VIII). There is no longer a risk in the United Kingdom and other developed countries where blood donations are screened and people who are at risk of HIV infection are discouraged from giving blood. It continues to be a risk in some parts of the world. Transmission by blood or blood products occurs mainly when needles and other equipment are shared by injecting drug users; this has been an important mode of transmission in some UK cities and in continental Europe, where up to 60 percent of HIV infections occur in injecting drug users or their partners. Transmission can also occur from infected women to their children, *in utero* or at delivery, or via infected breast milk after birth. None of these modes of transmission is likely to occur in the workplace, except in very specialized circumstances.

## Workplace transmission

The risk of transmission of HIV in the workplace is very low. The risks are confined to accidental exposures to material containing live virus, namely, inoculation injuries with contaminated sharp instruments or tissues (e.g., needle stick injuries), and contamination of broken skin or mucous membranes. It is clear that HIV is very much less transmissible than hepatitis B in these circumstances. Large prospective studies have found that the risk of transmission of HIV after a single infected needle stick is about 0.3 per cent,[2] whereas the equivalent risk for hepatitis B (e antigen positive source) is up to 30 per cent.

Up to October 1992, there were 146 cases of occupational transmission of HIV from contact with infected blood reported world wide, mostly related to needle stick or other percutaneous injuries (Table 22.4).[2] This may well be an underestimate of the actual number of occupational infections that have occurred, but nevertheless the number is very small in relation to the many thousands of procedures carried out on patients with HIV infection, including circumstances where infection control provisions are inadequate.

Occupational transmission in the health care setting includes transfer of the infection in both directions—from patients to health care workers or from health care workers to patients. There is only one reported case of the latter: a Florida dentist with AIDS who transmitted HIV to five of his patients in the course of his practice.[3] The exact mode of transmission is unclear. Clearly, the risk of

**Table 22.4**    Occupational transmission of HIV to September 1993

|                                                        | US  | Rest of world | UK  | Total |
| ------------------------------------------------------ | --- | ------------- | --- | ----- |
| Documented seroconversions (specific exposure incident) | 37  | 23            | 4   | 64    |
| Probable occupational infection (no lifestyle risks)   | 78  | 34            | 6   | 118   |
| *Totals*                                               | 115 | 57            | 10  | 182   |

From Heptonstall, J., Porter, K., and Gill, O.N. (1993). *Summary of published reports of occupational transmission of HIV*. Internal publication of the Public Health Laboratory Service. Colindale, London.

occupational infection to health care workers is far greater than the risk of an HIV-infected health care worker infecting patients or colleagues. The single reported case of HIV transmission to patients contrasts with the steady stream of clusters of hepatitis B infection contracted from infected health care workers, mainly surgeons and dentists.[4]

Prevention of occupational HIV transmission in the health care setting relies upon safe practice to avoid exposure to blood and body fluids.[5] Some people consider that a two-tier approach, with identification of infected patients and special precautions in their care, is feasible and cost-effective. However, it is now increasingly accepted that a 'universal precautions' approach should be adopted.[6,7] This means that all blood is considered infectious and precautions to avoid needle sticks and skin or mucous membrane exposures to blood are taken with all patients and with all blood and tissue samples. Local guidelines for safe practice in all situations where contact with blood or body fluids is possible should be drawn up; all employees who may have contact with blood or body fluids should be trained in these practices and the adherence to practice guidelines should be regularly reviewed. Protective equipment and clothing, such as gloves, gowns and eye protection, should be provided as necessary. Under the COSHH (Control of Substances Hazardous to Health) Regulations, employers are required to assess risks to health to employees and others of hazardous substances and take steps to reduce these risks. The Regulations include biological hazards, such as blood that could contain infectious agents. The level of precautions required for a particular procedure will depend on the likelihood of blood exposure during that procedure. In the health care setting the precautions taken to protect employees from infected patients will also serve to protect patients from any infected employees.

Despite all precautions, accidental exposures to blood will continue to occur in health care work and related occupations. Such exposures cause great anxiety to employees, especially if the blood involved is known to be infected with HIV. Procedures for reporting and managing blood exposure incidents should be set up and publicized to employees.[8,9] The use of prophylactic *zidovudine* in these circumstances is of unproven value and a number of seroconversions have been reported despite its use.[10] The drug should probably be available to employees who wish to use it after a significant exposure to HIV infected blood, but its use should not be a substitute for proper counselling of the employee.

One special case of occupational transmission of HIV is in relation to sex workers. Studies have shown varying prevalences of HIV infection among prostitutes in different parts of the United Kingdom. Prostitutes are clearly at risk of HIV infection, as well as other sexually transmitted diseases, as are their clients. Preventive measures (i.e., safer sex practices such as the correct use of condoms and avoidance of activities likely to cause trauma or bleeding) are particularly important for this group.

# Special work problems

## Dealing with prejudice

As indicated in the introduction to this chapter, the main problems in the workplace often arise from those employees who are not HIV infected rather than those who are.[11,12] Unreasonable and irrelevant demands may result from lack of accurate information, fear or prejudice. The demands can relate not only to known infected individuals but also to individuals perceived to be at risk of being infected. Examples of such demands have included refusal to work with HIV-infected employees, with haemophiliacs, with gay men, or those thought to be gay, and requests for separate work equipment, toilet facilities or canteens.

Many of these difficulties can be tackled successfully by a combination of a clear policy in the organization, supported by senior management, and a programme of education of employees at all levels. Action is most effective if taken before problems arise. Many UK companies now have policies relating to HIV infection. These policies usually include statements about confidentiality, employment rights and the non-acceptability of workplace discrimination against colleagues with known or suspected HIV infection and are accompanied by a programme of employee education.[13] To be effective, policies need to be implemented should the need arise, to the extent of taking disciplinary action.

---

**Elements of a policy on HIV in the workplace**
- Background information about modes of transmission, lack of risk in the workplace
- Employment policy regarding HIV pre-employment
- Statement on rights to confidentiality about all medical information, including HIV status
- Statement about rights of workers who become ill from any cause (e.g., to redeployment, medical retirement)
- Statement about non-acceptability of workplace discrimination on basis of known or suspected HIV status
- Statement on programme of education for staff about HIV issues
- Statement about arrangements for advising HIV-infected staff about any necessary work limitations in confidence (for health care setting only)

---

Workplace education programmes need involvement of all relevant personnel, such as occupational health professionals, human resources specialists, and others concerned with staff training. General public health campaigns in the United Kingdom have been designed to heighten awareness of the risks of transmission of HIV; in the workplace these messages need to be accompanied by more reassuring ones about the lack of risk from everyday activities at work. Programmes should be tailored to the level of the audience concerned and should include basic information about the nature of HIV and AIDS, the modes of transmission of HIV, the risks of transmission in different circumstances, and the need to treat colleagues with AIDS like anyone else with a serious illness. The opportunity can also be taken to inform employees about how to protect themselves from HIV infection in their own personal lives. This may be backed up by provision of, for example, condom vending machines in the company toilets.

Particular education is needed for employees who travel abroad as part of their work[12]. (See Appendix 5.) They need to be made aware of the risks of casual sexual encounters in countries where there is a high prevalence of HIV infection. They also need to know how to reduce the risk of having accidents which may result in the need for an emergency blood transfusion abroad; avoidance of excess alcohol before driving is important. Some companies have arrangements whereby employees stationed abroad act as a 'walking blood bank' for colleagues at nearby locations who may need transfusions. Employees travelling to areas with high endemic rates of HIV infection and poor health care facilities may wish to carry a travel kit containing sterile disposable syringes and needles, but should remember that these are of limited use should an accident occur that makes blood transfusion necessary.

Encouragingly, there is now evidence that programmes of education can improve knowledge and attitudes about HIV infection. In the authors' experience, there are now individuals with AIDS being given help and support by colleagues at all levels in an organization where there were cases of physical intimidation of employees suspected of being HIV positive a few years ago.

## Care of the HIV-infected employee

Modifications of working practices are not necessary to protect others from infection by HIV-infected workers, except in very special circumstances (see p. 425). Modifications may be needed to allow HIV infected individuals suffering physical and psychological problems to stay at work as long as possible. Individual workers with HIV infection should be able to discuss their diagnosis, in confidence, with an occupational physician and be given support and advice as necessary. The advice given will depend on the clinical stage of the disease and the individual's work circumstances. Liaison between the individual's clinical team and the occupational physician allows the best management. The consent of the worker for such communication is, of course, necessary.

In the asymptomatic stage, support in dealing with anxiety and depression is important. This can come from the clinical and counselling team concerned in the worker's care and from the occupational health services. Once symptoms of fatigue and malaise appear, it may be necessary to consider modified duties or reduced working hours. Work that involves heavy physical exertion or significant stress (such as time pressures or caring for sick patients) is usually best avoided if possible. Involvement of the immediate manager, with the individual's consent, is helpful. When AIDS has developed, the individual will need to visit hospital frequently for treatment and monitoring and there will be episodes of acute illness. It is difficult to maintain work in this phase but some form of flexible work arrangement that utilizes the skills of the individual can be beneficial to both the worker and the organization. Neurological deficits are frequent in more advanced forms of HIV disease and this will affect the work an individual is able to undertake. Careful assessment and monitoring is necessary to ensure that the individual remains capable of the work and is not unsafe because of, for example, impaired memory or difficulties with concentration.

When work is no longer possible, retirement on ill-health grounds should be arranged where this is available in the organization. In this respect AIDS is no different from any other progressive debilitating disease. In the authors' experience, it is useful to discuss with workers, while they are still relatively well, the work arrangements that can be made as they become ill. This should include the possibilities of part-time working and ill-health retirement. Such early discussions allow individuals to think about choices (for example about redeployment options) in advance and to feel more confident about what will happen as they become ill. This approach of dealing with 'dreaded issues' in advance is often used in general AIDS counselling.[14]

## Pre-employment screening and HIV testing

The idea of HIV antibody testing as a condition of employment is controversial.[15,16] In support of such a policy, it is argued that this enables the employer to reject prospective employees who are infected, thus avoiding the eventual problems associated with future morbidity or mortality as well as difficulties from other employees. A number of companies operate a policy of pre-employment HIV testing and this is legal provided that it is applied equally to men and women and to all races.

However, there are important ethical and other criticisms of pre-employment HIV screening[15,16] The test may be negative for up to three months after infection and tested employees may become infected after employment. This may lead to calls for exclusion of so-called high risk groups, such as haemophiliacs or homosexual men, with or without HIV testing. It could even extend to excluding people with many sexual partners. Being HIV-infected does not affect work capacity unless related disease develops and there is no accurate way of determining prognosis regarding work capacity. If the occupational pension scheme is a concern, there is no longer a requirement for an employee to belong to the company scheme. To be consistent, employers enacting a policy of pre-employment HIV screening should also consider excluding other individuals with a high risk of future morbidity, such as heavy smokers, or those who consume large quantities of alcohol.

Occupational physicians and nurses have a duty of care towards candidates for employment.[16] Screening for HIV offers little advantage to the employer and may have disadvantages to the candidate, both psychological and social. Any testing must always be preceded by competent and informed consent. The candidate must be informed of the test result, strict confidentiality maintained, and post-test counselling undertaken. *Routine pre-employment screening without adequate counselling both pre- and post-test is not ethically acceptable and occupational physicians should not lend themselves to such a policy.*[16]

Routine HIV screening of all donated blood is necessary to protect the safety of those requiring blood transfusions. However, it is important that those who have been at risk of acquiring infection do not donate blood; this reduces the risk of donations within the window period before antibodies appear. Blood donation sessions at work may lead to pressure on everyone to donate, including individuals who know themselves to have been at risk recently. Such undue pressure should be avoided. To help with this problem, the transfusion service will accept an individual's instruction in confidence to discard his or her donated blood if that individual is concerned about its safety.

## Infected health care workers

There is considerable public concern about the risk of transmission of HIV from infected doctors and other health care workers to their patients. There is evidence from observational studies in operating theatres of a high rate of sharps injuries during surgical procedures (up to 10 per cent in some specialties) with the sharp instrument re-contacting the patients' tissues in up to 30 per cent of injuries, so giving a potential for transmission of infection from operator to patient.[2] In practice, there is no evidence of transmission of HIV to patients during surgical procedures. More than 19 000 patients of HIV-infected health care workers have been followed-up, with no cases of transmission demonstrated.[17] In the few patients found to be HIV positive (as expected among 19 000), genetic sequencing indicated that they did not have the same strain of virus as the health care worker concerned.[17]

Official guidance about HIV-infected health care workers has recently been updated in both the United States and the United Kingdom.[18–20] In both countries the guidance is that health care workers who are infected with HIV should not carry out invasive procedures where there is a risk that their blood may contact the patient's open tissues. Situations likely to be particularly risky are those where the operator's hands are incompletely visible in a restricted space within the body cavity. This may occur, for example, during gynaecological procedures in the pelvis or during dental procedures. Importantly, in neither the United Kingdom nor the United States guidance is screening of health care workers for HIV recommended. However, health care workers who suspect that they may be infected are expected to have themselves tested. If testing confirms infection, they have an ethical duty to seek professional advice about any limitation of their practice that may be necessary and to act on that advice.[21] Current UK guidance states that a doctor caring for a health care worker who is HIV-infected and who does not take advice about ceasing to perform invasive procedures should inform the appropriate professional body and the employer.[19] An expert panel has been set up in the United Kingdom to provide advice about limitation of practice when this cannot be agreed locally.[19]

Occupational physicians with responsibility for health care workers have an important role in the management of HIV-infected workers, as emphasized in the latest government guidance on the issue.[19] They must encourage workers who suspect or know themselves to be infected to come to them for sensitive and confidential advice. If limitation of practice is necessary, the occupational physician should advise management accordingly but without revealing any clinical information and with the agreement of the individual concerned. Each case should be dealt with individually after taking expert virological and other advice as necessary. A blanket view that all infected health care workers will automatically be banned from all surgical procedures, even modern minimally invasive procedures, is unhelpful and is likely to discourage concerned health care workers from coming forward for testing and seeking advice. There is already disquiet that the present official guidance in the United Kingdom and United States may be a disincentive to health care workers to have themselves tested for HIV, since it could be seen as penalizing the conscientious.

Where possible, an infected health care worker who cannot continue with his or her normal duties should be redeployed without loss of income. This will require a sympathetic approach by management and the occupational physician has a role to protect the worker. If it seems likely that the HIV infection was occupationally acquired, health care workers should be able to claim DSS Injuries Benefit, even though HIV is not a Prescribed Disease, but clearly this would not compensate for loss of a career.

Confidentiality is of great importance when dealing with HIV infection, and health care workers have the same rights to confidentiality as anyone else.[15] Patients can be assured that the routine precautions taken in their care protect them from the minute risk of infection from their carers. Repeated routine screening of health care workers which is sometimes demanded by pressure groups cannot offer certain protection because of the window period before antibodies develop; it is neither justifiable nor feasible. The decision whether to notify and offer testing to patients who have been operated on by a surgeon found to be HIV-infected is a difficult one; incomplete follow-up investigations are of limited scientific value and the anxiety caused to the patients may outweigh any possible benefits. However, where health care workers known to be HIV-infected have been involved in invasive procedures, employers are now officially advised that they must contact the patients concerned and offer them counselling and HIV testing if they wish it.[20] They must endeavour to preserve the confidentiality of the worker concerned although, in practice, it will usually be difficult to prevent his or her identity from becoming public.

The risk of transmission of HIV to patients is not the only consideration in the occupational management of an infected health care worker. Such workers should be under regular medical supervision. If they become immunosupressed, they may be at risk of infections from patients and should not work in areas where such infections are frequently encountered; conversely, they may acquire infections, for example with mycobacteria, that could be transmitted to patients and colleagues. Liaison between the physician caring for the health care worker and the occupational physician is essential. (see also Appendix 6, p. 487)

### Hepatitis B and health care workers (see also Chapter 13)

Because of the similarities between HIV and hepatitis B in mode of transmission and occupational risks, mention should be made of the recently revised official guidance on hepatitis B-infected health care workers.[22] As with HIV, the guidance is that health care workers who are infectious carriers of hepatitis B indicated by the presence of the e antigen should not participate in invasive procedures. However, in view of the availability of an effective vaccine and the continuing evidence of transmission from health care workers to patients, the guidance also states that it should be a condition of employment for workers undertaking invasive procedures that they are immunized against hepatitis B and are not e antigen-positive. Fortunately, experience of a large programme of hepatitis B immunization and antibody testing among health care workers suggests that e antigen-positive individuals are rare. Occupational physicians should be involved in drawing up and implementing local policies in response to the new guidelines and should provide confidential advice to health care workers who are found to be e antigen positive.[22] Screening for hepatitis B e antigen in non-responders to immunization is justifiable but there are concerns that it may lead to renewed demands for screening of health care workers for HIV.

## Conclusions and recommendations

The background, natural history and risks to life associated with HIV infection and related disease have predisposed to discrimination within the workplace and stigmatization of perceived risk groups of individuals. Pre-emptive strategies to educate and inform people at work about HIV may prevent workplace problems and reduce stress for infected individuals and those at risk of infection. Occupational physicians have an important part to play in this process.

The continued employment of infected workers, with or without constitutional illness, is feasible. It is an important factor in the successful management of their condition and should be strongly encouraged. The modifications of work and environment which may be needed are, in principle, no different from those likely to be necessary for any employee with a progressive and debilitating condition. The possibility of neuropsychiatric manifestations requires consideration in certain occupations, particularly as they may appear relatively rapidly in a younger than usual age group. Particular considerations apply to the health care setting, both to reduce the small risk of occupational infection and to ensure that HIV-infected workers do not pose any risk of infection to patients.

Because of the fear and prejudice that are still associated with HIV infection, strict adherence to the normal professional duty of confidentiality is of particular importance for individuals with HIV infection, in both their clinical care and their occupational health management.

### Selected references and further reading

1. Mindel, A. (ed.) (1990). *AIDS: a pocketbook of diagnosis and management.* Edward Arnold, London.
2. Royal College of Pathologists (1992). *HIV infection: hazards of transmission to patients and health care workers during invasive procedures.* Report of a Working Group of the Royal College of Pathologists. Royal College of Pathologists, London.
3. Ciesielski, C. *et al.* (1992). Transmission of human immunodeficiency virus in a dental practice. *Ann. Int. Med.*, **116**, 798–805.
4. Heptonstall, J. (1991). Outbreaks of hepatitis B virus infection associated with infected surgical staff. *Communicable Disease Report*, **1**, R81–R85.
5. BMA (British Medical *Association*) (1990). *A code of practice for the safe use and disposal of sharps.* BMA, London.

6.   Centers for Disease Control (1988). Update: universal precautions for prevention of transmission of human immunodeficiency virus, hepatitis B virus and other blood borne pathogens in health care settings. *Morbid. Mortal. Wkly Rep.*, **37**, 377–388.

7.   UK Health Departments. (1990). *Guidance for clinical health care workers: protection against infection with HIV and hepatitis viruses*. HMSO, London.

8.   Oakley, K., Gooch, C., and Cockcroft, A. (1992). A review of incidents involving exposure to blood in a London teaching hospital, 1989–91. *Brit. Med. J.*, **304**, 949–51.

9.   Cockcroft, A. and Williams, S. (1993). Occupational transmission of HIV and management of accidental blood exposures. *Med. Int.*, **21**, 38–40.

10.   DOH (Department of Health) (April 1992). *Occupational exposure to HIV and use of zidovudine: a statement from the expert advisory group on AIDS*. (PL/CO(92)1). DOH, London.

11.   Department of Employment and Health and Safety Executive (1987). *AIDS and employment*. Central Office of Information, London.

12.   Society of Occupational Medicine (1992). *What employers should know about HIV and AIDS*. Society of Occupational Medicine, London.

13.   Williams, S. and Cockcroft, A. (1992) Policies for HIV and hepatitis B infected health care workers. *Occup. Hlth. Rev.* **36**, 12–14.

14.   Bor, R., Miller, R, and Goldman, G. (1992). *Theory and practice of HIV counselling: a systematic approach*. Cassell, London.

15.   Sieghart, P. (1989). *AIDS and human rights: a UK perspective*. BMA Foundation for AIDS, London.

16.   British Medical Association Foundation for AIDS (1992). *HIV infection and AIDS: ethical considerations for the medical profession*, (2nd edn). BMA Foundation for AIDS, London.

17.   Centers for Disease Control (1993). Update: investigations of persons treated by HIV-infected health care workers—United States. *Morbid. Mortal. Wkly. Rep.*, **42**, 329–37.

18.   Centers for Disease Control (1991). Recommendations for preventing transmission of human immunodeficiency virus and hepatitis B virus to patients during exposure-prone invasive procedures. *Morbid. Mortal. Wkly. Rep.*, **40**, (RR–8).

19.   UK Health Departments (March 1994). *AIDS–HIV infected health care workers: guidance on the management of infected health care workers*. DOH, London.

20.   UK Health Departments (April 1993). *AIDS–HIV infected health care workers: practical guidance on notifying patients*. DOH, London.

21.   GMC (General Medical Council) (1993). *HIV infection and AIDS: the ethical considerations*. GMC, London.

22.   UK Health Departments (August 1993). *Protecting health care workers and patients from hepatitis B*. DOH, London.

# Appendix 1

# Driving

*J.F. Taylor*

STANDARDS OF FITNESS REQUIRED FOR BRITISH DRIVING
LICENCE HOLDERS AND APPLICANTS

### Driving licences

The licensing authority for driving licences is the Secretary of State for Transport and he delegates his function to the Driver and Vehicle Licensing Agency (DVLA). The medical assessment of drivers is made by the Agency's Drivers Medical Branch advised by the Medical Advisory Branch comprising a team of doctors. The Road Traffic (Driver Licensing and Information System) Act 1989 amended the Road Traffic Act 1988 so that the DVLA now issues all driving entitlements, and these are shown in an EC Model Licence in terms of categories. Previously heavy goods and public service vehicle drivers had to have separate licences issued by the Traffic Commissioners.

### The duty of applicants for licences

The application for a licence is made on Form D1 obtainable from a Post Office. An application for a bus or lorry licence (PCV/LGV) has to include a medical report form (DTP 20003) also obtainable from Post Offices. The address for medical enquiries is The Driving and Vehicle Licensing Centre, DVLA, Swansea, SA99 ITU. Telephone enquiries on medical aspects for fitness to drive should be made on 01792 304747 (01792 304212 after hours). A leaflet explaining the medical and other aspects of driver licensing (D100) is also available from Post Offices.

### Duration of driving licences

The motorcar and motorcycle driving licence currently covers light goods vehicles and minibuses and is normally valid until the driver is aged 70, but persons with medical conditions likely to be progressive or intermittent may, at the discretion of the licensing authority, have their licences restricted to one, two or three years. After the age of 70 these licences are renewable, normally on a three-yearly basis on payment of a fee. A fee is not charged for medically restricted short-period licences. Large goods vehicles (LGVs) currently are those with a laden weight of, or in excess of, 7.5 metric tonnes. From 1 July 1996, when the second EC Driver Licensing Directive comes into force, new light goods vehicle and minibus drivers will require an LGV or PCV licence to drive goods vehicles of 3.5 metric tonnes laden weight or more, or passenger-carrying vehicles (PCVs) having nine seats or more, but a PCV licence will not be required for vehicles operated by certain voluntary groups.

Ambulances, taxis and police cars are not specifically singled out in driver licensing legislation but taxi drivers are licensed by local authorities under local government legislation. The Medical Commission on Accident Prevention recommends that the higher LGV/PCV public standards should be applicable to drivers of these vehicles. In the main, the minimum age for holding an LGV or PCV licence is 21, although in certain circumstances it can be 18. These licences normally expire after the licence holder's 45th birthday and are renewable every five years up to the age of 65 and annually thereafter. Each application has to include a medical report on form DTP 20003 completed by a registered medical practitioner, most commonly the general practitioner. If company doctors are not familiar with an applicant's medical history they are advised to consult the patient's GP.

## Duties of the applicant and licence holder

Relevant disabilities are those where a person is unfit to drive and where the licensing authority is bound to refuse or revoke the application or licence. Relevant disabilities are prescribed in law or alternatively comprise **any other medical disease or disability likely to cause the driving of a motor vehicle by the applicant or licence holder to be a source of danger to the public.**

The following bar disabilities are prescribed in relation to motorcar and motorcycle drivers (Group 1 in the terms of the EC Directive):

(1)  a person who is suffering from epilepsy and is not free from any attack for at least two years or alternatively has not established a pattern of attacks asleep and not awake for more than three years or thirdly is likely to be a danger to the public when driving;

(2)  severe mental handicap (in Scottish terminology, mental deficiency) such that a person is incapable of leading an independent life or of guarding against serious exploitation;

(3)  liability to sudden attacks of disabling giddiness or fainting caused by any disorder (but if they are caused by a heart disorder which can be controlled by an implanted pacemaker, this bar is lifted subject to the person undertaking to have regular pacemaker checks at a clinic and having a three-year licence);

(4)  inability to read in good daylight (with the aid of glasses or contact lenses if worn) a registration mark fixed to a vehicle containing figures and letters 79.4 millimetres high at a distance of:
    (a) 20.5 metres, in any case except that mentioned below; or
    (b) 12.3 metres, in the case of an applicant for a licence authorising the driving of pedestrian controlled vehicles (e.g., milk floats or motor-propelled mowing machines);

(5)  in addition, as mentioned above, the person must not suffer from any other disease or disability likely to cause him or her to be a source of danger to the public when driving or in pursuance of a driving licence.

LGV/PCV prescribed disabilities (Group 2 requirements in the EC Directive) include all those above in Group 1, and, in addition, the following:

(1)  any liability to epileptic seizures, which will usually be interpreted as positive if:
  (i) the applicant has had any epileptic attack in the last 10 years; or
  (ii) the applicant has taken any medication to prevent epilepsy in the last 10 years; or
  (iii) a consultant has confirmed there is a continuing liability to epileptic seizures;

(2)  abnormal sight in one or both eyes where:
  (a) in the case of a person who held an existing licence on 1 January 1983 and who holds such a licence on 1 April 1991, the visual acuity is worse than 6/12 with the better eye and worse than 6/36 with the other eye and, if corrective lenses are worn, the uncorrected acuity in each eye is worse than 3/60; or
  (b) in any other case, the visual acuity is worse than 6/9 in the better eye and worse than 6/12 in the other eye and, if corrective lenses are worn, the uncorrected acuity in each eye is worse than 3/60;

(3)  sight in only one eye unless:
  (a) in the case of a person who held an existing licence on 1 January 1983 and who holds such a licence on 1 April 1991 the traffic commissioner in whose area he resides or the traffic commissioner who granted the last-mentioned licence knew of the disability before 1 January 1991 and the visual acuity in that eye is no worse than 6/12; or
  (b) in the case of a person who did not hold an existing licence on 1 January 1983 but who held an existing licence on 1 April 1991 the traffic commissioner in whose area he resides or the traffic commissioner who granted the last-mentioned licence knew of the disability before 1 January 1991 and the visual acuity in that eye is no worse than 6/9;

(4)  diabetics subject to insulin treatment unless the person in question held, on 1 April 1991, an existing licence and the traffic commissioner in whose area he resides or the traffic commissioner who granted the licence knew of the disability before 1 January 1991.

In this regulation measurements of visual acuity refer to visual acuity measured on the Snellen scale.

### Notification of disabilities to the licensing centre

The Road Traffic Act 1988 places a statutory obligation on driving licence holders and applicants to notify any disability likely to affect safe driving either now or at some future date to the DVLA as soon as the person becomes aware of the condition. Awareness normally involves being told by a medical practitioner that it is relevant or prospectively relevant. Only temporary disabilities such as fractured bones not expected to last more than three months are excluded from this obligation. However, conditions such as strokes—with underlying cerebrovascular disease—or conditions such as sleep apnoea unless permanently cured by surgery are not exempt from this three-month rule. Licence holders are also required to notify to the licensing centre any disability, already notified, which has become worse.

**Procedure for medical assessment**

When it receives information about a disability from an applicant/licence holder or third party, the DVLA may require the applicant or licence holder to authorize his or her doctor to make available information about the disability to the Medical Advisory Branch at the centre. If the applicant or licence holder fails to do so, or if the information available from the doctor is not conclusive in relation to fitness to drive, the Agency may require him or her to have a medical examination by a nominated doctor or doctors. If necessary, to establish the effect of the disability on ability to drive, the Agency may require him or her to take a further driving test. Failure of a licence holder or applicant to give consent to their medical practitioner to make reports to the DVLA or failure to attend a medical examination without reasonable excuse, will usually lead to a driving licence being withheld or withdrawn.

**Loss of a limb due to trauma**

Applicants for licences suffering from a static limb disability have an automatic right in Great Britain to a provisional driving licence for the purpose of taking a driving test to prove their ability to drive. Normally provisional licences are valid until the applicant's 70th birthday, except in the case of motorcycle entitlement which is only valid for two years and cannot be renewed until a year has elapsed unless a test has been passed.

**Doctor notification without the patient's consent**

Circumstances sometimes arise where a doctor who has told a patient not to drive and to report a relevant disability to the DVLA finds that the patient has disregarded the advice and is continuing to drive to the danger of the public. In such cases it is advisable for the doctor to repeat the advice to the patient in writing and at the same time seek the medical opinion of his professional indemnity association. The professsional indemnity associations normally advise direct notification without the consent of the patient at the same time as informing the patient of the action taken. The authoritative document for reference is the General Medical Council pamphlet 'Professional conduct and discipline; fitness to practice'. For the address of the General Medical Council see Appendix 9, p. 518.

**Medical appeal provisions**

Where a driving licence is refused or revoked on medical grounds or restricted in period of duration, there is a right of appeal to a Magistrates Court in England and Wales or to a Sherriffs Court in Scotland.

**Medical aspects of fitness to drive**

More detail on medical fitness to drive and British driver licensing standards are contained in 'Medical aspects of fitness to drive'[1], a guide for medical practitioners published by the Medical Commission on Accident Prevention. (For the address see Appendix 9.) For details of the assessment of cardiac fitness for vocational driving see Annex A to Chapter 14 (p. 282).

[1] Raffle, P.A.B. Medical aspects of fitness to drive, (4th edn). Medical Commission on Accident Prevention. HMSO, London

# Appendix 2

# Civil aviation

*G. Bennett*

---

### Introduction

There are two fundamentally different requirements for medical standards in the aviation industry. Because of the very high cost of training, say, a Boeing 747 pilot, an employer seeks not only short-term safety and effectiveness but also the probability of the employee remaining fit through a long-term career. On the other hand the national authority responsible for air safety—in the United Kingdom, the Civil Aviation Authority (CAA)—can only be concerned with the probability that a licence holder will be able to function effectively and will not be likely to suffer sudden incapacitation during the short period (six months to one year) for which his or her medical certificate is valid. A young man with a progressive disability might be given a licence subject to regular reviews but would not be hired by a major airline. Counselling is needed and would be given by the CAA.

Risk management is the main principle of aviation licensing. A zero defect policy is not attainable. The best airlines operating the best aircraft achieve a fatal accident rate of one in 2 million flights[1] and the CAA sets a safety target of one fatal accident in 10 million flights. Many factors may cause accidents, so the medical-cause safety target is better than one in 100 million flights.[2]

### Pilots

The medical standards for pilots (and for flight engineers and air traffic control officers) are internationally agreed and are contained in Annex 1 to the Convention on International Civil Aviation.[3] A few, such as the visual requirements, are specific but many are couched in such general terms as 'cases of metabolic nutritional or endocrine disorders likely to interfere with the safe exercise of the applicant's licence privileges shall be assessed as unfit'. There is also a waiver clause which allows a national authority to issue a licence if it believes it is safe to do so even if the standards are not met. The International Civil Aviation Organization, a United Nations organization, therefore issues a manual of guidance material[4] on the interpretation of the standards.

Possible exposure to a harsh environment, notably hypoxia, accelerations, and sudden pressure and temperature changes, requires very good cardiovascular function and freedom from conditions likely to be aggravated by such sudden changes—middle ear and sinus disorders, lung bullae, herniation, etc.

The special senses, especially vision, are clearly important. Uncorrected distant visual acuity must in some countries be 6/60 (20/200) or better. Correction to 6/9 (20/30) or better is required, and there are near and intermediate visual requirements. Normal colour vision is not always necessary provided the candidate can reliably distinguish signal red, white, and green. Experienced pilots who lose an eye can often continue to fly satisfactorily by day but may have difficulty landing at night.

Pilots with disabilities resulting from orthopaedic or neurological conditions are given a practical test in each aircraft type they wish to fly.

The lifestyle of a professional pilot is necessarily irregular and this excludes applicants with some gastrointestinal and metabolic disorders. Diabetes requiring insulin is absolutely disqualifying and oral therapy is usually so.

Because the continual exercise of judgement and self-discipline is so vital to the pilot's task, significant mental and personality disorders are unacceptable. A history of psychosis is permanently disqualifying. Neurotic illness is assessed on the probability of recurrence, as is alcohol and drug abuse. HIV infection may first manifest itself with neuro-psychiatric symptoms and is considered disqualifying in many countries.

Conditions likely to cause incapacitation, either sudden or subtle, are usually disqualifying. Passenger aircraft smaller than 5700 kg (air-taxi size) sometimes only carry one pilot, whose incapacitation would inevitably result in an accident. Larger aircraft must carry two pilots and accident experience and simulator research indicates that on only one occasion in a hundred of sudden pilot incapacitation this may result in an accident.[5] Pilots with medical conditions carrying a sudden incapacitation risk of 1 per cent per year can continue to be licensed to fly larger aircraft; the safety target will still be met.[6]

A pilot's licence is temporarily suspended on presumption of pregnancy but flying in a two-pilot aircraft is usually possible in the middle trimester.

Commonly used therapeutic agents are often unacceptable because of their side-effects. Performance testing in a flight simulator may be carried out if necessary. In many cases the disorder requiring the therapy will be disqualifying, at least temporarily.

Experience indicates that accident risk increases directly with the total number of medical disabilities. It also falls dramatically with increasing age and experience up to age 60, when most professional pilots retire. Unnecessary removal of middle-aged pilots on medical grounds means their replacement by younger, less experienced pilots and is positively detrimental to air safety.

The medical standards for pilots engaged in flying instruction and non-passenger-carrying activities, such as banner-towing, are at present somewhat more relaxed than the standards above but this is not likely to be the case after European standards are harmonized.

The initial medical examination for a professional pilot's licence (and flight engineer's and air traffic control officer's) is carried out in the United Kingdom by the CAA. Airline Transport pilots are then examined at six-monthly intervals

by medical examiners authorized by the CAA who have had postgraduate training in aviation medicine. Commercial pilots below the age of 40 are examined
annually, and six-monthly above the age of 40.

### Flight engineers

Flight engineers play an important role in monitoring the actions of the pilots as
well as controlling the aircraft's systems. Their medical standards are therefore
essentially similar to those of pilots. Because they are not physically handling the
flying controls at critical stages of flight, their sudden incapacitation does not
present the same threat to safety as does the pilots'. They may, therefore, continue
to fly with conditions which present a somewhat greater risk of incapacitation.

### Air traffic control officers

The increasing congestion of air traffic means that the role of air traffic control
officers in maintaining safety is almost on a par with that of pilots. Their
medical standards are therefore similar. Some controllers work in teams and in
these a risk of incapacitation comparable to that for pilots of larger aircraft may
be accepted.

### Cabin crew

Stewards and stewardesses do not hold licences and formal medical standards
are not laid down. The CAA merely requires airlines to ensure by medical examination that they are fit to carry out their assigned duties. Good cardiorespiratory
function and freedom from conditions aggravated by pressure changes and the
effects of irregular working and world-wide travel are important. Uncorrected
distance vision of 6/60 (20/200) or better is necessary, as spectacles and contact
lenses may be lost in an accident where the cabin crew's effectiveness is vital to
passenger survival.

### European harmonization

A European Community (EC) Regulation effective in 1993 requires EC states to
harmonize their aviation medical requirements and accept each others licences
by 1997. Most of the non-European states have joined in the harmonization
process and the Joint Aviation Authorities (JAA) have produced a set of
European medical standards.

  These are similar to the international standards but limit national authorities'
discretion under the 'waiver' clause and call for additional specialist ophthalmological, pulmonary function, and cardiovascular risk assessment at periodic
intervals related to age.

  N.P.  An age limit of 65 is proposed for two-pilot and multi-crew operations.

**Selected references and further reading**

1. Bennett, G. (1992). Medical-cause accidents in commercial aviation. In First European workshop in aviation cardiology, (ed. M. Joy). *Eur. Heart J.*, **13**, (Suppl. H), 13–15.
2. Chaplin, J.C. (1988). In perspective—the safety of aircraft pilots and their hearts. *Eur. Heart J.*, **9**, (Suppl. G), 17–20.
3. International Civil Aviation Organization (1988). *Annex 1 to the Treaty on International Civil Aviation*, (8th edn). International Civil Aviation Organization, Montreal.
4. International Civil Aviation Organization (1985). *Manual of civil aviation medicine*, (2nd edn). International Civil Aviation Organization, Montreal.
5. Bennett, G. (1988). Pilot incapacitation and aircraft accidents. *Eur. Heart J.* **9**, (Suppl. G), 21–4.
6. Tunstall Pedoe, H. (1988). Acceptable cardiovascular risk in aircrew. In Second United Kingdom workshop in aviation cardiology, (ed. M. Joy and G. Bennett). *Eur. Heart J.*, **9**, (Suppl. G), 9–11.

# Appendix 3

# Seafarers

## *D. Dean*

MEDICAL AND VISUAL STANDARDS FOR ENTRY INTO THE MERCHANT
NAVY AND FOR SERVING SEAFARERS

### Introduction

The Department of Transport is responsible for the statutory medical standards for seafarers which were introduced under The Merchant Shipping (Medical Examination) Regulations 1983, SI 1983, No. 808. The current revised standards are contained in Merchant Shipping Notice No. MI331. These standards apply throughout to serving seafarers and provide the legal basis for the issue of medical certificates in accordance with Article 3 of ILO Convention 73.

The standards existing before the introduction of the statutory requirements were revised in 1976 by a panel of senior doctors working in the British shipping industry. Seafarers employed by member companies of the then General Council of British Shipping were examined voluntarily to these standards by agreement with the seafaring trade unions. After being given the force of law the specific medical standards for serving seafarers were revised in 1984 by a working party drawn from the Faculty of Occupational Medicine. In 1991 the General Council of British Shipping (GCBS) reverted to its former title of the Chamber of Shipping (CoS).

The industry medical standards still make provision for the examination of all entrants to the Merchant Navy, including former merchant seafarers applying for re-entry. The Department of Transport did not assume responsibility for these standards, but states in the General Introduction to Merchant Shipping Notice No. M1331 that:

Seafaring is a potentially hazardous occupation which calls for a high standard of health and fitness in those entering or re-entering the industry.

It is better, therefore, at an initial examination, to exclude an applicant if there is any doubt about his continuing fitness.

The provision of a right of appeal in cases where a person is found permanently unfit, or fit for restricted service, only applies to serving seafarers. The initial decision as to the fitness of an applicant on entry rests solely with the examining doctor, who, therefore, bears a heavy responsibility to the applicant, future shipmates, the employer, and for the safety of the ship.

The introduction to Notice No. M1331 notes that 'it would be unsafe practice to allow seafaring with any known medical condition where the possibility of serious exacerbation requiring expert treatment could occur as a calculated risk'. In this reference the term 'expert treatment' includes not only treatment which the medical profession would regard as secondary or tertiary care, but also the primary care provision which is taken for granted ashore. Treatment aboard ship will almost always be provided by designated ships' officers whose training enables them only to give first aid and emergency care based upon elementary instruction in diagnosis and treatment. They are not trained for and cannot be expected to provide the degree of responsibility in medical matters which is given by professionally qualified staff.

In order to provide a uniform standard for examining doctors who are required to assess fitness for seafaring, CoS accepts the current entry standards as both necessary and sufficient. They are compatible with the later application of the statutory standards which apply to serving personnel. It would be unjust were recruits at different centres to be examined to varying standards, as well as being potentially prejudicial to the safety of the vessel and to the quality of the service which the Department of Transport is entitled to expect from approved doctors.

The reasons for exclusion on medical grounds are rigorous in view of the need for seafarers to be available for service anywhere in the world, in some cases with minimal medical services even when ashore. The Master of a ship must be able to rely upon his crew at all times, and it is the duty of the examining doctor to ensure that seafarers are physically and emotionally able to cope with severe conditions. Exceptions cannot be made on grounds such as service being expected only under specified conditions; once an entrant seafarer has an unrestricted certificate of fitness he may be assigned anywhere without further medical review.

Although it is not a part of the examination, doctors should, if possible, also take the opportunity to advise about health precautions which may be necessary, such as vaccination, and may wish to provide simple lifestyle counselling in regard, for instance, to diet or the use of alcohol and tobacco. It is important where possible to emphasize the technically skilled nature of work at sea in a modern ship, which requires a disciplined attitude to ensure the safety of all on board.

Shipping is an international business and so AIDS has from an early stage been kept under review with particular reference to seafarers. This is not because seafarers are considered a high-risk group but by virtue of the world-wide nature of their occupation they are more likely to be exposed to AIDS in their job than UK-based workers.

From as early as 1985, guidance notes and other material have been circulated to the shipping industry and regularly updated by the CoS with the support and co-operation of the seafaring trade unions.

The Department of Transport has also circulated notice M1301 'General advice to seafarers', and notice M1302, an insert on AIDS for inclusion in the Ship Captain's Medical Guide. The CoS has additionally widely distributed to seafarers the government publications 'Don't Die of Ignorance' (DHSS) and 'AIDS and employment' (DE./HSE).

The specific medical standards are that on entry candidates who are HIV positive or have AIDS would be rejected, while serving seafarers who are HIV positive may continue at sea subject to medical surveillance to assess progress but are certified permanently unfit on developing confirmed AIDS.

**Employment Standards and Administrative Procedures**

1.  (a) All seafarers below the age of 18 shall have a yearly medical examination.

   (b) Seafarers between the ages of 18 and 40 shall be examined at intervals not exceeding five years.

(c) Seafarers aged 40 years and over shall be examined at intervals not exceeding two years.

(d) Seafarers serving on bulk chemical carriers shall be subject to annual examinations and blood tests at yearly or more frequent intervals, according to the nature of the cargo.

2. The value of medical surveillance, after sickness absence, in maintaining the health of the seafarer should not be forgotten, particularly after illness ashore lasting for a month or more.

3. Disposal in accordance with the medical and visual standards for seafarers is as follows:

The standard has been met:

A.   for unrestricted sea service

*Note*: Category 'A(T)' may be used where a serving seafarer can be considered fit for all shipping trades, geographical areas, types of ships, or jobs but where medical surveillance is required at intervals. The medical certificate (ENG 1) should be validated only for the appropriate period which would take into account the expected duration of the tour of duty.

E.   for restricted service only
     Restriction .................

The standard has not been met:

B.   permanently

C.   indefinitely: review in ................. months

D.   temporarily: review in ................. weeks

Approved doctors should make full use of categories E, C, and D before declaring a serving seafarer permanently unfit.

It is the responsibility of the employer, or those authorized to act on his behalf, to ensure that the category recommended by the approved doctor is taken fully into account when the engagement or the continued employment of a seafarer is under consideration.

4. Article 4 of ILO Convention 73 states that 'when prescribing the nature of the examination, due regard shall be had to the age of the person to be examined and the nature of the duties to be performed'. In addition, Article 3 of the Convention states that a serving seafarer should have a medical certificate 'attesting to his fitness for the work for which he is to be employed at sea'.

In reaching his conclusion, the doctor should therefore consider any medical conditions present, the age and experience of the seafarer, the specific work on which he will be employed and the trade in which he will be engaged — where this can be determined.

If a seafarer is found to be fit to continue in his present job but does not meet the full category 'A' standard, a restricted service certificate must be issued stating the restrictions applicable.

5. The standards are framed to provide the maximum flexibility in their interpretation compatible with the paramount importance of maintaining the safety of vessels at sea

and the safe performance of the serving seafarer's duties while, at the same time, protecting his health.

Conditions not specified in the standards, which interfere with job requirements, should be assessed in the light of the general principles outlined above.

6. It may be necessary on occasion and, with the seafarer's consent, for the approved doctor to consult the general practitioner. When it is necessary to consult with other doctors the usual ethical considerations will pertain, but it should be clearly understood that the decision on fitness in accordance with the required medical standard rests with the approved doctor, subject to the medical appeal machinery.

7. Full clinical notes should be kept of any detailed medical examination. All sections of the approved form of report should be completed without exception and the form retained for six years.

*Restricted service*

8. Restricted service means that the serving seafarer's employment is restricted to certain shipping trades, geographical areas, types of ships, or jobs for such periods of time as may be stipulated by the approved doctor. The type of restriction and the length of time it will operate should be made clear. The requirements of an advised treatment regimen should never be set aside.

9. Unlike many industries, there is no light work at sea — although the physical requirements may vary between different types of ships, their departments, and individual jobs in them, all jobs need an acceptable degree of fitness, in accordance with these standards, which is uniform for all shipping trades. For instance, coastal and ferry work can be arduous and uncomfortable even though the voyages may be short. Therefore, restriction to these types of work should be advised only if the shortness of the voyage will permit adequate treatment and/or surveillance of a condition which is not affecting the performance of the seafarer's duties.

*Permanent unfitness*

10. In a serving seafarer, a decision of permanent unfitness should be reached only after a full investigation and consideration of the case and should be fully discussed with the seafarer. The seafarer's general practitioner should be informed of the decision and the reasons for it in the context of the medical standards, provided permission to do so has been obtained from the seafarer.

*Medical appeals*

11. All serving seafarers found permanently unfit or fit only for restricted service have a right of appeal to an independent medical referee appointed by the Department of Transport. Wherever possible, medical referees should be assisted by the disclosure, in confidence, of any necessary medical information.

12. Medical referees are empowered, while working to the same standards, to:

– ensure that the diagnosis has been established beyond reasonable doubt, in accordance with the medical evidence on which the approved doctor reached his decision and, normally, with the assistance of a report from a consultant in the appropriate specialty;

– determine whether the standards have been properly interpreted; and

– consider the possibility of a seafarer, previously declared permanently unfit, returning to sea.

In cases not provided for in the medical standards or for category 'B' conditions where exceptional medical considerations apply, the medical referee should decide an appropriate disposal after consultation with the approved doctor involved and consideration of all the evidence presented to him.

MEDICAL STANDARDS FOR SEAFARERS

*Note:* for conditions marked with an asterisk, acceptance after a successful operation would be considered.

| Standards for entrants and re-entrants for seafarers | Standards for serving seafarers required by the marine division of the department of transport[1] |
| --- | --- |
| *1. General appearance* | |
| General appearance and physique must be adequate. Weight should be compatible with age, height and build. Weight greater than 20% above that recorded in the Metropolitan Life Tables should exclude the applicant at that time. | It is essential that seafarers should not have any physical disability or defect which might interfere with the discharge of their duties. Weight in excess of 25% of figures quoted in Metropolitan Life Tables is not allowed otherwise a degree of obesity not adversely affecting health, exercise tolerance, and mobility is permitted. Seafarers with infectious diseases must be treated satisfactorily before resuming service. All confirmed cases of AIDS are permanently unfit. All malignant diseases must be carefully assessed and no unrestricted grading allowed within 5 years of the completion of treatment except in cases of neoplasm of the skin. |
| *2. Disability and deformities* | |
| There must be no deformity of body or limbs which could give rise to disability. | Seafarers should not have any defect of the musculoskeletal system which would impair the satisfactory performance of their job. |
| A limb prosthesis is not acceptable. | Ditto |

[1] Further details may be obtained from merchant shipping notice M1331 available from HMSO

| Entrants and re-entrants | Serving seafarers |
| --- | --- |
| **3. Musculoskeletal** | |
| There must be no chronic or recurrent disease of muscles, bones, or joints. There must be no defect affecting balance or co-ordination. | Muscular power, balance, mobility and co-ordination should be unimpaired. |
| **4. Hernia** | |
| Any hernia,* even if controlled by a truss, will cause rejection. | Seafarers with a hernia are unfit for service until it has been satisfactorily surgically repaired. |
| **5. Speech** | |
| There must be no speech defect or stammer sufficiently serious to render the applicant incapable of carrying out his or her duties efficiently | A speech defect likely to interfere with communication would result in the seafarer being declared permanently medically unfit |
| **6. Sexual Development** | |
| Immature sexual development will cause rejection. The testes should be fully descended.* A hydrocoele* will cause rejection. | Any abnormality of the primary or secondary sexual characteristics must be investigated and the fitness decision based on the outcome. A symptomless small hydrocoele is permitted but a large or recurrent condition must be treated |
| **7. Cardiovascular** | |
| There must be no past history nor present evidence of disease of the cardiovascular system nor congenital defect. The blood pressure should always be recorded and must be within accepted normal limits. | The cardiovascular system must be free from acute or chronic disease causing significant disability. Seafarers developing coronary thrombosis, angina, disorders of rhythm, or a cerebrovascular condition are permanently unfit for further service. Cases of hypertension are allowed provided the blood pressure can be maintained below 170/100 mm with treatment not causing significant side effects. |

| Entrants and re-entrants | Serving seafarers |
|---|---|
| **8. *Vein conditions*** <br> A material degree of varicose veins* or any leg ulceration, or varicose eczema, will cause rejection. <br> A varicocoele* or haemorrhoids* causing symptoms or thought to be troublesome will cause rejection. | Serving seafarer standards for cases with varicose veins, varicose ulceration, varicocoele or haemorrhoids permit continuing service if symptomless. But if otherwise, not until satisfactorily treated. |
| **9. *Haemopoietic System*** <br> There must be no disease of the haemopoietic organs. | Ditto |
| **10. *Genito-urinary*** <br> The kidneys, ureters, bladder and urethra must be healthy. Urine should be free from abnormal constituents. <br><br> Applicants having proteinuria or glycosuria or other urinary abnormality should be referred for investigation. | Ditto. The fitness categorization should be based on the result of the investigations. <br><br> Those with subacute or chronic renal disease should be similarly assessed and the developed condition would normally preclude seafaring service. |
| **11. *Renal*** <br> The loss of one kidney, prostatic disease or enlargement, urinary obstruction from any cause or a history of recurrent stone will cause rejection. | Seafarers with a normally functioning single kidney would be unsuitable for service in tropical climates or work in a high temperature environment. Cases of renal or ureteric calculus should be investigated and return to sea after satisfactory treatment is possible, provided there is normal |

| Entrants and re-entrants | Serving seafarers |
|---|---|
| | renal function and no remaining calculi. Those with recurrent stone formation are permanently unfit. Seafarers developing an enlarged prostate should be investigated and appropriately treated. |
| **12. Urinary incontinence** | |
| Any incontinence of urine will cause rejection. | Incontinence of urine cases should be referred for investigation and, if irremediable, are permanently unfit for service. |
| Boys who have suffered nocturnal enuresis should have been dry for at least 2 years. | |
| **13. Endocrine** | |
| There must be no disease of the endocrine glands. | Seafarers with thyroid or other endocrine disease should be investigated and the fitness category decided on the case assessment. Cases of diabetes mellitus are allowed 6 months to achieve stabilization with treatment. If insulin is required they are permanently unfit for further service. Where control is achieved by diet alone or in combination with oral therapy, in the absence of complications seafaring may be resumed, subject to review every 6 months. |
| **14. Skin** | |
| Skin must be healthy and there must be no communicable disease. Applicants with a history or signs of any recurrent disabling skin disease or signs of skin sensitivity will be rejected. | Seafarers with acne or psoriasis may continue seafaring if satisfactorily controlled and treated. Severe and resistant cases, however, are permanently unfit for service. |

| Entrants and re-entrants | Serving seafarers |
| --- | --- |
| Any condition liable to be aggravated by heat, sea air, oil, caustic, or detergents should be rejected. | Special care is required in assessing seafarers with skin conditions for service in tropical climates or if there is likely to be aggravation by heat, sea air, oil, caustics, detergents, or specific occupational allergens. |
| Catering staff in particular should have no focus of skin sepsis. | Ditto |
| Those dealing with passengers should have no objectionable lesions, however harmless, on the exposed parts of the body. | Skin infections, dermatitis, and eczema should be treated and service resumed when the skin is healthy. |
| **15. Respiratory** | |
| There must be no organic disease of the respiratory system and there must be no history of tuberculosis nor of recurrent bronchitis. | The respiratory system should be free from acute or chronic disease causing significant disability. |
| Adult sufferers from bronchial asthma are unacceptable. An adolescent having a childhood history of bronchial asthma must be symptom free for 5 years without any treatment. | Uncomplicated cases of chronic bronchitis and/or emphysema with good exercise tolerance may continue seafaring but more serious cases with recurring illness and significant disability are permanently unfit. Seafarers with bronchial asthma occurring after 16 years of age are also permanently unfit. Seafarers with active pulmonary tuberculosis should not return to service until a chest physician has advised that a course of treatment has been completed and the lesion fully healed. On-going surveillance would also be necessary. |

| Entrants and re-entrants | Serving seafarers |
|---|---|
| **16. *Alimentary*** | Seafarers developing peptic ulceration should be referred for investigation and treatment and not resume seafaring until symptom free with gastroscopic evidence of healing and on an ordinary diet without treatment for at least 3 months. Cases having sustained gastrointestinal bleeding, perforation, recurrent ulceration, or an unsatisfactory operation result are permanently unfit for seafaring. |
| The alimentary system must be normal. Teeth and gums must be healthy. Dentures must be adequate and well fitting. Tonsils must be healthy. A past history of peptic ulceration or any other significant disorder of digestion will cause rejection. Faecal incontinence will cause rejection. | |
| | Dental defects and conditions of the tonsils, mouth, and gums should be satisfactorily treated before seafaring is resumed. Oesophageal, hepatic, pancreatic, and gall bladder disease must be investigated and treated and fitness determined on case assessment. Those cases where alcohol is an aetiological factor are usually permanently unfit for service. |
| **17. *Nervous system and mental disorders*** | Seafarers with organic nervous disease especially if causing defects of muscular power, balance, mobility and co-ordination are permanently unfit for service. |
| There must be no organic disease or functional defect of the nervous system. There must be no history of epilepsy, major fits, or petit mal. A past history of mental disorder or psychoneurosis will cause rejection. A history of intemperate use of alcohol affecting health or abuse of drugs will cause rejection. | |

| Entrants and re-entrants | Serving seafarers |
| --- | --- |

Similarly the incidence of an acute psychosis, recurrent psychoneurosis or drug abuse within the last 5 years and alcohol misuse affecting health or causing a behaviour disorder would result in permanent unfitness certification.

Any type of epilepsy after the age of 5 years precludes seafaring service although a seafarer with controlled epilepsy without fits for 2 years may be considered for service on a vessel carrying a medical officer provided there is no involvement with the safety of the ship or any passenger. A single fit in a serving seafarer should be referred for investigation and a resumption of seafaring is allowed provided that the past history is clear, no abnormality is discovered, and 1 year has elapsed without treatment.

### 18. Ears and Hearing
There must be no material defect of hearing. Tympanic membranes must be intact and healthy. There must be no evidence of disease of the external auditory meati.
Hearing should be assessed and recorded audiometrically.

A serving seafarer with impaired hearing should be referred for specialist investigation and opinion. Audiometry is required when there is clinical evidence of hearing impairment. A degree of impairment of hearing sufficient to interfere with communication under shipboard conditions precludes further service. The use of a hearing aid by personnel in the deck or engine room departments is not permitted although hearing aids may be

| Entrants and re-entrants | Serving seafarers |
|---|---|
| | acceptable for catering staff if failure to hear an instruction would not endanger the seafarer or shipmates. External and middle ear conditions should be treated and completely resolved before a resumption of seafaring is permitted. |
| *Ménières disease and transient ischaemic attacks* Not suitable. | Permanently unfit. |
| 19. *Gynaecological Conditions & Pregnancy* Female seafarers should be free of any significant gynaecological disorder or disease. | There should be no gynaecological disorder or disease likely to cause trouble at sea or affect working capacity. |
| | A serving seafarer with a normal pregnancy may be permitted to work at sea until the 28th week on short-haul trips or on longer voyages if a medical officer is carried as a crew member. |
| Employment is not permitted after week 28 of pregnancy until at least 6 weeks after delivery. | Ditto |
| 20. *Eye disease and visual defects* See Annex A | See Annex B. |

ANNEX A

**Entrants visual standards for the Merchant Navy**

1. *Deck department*

| | Better eye | Other eye | Both eyes | Colour vision (Ishihara plates) |
|---|---|---|---|---|
| (a) Where aids to vision are not used | 6/6 | 6/9 | 6/6 | Normal |
| (b) Where aids to vision are used | | | | |
| (i) Under 22 years of age | | | | |
| Aided vision | 6/6 | 6/9 | 6/6 | Normal |
| Unaided vision not less than | 6/12 | 6/12 | 6/12 | Normal |
| (ii) 22 years of age and over | | | | |
| Aided vision | 6/6 | 6/9 | 6/6 | Normal |
| Unaided vision not less than | 6/12 | 6/24 | 6/12 | Normal |

2. *Engine Room*

| | Better eye | Other eye | Both eyes | |
|---|---|---|---|---|
| Aided vision allowed if necessary | | | | Pass Engineers Modified |
| Not less than | 6/12 | 6/60 | 6/12 | Bar or Trade test |

3. *Electrical or radio staff*
   A visual acuity with glasses if required sufficient to carry out duties efficiently Less than 6/60 in other eye is not acceptable.

   Pass Engineers Modified Bar or Trade test

4. *Catering Department, Surgeon etc.*
   Visual acuity standards as for (3).

   Not required

ANNEX B

**Serving seafarer visual standards for the Merchant Navy**

1. No person should be accepted for training or sea service if any irremediable morbid condition of either eye, or the lids of either eye, is present and liable to the risk of aggravation or recurrence.

2. Binocular vision is necessary for all categories of seafarers. However, the following monocular seafarers should be allowed to continue at sea:
   (a) seafarers in deck department employment with a satisfactory record of service prior to 1 September 1976 and not requiring visual aids;
   (b) seafarers in non-deck employment with a satisfactory record of service prior to 1983.

3. In all cases where visual aids (spectacles or contact lenses) are required for the efficient performance of duties, a spare pair must be carried when seafaring. When different visual aids are used for distant and near vision a spare pair of each must be carried.

4. The distant vision standard for the watchkeeping deck department personnel is identical to the requirement of the Department of Transport letter test for applicants to enter the examination for a certificate of competency. The Department of Transport requirements are contained in Merchant Shipping Notice No. M961. The Department's tests are carried out at designated Department of Transport sight testing centres.

*Colour vision*

5. The methods of testing colour vision differ; the Department of Transport currently uses a lantern test but the industry uses Ishihara plates. Where examination results conflict, the Department of Transport's test is accepted as the definitive test.

6. Colour vision for deck officers and ratings may be regarded as normal, when using the Ishihara method, if plates 1, 11, 15, 22 and 23 are read correctly.

7. A seafarer with a record of efficient service who is required to pass the modified colour vision test but fails should be given the opportunity to pass a suitable trade test.

| Officers, cadets, apprentices and ratings | Distant vision | | | Near vision both eyes together aided or unaided vision | Colour vision |
|---|---|---|---|---|---|
| | Better eye | Other eye | Together | | |
| *Deck department* | | | | | |
| 1. Seafarers required to undertake lookout duties and under the age of 40 years | | | | A visual acuity sufficient to carry out duties efficiently | Normal |
| With or without glasses or contact lenses | 6/6 | 6/9 | 6/6 | | |
| Unaided vision not less than | 6/12 | 6/24 | 6/12 | Ditto | Ditto |
| 2. Seafarers required to undertake lookout duties and over the age of 40 years | | | | | |
| With or without glasses or contact lenses | 6/6 | 6/12 | 6/6 | Ditto | Ditto |
| Unaided vision not less than | 6/24 | 6/24 | 6/24 | Ditto | Ditto |
| 3. Seafarers required to operate lifting plant of type used in dockwork etc. | | | | | |
| With or without visual aids | 6/9 | 6/12 | 6/9 | Ditto | Ditto |
| Unaided vision not less than | 6/60 | 6/60 | 6/60 | Ditto | Ditto |
| 4. Seafarers not required to perform the duties in 1, 2 or 3 above | | | | | |
| Aided vision if necessary | 6/18 | 6/60 | 6/18 | Ditto | Ditto |

| | Distant vision | | | Near vision both eyes together aided or unaided vision | Colour vision |
|---|---|---|---|---|---|
| | Better eye | Other eye | Together | | |

*Other departments*

| | Better eye | Other eye | Together | | |
|---|---|---|---|---|---|
| Engine room: aided vision if necessary | 6/18 | 6/60 | 6/18 | A visual acuity sufficient to carry out duties efficiently. | Personnel should pass the modified colour test on charts supplied. |
| Radio officer, electrician officer | A visual acuity (aided if necessary) sufficient to carry out duties efficiently Less than 6/60 in the 'other eye' is unacceptable. Monocular sight: Normally permanently unfit but see 2. above. | | | | These officers should pass the modified colour test as for engine room department. |
| Catering department and miscellaneous (including surgeon, purser, etc.) | A visual acuity (aided if necessary) sufficient to carry out duties efficiently. Less than 6/60 in the 'other eye' is unacceptable. Monocular sight: normally permanently unfit, but see 2. above. | | | | Not tested |

# Appendix 4

# Offshore workers and divers

*E.M. Botheroyd and N.K.I. McIver*

OFFSHORE WORKERS

## Introduction

The assessment of fitness is made on consideration of any medical condition identified. This includes the nature, prognosis, management, and likely requirement and significance of therapy for any such conditions. Every attempt is made to match the employee to his employment, taking account of the location, rather than declaring a candidate unfit whenever any abnormality is discovered. To reach a decision it may be necessary to consult the operator's medical adviser, inspect the work location and its accessibility, and balance the risk to the employee's health against his value at that worksite. The patient's general practitioner, other relevant specialists, and even insurers may need to be consulted. Occupational physicians with experience of the offshore industry can be of benefit to both the employees and employers by screening the offshore workforce and offering well-informed medical advice. The aim is to reduce risk to the patient and his colleagues, and to avoid any medical condition which may jeopardize his or their health and safety. A further benefit of regular health surveillance is the detection of long-term health hazards.

The Medical Advisory Committee of the United Kingdom Offshore Operators Association (UKOOA MAC) has drawn up guidelines of medical standards of fitness for offshore work.[1] Companies which have workers offshore and physicians who may need to assess such workers should obtain a copy of this document.

Examinations are required at the following frequencies:

| up to 39 years | 3-yearly |
| aged 40–50 years | 2-yearly |
| aged 51 and over | annually |

The importance of re-assessing all individuals' medical fitness following absence due to illness or injury is emphasized but does not automatically involve formal medical examination.

While the UKOOA MAC has drawn up guidelines for the operators which any of the sub-contracting companies may use in the UK sector of the North Sea, some companies have their own individual medical policies. The underlying philosophy is to improve the fitness and efficiency of the offshore workforce by selection of suitable individuals and excluding those with conditions which may be detrimental to themselves or to others and may lead to reduced efficiency, possible danger, or the need for urgent medical evacuation. The latter has, on occasion, led to considerable risk. There is an increase in naturally occurring morbidity in an ageing workforce and there are now people who have been working in offshore oil and gas fields for more than 20 years; hence the importance of more frequent medical examinations with increasing age.

Unfortunately there is no universally recognized medical policy, which means that some workers are required to undergo a separate medical examination each time they change company or move across national boundaries. In Norway and in the Netherlands there are unified standards of fitness for offshore workers. In the Netherlands workers are issued with a log book which they carry wherever they travel.

All grades of offshore employees must complete a survival course involving immersion, and some may be required for firefighting duties, both of which require a high standard of general fitness. Some groups, such as divers, are covered by statutory medical examinations (see p. 462); others may only be temporary visitors, but no person on an offshore rig must be a physical or mental liability to himself or others.

The certifying physician should have a thorough knowledge of the offshore workplace acquired by personal experience. While most operating companies have occupational medical departments, many sub-contracting companies have no regular occupational medical support and depend for advice on physicians who may have no first-hand experience of the offshore work site.

The offshore working environment may be hazardous and medical management or evacuation is on occasion governed by bad weather conditions—in particular by fog. Fitness for work offshore has an additional dimension as it will require the exclusion of persons with any medical conditions which may require urgent medical attention and, thus, emergency evacuation.

In the following paragraphs attention is drawn to those areas which are the source of greatest uncertainty in the assessment of offshore workers.

**General points**

There are no statutory standards for offshore workers in the United Kingdom, where each company must set its own standards based on the UKOOA guidelines and the advice of its own physician. The final decision regarding the acceptability of an employee must rest with the employer.

When a candidate first presents himself to a new medical examiner the importance of an accurate and complete history must not be underestimated. Undeclared (undetectable) medical problems may otherwise not be picked up (e.g., epilepsy). A report of previous history may be sought from the candidate's own general practitioner.

In addition to a detailed medical and occupational history, a physical examination and, in some cases, ancillary investigations are required. There may be higher grades of fitness required for specialist workers, such as those on the drilling rig floor, while others may require specialized examinations, such as more detailed visual assessment for crane operators. A suitable physical examination form for offshore work is included at the end of this appendix (Annex B, p. 468).

All employees must be fit enough to participate in survival training which includes escaping from a submerged helicopter, and in some cases firefighting. They must be able to get to and from the worksite safely whether by sea or helicopter and to take care of themselves and to help rescue others in an emergency. This requires general soundness of wind and limb.

The average age of the offshore workforce is increasing and there is an associated increase in morbidity. Health promotion is important and enquiries should be made concerning the family history, and appropriate advice given in respect of other risk factors, such as smoking, exercise, alcohol, and obesity. In some patients a random cholesterol level may be helpful if other risk factors are present.

**Dental fitness**

Dental emergencies are a common reason for evacuation from offshore.[2] An oral inspection will give an indication of oral hygiene and obvious deficiencies will require dental attention before proceeding offshore.

**Infection**

The confines of an offshore installation mean increased risk of transfer of infectious disease through closer contact and shared living facilities. Influenza and infectious enteritides have serious consequences in an offshore community while Hepatitis A is potentially disastrous, especially in food-handlers.

**Digestive system**

The more common problems include irritable bowel syndrome, gastro-oesophageal reflux and peptic ulceration. While a patient with a proven peptic ulcer may be symptom-free on therapy, endoscopic evidence of healing is a prerequisite to returning offshore. For duodenal ulcer eradication of *Helicobacter pylori* with antibiotics should be tried. The presence of a stoma may be socially embarrassing in a shared cabin and communal washroom facilities.

**Liver and pancreas**

Some workers drink heavily immediately before going to work offshore; some companies require a pre-flight breathalyser test and anyone with a reading exceeding 35 μg per 100 ml of breath will be barred until the reading is below that level. Most companies make employee assistance programmes available to any workers with drink problems without major sanctions in the first instance. As offshore workplaces are 'dry' there must be vigilance for the occasional undetected drinker who is deprived suddenly on returning to work offshore, and presents acute withdrawal symptoms.

**Screening for drugs of abuse**

Drugs of abuse have major safety implications offshore. Arrangements for urine screening with proper procedures to ensure confidentiality, supervised chain of custody, and confirmation of positive results by specialist laboratories are being introduced. This appears already to have reduced the incidence of drug abuse in offshore workers. The number of positive detections has dropped as drug testing has become more widely introduced. Some companies insist on screening for drugs and alcohol in the event of an accident, but hospital staff may be reluctant to obtain such samples in cases of serious injury.

**Cardiovascular system**

Cardiovascular assessment is particularly important. Any symptomatic valvular or myocardial disease, ischaemia, infarction, or cardiac dysrhythmia should be cause for rejection. However, a patient who has had successful surgical correction of valvular or congenital heart disease could be considered acceptable. While there are some sedentary duties offshore, everyone has to practise regular emergency evacuation drills which involve considerable exertion. This is particularly relevant when a patient is re-assessed after myocardial infarction which would normally be unacceptable, except in rare cases when a patient may be able to pass an exercise tolerance test and suitable employment can be agreed by the operator's medical advisers at review not less than one year after the infarction. Such patients are unacceptable for certain critical occupations such as crane operators, for example.

Coronary artery bypass surgery does not guarantee freedom from recurrent stenosis and is normally cause for rejection. However, some patients, if free of all symptoms after surgery, and without electrocardiographic evidence of myocardial ischaemia, may be passed fit subject to stringent and regular review. Each case must be individually assessed and the final decision should rest on the recommendation of the operator's medical adviser.

The doctors who provide emergency medical support to the offshore industry can now rely on the superior quality of medical skills and statutory training of offshore rig medics. In many cases electrocardiograms (ECGs) can be transmitted ashore for interpretation, although the management of the case will still depend largely on the clinical picture. Immediate assistance is quicker for installations closer to shore where evacuation times of approximately an hour can be achieved. In more remote locations and in poor weather this is not possible, and the rig medic may have to treat the patient on site. Some physicians with responsibility for offshore personnel believe that no patients with a history of previous cardiovascular disease should be allowed offshore.

### Hypertension

Treated hypertensives without target organ damage and who do not show sustained blood pressure levels above 160/90 may be acceptable. Risk factors do remain and regular screening and follow-up are important. Annual review would be appropriate. The therapy hypertensives are receiving must be without significant side-effects.

### Respiratory system

Pulmonary embolism would be a difficult emergency offshore and even one episode would require careful assessment to eliminate the cause before return.

Spontaneous pneumothorax may be recurrent. After one year without recurrence or after successful surgical treatment the patient may be acceptable.

Symptomatic, restrictive obstructive airways disease even if reversible and only on response to exertion is unacceptable. Assessment by standard spirometery giving readings of forced vital capacity (FVC) below 70 per cent of predicted and forced expiratory volume in one second ($FEV_1$) below 65 per cent would indicate a significant disability.

### Asthma

A history of asthma beyond the age of five should be carefully evaluated. Those mild asthmatics who only take occasional bronchodilators or who are advised to take low-dose inhaled corticosteroids on a regular basis and have a proven record of stable health onshore may be capable of working offshore without undue risk. Patients on regular therapy must continue to take it when they are offshore and must carry adequate supplies. Patients with an unstable asthmatic history requiring oral steroids or emergency intervention are not acceptable. Chronic conditions leading to reduced performance and fitness, such as pulmonary fibrosis, active sarcoid, or any acute inflammatory condition would exclude until stabilized.

### Occupational asthma

Any element of reversible airways obstruction should be identified at the pre-employment assessment and the situation monitored for precipitating causes in the offshore environment.

The rig medic may monitor the patient's respiratory function with a peak flow meter to detect any changes related to occupational exposure to dusts, irritants, or sensitizers.

## Ear, nose, and throat

Acute infections require treatment before acceptance. Any symptomatic chronic disease or vertigo is unacceptable. Dry perforations may be acceptable but active or chronic middle-ear disease is a bar. Significant symptomatic nasal airway obstruction or recurrent or chronic sinus infection would be unacceptable until corrected. Hayfever which responds to therapy (without side-effects) would usually be acceptable. Many offshore workers show a progressive noise-induced hearing loss but hearing conservation programmes have improved this situation. Regular audiometric testing is advised at pre-employment and periodic medical examinations. The ability to interpret speech and to detect audible alarms is essential.

## Haematology

A routine full blood count is a useful screening procedure. Of the conditions identified some may require further investigation while some may be immediately treatable and curable, such as pernicious anaemia, although this is rare among the normal age groups offshore.

### Anaemia

Anaemia is the most commonly discovered condition and must be investigated to ascertain its cause. Iron deficiency anaemia due to unsuspected gastrointestinal blood loss may cause reduced work capacity and productivity and will need full investigation; whether the patient will be fit for offshore employment will depend on the underlying cause.

### Polycythaemia

Primary and secondary polycythaemia characterized by an elevated packed cell volume (PCV) are associated with transient ischaemic attacks, visual disturbances, and peripheral vascular disease which would be hazardous in the offshore situation. Elevated mean cell volume (MCV) is caused by vitamin $B_{12}$ and folic acid deficiency as well as excessive alcohol intake. Patients with the former when treated are acceptable for offshore work. Patients with a raised MCV due to alcohol intake require further investigation and review.

*Malignant diseases*

Leukaemia, lymphomas, and multiple myeloma require individual assessment. Acute leukaemia may, unlike other forms of disseminated malignancy, have remission phases when the patient is free of all symptoms, while chronic lymphatic leukaemia may be almost benign. Fitness for work must be assessed individually, although patients on treatment with cytotoxic or immunosuppressive agents would not normally be considered fit for offshore work.

*Thalassaemia and haemoglobinopathy*

Thalassaemia major and sickle cell disease would be contraindications for offshore work. Individuals with thalassaemia trait and sickle cell trait would be considered fit for work offshore, but not for diving.

*Coagulation disorders (Haemophilia A and Haemophilia B—Christmas disease)*

Haemorrhage at work has been shown to be usually a result of accidental trauma. The facility for emergency treatment with Factor VIII (a sick bay with refrigeration facility) may be available offshore, but the risk of isolation through bad weather or transport being unavailable would usually make these conditions contraindications for offshore work.

## Mental disorders

Any acute or chronic psychosis or neurosis is not acceptable unless the patient is fully recovered, off all therapy, and free of all symptoms for one year. A history of alcohol or drug abuse is not acceptable.

*Stress*

Offshore workers are separated from their families and may be additionally stressed by living and working at a remote, isolated, and sometimes environmentally hostile location. Additionally there is the enforced proximity of colleagues whether at work or off duty. Twelve-hour working shifts are commonplace with an on-call out-of-hours commitment in addition, and the only mode of transport to the shore is by helicopter which may be a stressful experience for some people. The offshore worker must be able to cope with close confinement, noise, and constant artificial light. Some workers are expected to work at considerable heights above the sea. Add to this the constant threat of perceived danger and it is clear that patients with a tendency to anxiety or undue sensitivity are not likely to be suitable for offshore work.

Thirteen of 531 evacuations for medical conditions were for 'mental disorders' (2.5 per cent).[3] Norman[4] showed that 42 (2 per cent) of 2162 evacuations over an eight-year period were a result of mental disorders; this group included neuroses (22 cases), alcoholic psychoses (five cases) and organic psychoses (four cases).

Stress and psychological factors may be a cause of poor work performance long before overt symptoms appear. The examining doctor must pay particular attention to the mental state of any potential offshore worker and exclude any with evidence of an organic psychosis which could have potentially catastrophic consequences offshore. The employee must be mentally prepared for immersion training, firefighting and emergency evacuation exercises in bad weather.

**Central nervous system**

Any employee with an acute or chronic neurological problem, motor or sensory deficit, or impairment of special senses is likely to be unacceptable.

Patients with established epilepsy are unacceptable for offshore work. Following a single seizure the incidence of further convulsions ranges from 27 to 71 per cent in various studies.[5] An employee having had a single seizure may be acceptable provided at least five years have elapsed.

**Musculoskeletal system**

There must be normal mobility, agility, and strength in the spine and all limbs. Clearly a patient with a limb prosthesis is not generally acceptable for offshore work; exceptions may be considered very rarely by an occupational physician who is familiar with the job and the particular offshore worksite. In the great majority of cases, limb prostheses are not compatible with safe working and emergency procedures offshore.

**Morphology**

Offshore workers have been shown to have greater body mass than equivalent groups onshore.[6] Obesity can hamper evacuation procedures and is difficult to reduce permanently. The calculation of body mass index as an assessment of obesity (see Annex A, p. 467) with a generous, but absolute cut-off (defined in the UKOOA guidelines) of 35 kg/m$^2$ has helped to persuade workers to undertake urgent weight reduction to permit employment as well as benefiting the employee's general health.

**Endocrine and metabolic**

Some individuals with treated hypo- and hyperthyroidism have worked successfully off-shore after careful assessment and with careful monitoring of their therapy.

Diabetics are, in general, unacceptable. However, individual cases—stable, controlled on diet alone, or monitored on oral therapy—may be considered. Patients with other endocrine disorders are unlikely to be passed fit.

DIVERS

**Introduction**

Most employed divers are covered by the Diving Operations at Work Regulations 1981, SI 1981, No. 399. These regulations stipulate that no person shall take part in any diving operation as a diver unless he has a valid certificate of medical fitness to dive (Regulation 7(1)(c)). This certificate can be issued only after a medical examination in accordance with the Health and Safety Executive (HSE) guidelines, performed by a doctor approved by the HSE (Regulation 11).

The Regulations also impose a duty on persons who have responsibility for, or control over, diving operations to ensure that diving is safe so far as is reasonably practicable and the diver has a responsibility to declare if he is unfit to dive on any diving operation.

## The examination and certification mechanism

A network of doctors approved to carry out diving medical examinations, and issue certificates of fitness where appropriate, extends throughout the United Kingdom and some foreign countries. Such certificates are entered in the diver's personal log-book and their validity must not exceed 12 months. Before approval as an examining doctor by the HSE, a doctor must demonstrate knowledge and experience of diving medicine, have attended a recognized course in the subject, and show that he meets the clinical requirements of the Director of Medical Services of the HSE and has access to the necessary equipment for special examinations including electrocardiography and audiometry. Once approved the doctor will receive comprehensive guidance from the HSE in the form of document MA1 The Medical Examination of Divers (last fully revised August 1987), the chief features of which are set out below.

A diver who is found unfit to dive, or fit subject to limitations, has the statutory right to apply to the HSE for a review of the approved doctor's decision. Additional information will be gathered and a further examination may be arranged by the HSE who will then take the final decision. In the event of illness, injury, or treated acute decompression illness, the diver is advised to consult an approved doctor before returning to diving.

Although some countries have adopted UK standards, examiners should bear in mind that others may apply quite different ones. An alignment of standards within Europe is being sought. Copies of MA1 are available to approved examiners and on request from HSE Area Offices or by post from the Employment Medical Advisory Service. (For the full address see Appendix 9.)

## Medical considerations

Diving requires superior levels of physical fitness, self-reliance, and aptitude with reserves to cope in an emergency. The effects of immersion, increased breathing resistance, and exercise at depth produce physiological changes which require training for optimal performance. Once the diver descends to his worksite the work he must perform may require strength, agility, judgement, observation, and accuracy without distraction. These requirements are reflected in the demanding standards of fitness required for pre-employment selection to a career in diving. In general, this standard is applicable to all divers. However, there may be divers who, although not meeting these standards fully, are fit for restricted diving, e.g., short dives at shallow depths. Where an examining doctor is in doubt about a diver's fitness he is recommended to obtain a further opinion from a second approved doctor or advice from a specialist on any particular medical aspect. Great importance is attached to the initial baseline medical examination and the MA1 document makes a number of tests mandatory at that stage. Updated guidance is issued to approved doctors from time to time. MA1 should not therefore be taken in isolation as indicating the current position.

The HSE does not specify any minimum age limit for diving work, although approved doctors are advised that it is unlikely that anyone under 18 would be suitable. Nor is any upper age limit specified, provided that all the medical standards can be met.

The same general fitness criteria apply to both male and female divers, apart from relating size and strength to the type of professional diving involved. Available evidence, however, supports the view that no pregnant female should dive.

## The medical examination

The MA1 guidance note is a comprehensive and fairly detailed document. The commoner medical conditions which may cause problems are discussed in this appendix but readers are advised to consult the HSE if they want more information about particular conditions in relation to diving. MA1 provides specific guidance to approved doctors under the following main headings:

Skin
Ears
Respiratory system
Dental
Cardiovascular system
Exercise testing
Alimentary/peptic conditions
Genito-urinary system
Endocrine system
Musculoskeletal system
Central nervous system
Head injury
Psychiatric or psychological illness
Vision
Haematology

It is, however, made clear in MA1 that approved doctors have wide discretion in most of these areas.

## Medical history

There should be a standard enquiry into past and current health, occupational history, social history (including smoking and alcohol), and any details of past decompression illness.

The entry age should be not less than 18 years and the candidate should be assessed for maturity and robustness before entering diver training.

## Examination by system

An assessment of aerobic capacity (step-test and pulse score), body mass index (see Annex A, p. 467), static and dynamic mobility, agility, and strength is made as described in the MA1 document.

A commercial diver must not be obese, must be physically fit and trained for hard work. The effects of immersion, cold, and increased work of breathing make aerobic fitness more important.

### Ear, nose, and throat

In addition to normal clinical examination, hearing is assessed by audiometry and eustachian patency by observation of the tympanic membranes on performance of a Valsalva manoeuvre. The tympanic membranes should be intact.

### Vision

Although vision underwater is limited, binocular vision is necessary. Requirements at the surface are for corrected binocular vision (distance) 6/9 (20/30) or better, near vision N5. The fundi should be examined and visual fields should be full to confrontation.

Any history of glaucoma, uveitis, or optic neuritis requires specialist assessment. Colour vision should be recorded at the initial examination and impairment noted. Trade tests may be performed on location.

### Dental fitness

The teeth should be in good order. There should be no caries, no significant gaps, and no unfixed dentures.

### Respiratory system

There must be general fitness for vigorous swimming on the surface, and no conditions likely to lead to localized air trapping and barotrauma on ascent. Fibrotic lung disease, chronic obstructive airways disease, and reversible airways obstruction are absolute contraindications.

A history of childhood asthma needs full evaluation, as does exertion-induced bronchospasm.

Pneumothorax is a contraindication because of the risk of recurrence. Lung cysts and bullae are contraindications. A diver should avoid extremes of maximal voluntary ventilation, especially when ascending. Full-size posteroanterior (PA) and lateral chest radiographs are required on initial examination and spirometry at every examination.

### Cardiovascular system

A history, or discovery at examination, of ischaemic valvular or myocardial heart disease would be a bar. The assessment should include an electrocardiograph (ECG) at rest. Any variation from normal on examination or investigation, including disorders of rhythm, should be referred for specialist cardiological review and if risk factors such as poor family history, smoking, and obesity are present a supervised monitored exercise tolerance test should be performed with oxygen uptake if possible.

Such a test may on occasion demonstrate unsuspected imbalance between myocardial oxygen requirement and delivery via the coronary arteries. Any subject with risk factors for coronary artery disease should be tested to an equivalent of stage IV on the Bruce protocol (13 mets).

Conditions which permit intracardiac shunting from right to left, such as an atrial septal defect, may be cause for rejection, particularly if unexplained acute decompression illness has occurred.

The resting blood pressure (BP) should not be greater than 140 mmHg systolic or 80 mmHg diastolic (fifth phase). Patients on medication for hypertension are not acceptable.

## Gastrointestinal system

Any peptic ulceration, symptomatic oesophageal reflux, hiatus hernia, or active inflammatory bowel disease is a contraindication to diving. If asymptomatic and with endoscopic evidence of healing then return may be considered.

While an ostomy or stoma is not an absolute bar there are clearly difficulties with diving and careful individual assessment is needed. All abdominal wall hernias should be repaired before diving.

## Neurological

The more subtle and more serious forms of acute decompression illness may involve the central nervous system (CNS). Particular attention should be paid to a history of head injury or any CNS disorder. Examination should include the diver's attitude, speech, cerebration, verbal and intellectual response, and gait. Cranial nerves and special senses must be assessed.

Causes for rejection would include:

(1)  claustrophobia, severe motion sickness;

(2)  any unprovoked loss of consciousness, recurrent fainting, or epilepsy including single seizure (other than febrile convulsions occurring up to the age of five years);

(3)  migraine with neurological symptoms or signs;

(4)  any intracranial surgical procedure or depressed skull fracture;

(5)  head injury with loss of consciousness greater than 10 minutes or with focal localising signs; and

(6)  a period of post-traumatic amnesia greater than one hour.

Any evidence of cerebrovascular accident, significant spinal cord trauma, spondyloses with myelopathy, demyelination (multiple sclerosis), or neurodegenerative disease (Parkinson's disease) would be cause for rejection.

## Psychiatric or psychological

Any history or evidence of past or present mental disorder (including abuse of drugs and alcohol) should be cause for rejection unless of a trivial nature and unlikely to recur. Specialised assessment may be needed in cases where there is suspicion of latent brain damage.

## Haematology

Anaemia should be investigated; most blood dyscrasias will be cause for rejection and frank haemoglobinopathies should be excluded. Sickle cell trait may be permitted if asymptomatic and investigation by electrophoresis demonstrates a percentage of HbS below 40.

## Genitourinary system

A history of renal disease or of urinary tract investigation will be reason for more detailed questioning and examination. Dipstick urine analysis for glucose, protein, and blood should be undertaken routinely. Venereal disease will debar until adequately treated. The presence of kidney stones and other genitourinary diseases are usually a cause for rejection. (Cases of renal colic may not necessarily be so, but should be judged on an individual basis after specialist investigation.) The presence of a single kidney which is normally functioning will be acceptable for diving work.

## Malignancy

This is assessed on an individual basis.

## Infection control

The examining doctor must be satisfied that the diver is not suffering from a communicable disease. All such cases should be excluded from diving until treated. Separate guidance on the desirability of screening for HIV antibody and the management of divers having AIDS has been issued by the HSE.[7]

Investigations which may be required at the medical examination are: full blood count, HbS assessment, urinalysis, audiometry, chest X-ray (on entry only), ECG (with or without exercise), pulmonary function testing ($FEV_1$, FVC), and, for deep diving, electronystagmogram (ENG) and long-bone X-rays.

## Radiography

Routine pre-employment long-bone radiography is no longer required. Neither is routine radiography of long bones prior to Part I, Part III or Part IV training. However, radiography of the hips, shoulders, and knees should be carried out before the commencement of Part II training, and of the hips and shoulders at intervals thereafter while the diver is still engaged in mixed-gas or saturation diving.

ANNEX A    BODY MASS INDEX

The Body Mass Index is measured as follows: weight in kilograms divided by height in metres$^2$:-

$$\frac{\text{Wt (kg)}}{\text{Ht (m}^2)}$$

| Readings | Implications |
|----------|--------------|
| 18 kg/m$^2$ or less | Underweight. |
| 19–25 kg/m$^2$ | Healthy. A desirable BMI figure indicating a healthy weight. |
| 26–30 kg/m$^2$ | Overweight, health could suffer. Some weight loss should now be considered. |
| 31–40 kg/m$^2$ | Obese. Health is at risk. Losing weight now should be seriously considered. |
| 41 kg/m$^2$ or above | Very obese. Health is seriously at risk. Losing weight immediately is essential. |

From Garrow, J.S. (1988). Obesity and related diseases 1988. In *Human obesity*, (ed. G.A. Bray). Churchill Livingstone, Edinburgh.

## ANNEX B

| SURNAME: | GIVEN OR FORENAMES: | DATE OF BIRTH: |
|---|---|---|
| ADDRESS:<br><br>TELEPHONE: | | Married / Single /<br>Separated / Divorced |
| COMPANY: | EMPLOYMENT AS: | |

NAME AND ADDRESS OF FAMILY DOCTOR:

| PLEASE √ IN THE APPROPRIATE COLUMN | YES | NO |
|---|---|---|
| 1. Have you had any serious illness? | | |
| 2. Have you ever been in hospital? | | |
| 3. Have you had any operations performed? | | |
| 4. Have you been off work with illness or injury in the past two years? | | |
| 5. Have you had any ear trouble or discharge? | | |
| 6. Have you had ulcers or indigestion? | | |
| 7. Have you ever had diarrhoea lasting more than one week? | | |
| 8. Have you ever had heart trouble? | | |
| 9. (a) Have you ever had chest trouble or wheeze (e.g. asthma, bronchitis)?<br>(b) Have you ever taken steroid tablets for asthma? | | |
| 10. Do you have diabetes? | | |
| 11. Have you had any skin diseases or allergic rashes? | | |
| 12. Have you had any back trouble? | | |
| 13. Have you ever had arthritis or joint troubles? | | |
| 14. Have you had any accidents? | | |
| 15. Have you had any broken bones? | | |
| 16. Have you had any 'nerve trouble?' | | |
| 17. Have you ever had epilepsy or fits? | | |
| 18. Have you had any tropical disease? | | |
| 19. Have you ever had a life insurance refused or loaded? | | |
| 20. Have you ever failed a medical examination? | | |
| 21. Have you been in the Services? | | |
| 22. If 'Yes' were you discharged fit? | | |
| 23. Have you taken tablets, medicines or injections regularly at any time? | | |
| 24. Is there any serious illness in the family? | | |
| 25. How much do you smoke daily? | | |
| 26. How much alcohol do you drink each week? | | |
| 27. Have you had exposure at work to: Noise /Radiation /Chemicals? | | |
| 28. At work have you worn protective clothing /breathing apparatus or masks /or a Radiation Exposure Meter? | | |
| 29. At work have you used barrier creams to protect your skin? | | |

FOR WHAT COMPANIES HAVE YOU BEEN EMPLOYED IN THE LAST FIVE YEARS?

I have read and understood the above questions and I have given a full and truthful answer to them all. I give permission to Dr........................................................

to examine me on behalf of ..............................................................................................................................and convey to them a copy of his findings.

Date: ........................................................  SIGNED:........................................................

| Height: | | | cms. | Weight: | | | kgs. | BMI: | |
|---|---|---|---|---|---|---|---|---|---|
| Temp: | | | | Pulse: | | | | BP: | |

| Distant Vision: | Right 20/ | Left 20/ | Near Vision: | Right | Left | | Visual Fields: | Right | | Left |
|---|---|---|---|---|---|---|---|---|---|---|
| With glasses: | Right 20/ | Left 20/ | | Right | Left | | Colour Vision: | Ishihara | | City |
| Urine: | Albumen | | Sugar | | | Blood | | Sp. Gr. | | |

| | | Normal | Abnormal | COMMENTS |
|---|---|---|---|---|
| 1. | Personal hygiene | | | |
| 2. | General appearance | | | |
| 3. | Skin | | | |
| 4. | Indentification marks | | | |
| 5. | Eyes | | | |
| 6. | Ears | | | |
| 7. | Nose and sinuses | | | |
| 8. | Teeth and gums | | | |
| 9. | Throat | | | |
| 10. | Thyroid and neck | | | |
| 11. | Lymph glands | | | |
| 12. | Chest | | | |
| 13. | Breasts | | | |
| 14. | Abdomen | | | |
| 15. | Heart | | | |
| 16. | Circulation: Arterial | | | |
| | Venous | | | |
| 17. | Hernial Orifices | | | |
| 18. | Gluteal cleft | | | |
| 19. | Perineum | | | |
| 20. | Genitals | | | |
| 21. | Spine | | | |
| 22. | Joints | | | |
| 23. | Limbs | | | |
| 24. | Central nervous system | | | |
| 25. | Personality | | | |

**INVESTIGATIONS:**       Specify       Results

Blood tests

Chest X–rays

Other X–rays

E.C.G.

Audiometry

Vitalograph

Other investigations

EXAMINING DOCTOR'S COMMENTS

RECOMMENDATIONS

1. Acceptable for proposed employment without restriction

2. Acceptable for employment in a restricted capacity (Specify)

3. Unfit for proposed employment until defect corrected (Specify)

4. Unfit for the proposed employment.       Signed: ..................................................................................................

## Selected references and further reading

1. UKOOA (UK Offshore Operators Association) (1992). *Medical aspects of fitness for offshore work. A guide for examining physicians*. UKOOA, London.
2. Hahn, M.J. (1987). The dental status of workers on offshore installations in the UK oil and gas industry. *Brit. Dent. J.*, **163**, 262–4.
3. Phillips, J.C. (1987). Medical support by a team of doctors to offshore paramedics. *J. Roy. Coll. Gen. Pract.*, **37**, 168–9.
4. Norman, J.N. *et al.* (1978). Medical evacuations from offshore structures. *Brit. J. Indust. Med.*, **45**, 619–23.
5. Reynolds, E.H. (editorial) (1988). A single seizure. *Brit. Med. J.*, **297**, 1422–3.
6. Light, I.M. and Gibson, M. (1986). Percentage body fat and prevalence of obesity in a UK offshore population. *Brit. J. Nutrit.*, **56**, 97–104.
7. HSE (Health and Safety Executive) (1991). HIV infection and diving. IND(G), 101L C150 3/91. Medical Division of Health and Safety Executive. HSE, Bootle.
8. Cox, R.A.F. (ed.) (1987). *Offshore medicine*. Springer Verlag, London.

# Appendix 5

# Working overseas

## *R.A.F. Cox*

While most of the comments in this appendix apply to companies and their employees overseas, it must be remembered that many people are working overseas, often in hostile areas, without any support from parent organizations. Such people may include the self-employed, academics, missionaries, students, and professional adventurers. An excellent and fascinating account of the hazards facing anthropologists is given by Howell.[1] Any person planning to work overseas should, before departure, make careful preparation for the preservation of his health and the provision of medical care in the event of illness.

For the addresses of centres from which essential medical advice can be obtained see Appendix 9, p. 517. A list of useful books which may be consulted during the planning of an overseas assignment can be found at the end of this appendix.

Companies who send employees overseas, however long or short the assignment may be, retain a responsibility for them while they are abroad. It is, therefore, essential that employers ensure, as far as possible, that potential expatriates are fit for their overseas duties and that proper arrangements are in place to take care of them if they are ill or injured.

There are a great number of factors to be considered when a company is planning an overseas operation and consideration of the medical implications tends to have a very low priority even though concerns for general health will be a major anxiety of any potential expatriate and his family.

The company must, therefore, find out not only about diseases and medical conditions which may be prevalent in the area of their operation, but it must also review the local medical and hospital facilities and services and appoint a local doctor to act on its behalf. In many areas of the world this will require a visit by a doctor from the home country on behalf of the company.

Any company which embarks on overseas operations should appoint a doctor at its home base, if it does not already have its own occupational physician. This is necessary not only so that he can determine whether employees are fit to transfer overseas, but to liaise with the local overseas doctor and to advise on the numerous health queries which will inevitably arise in the course of a foreign operation.

No matter how thorough the pre-departure medical screening and examinations may have been, some illness will still occur, requiring decisions regarding treatment, possible repatriation and liaison with doctors and relatives in the home country. Even if illness does not occur, injury, especially from road accidents, is a constant risk and the most common reason for emergency repatriations. Policies and procedures for dealing with such contingencies must be in place before the operation begins. It may be fatal to wait until such an emergency arises. Such policies must include the mechanism by which the costs of local medical care are to be met. It is essential that all overseas assignees and regular travellers have adequate medical insurance cover, which is available from any of the major health insurers. In most countries this has to be purchased and in many places payment, or a guarantee of payment, is required before admission to hospital can be arranged or treatment can commence.

There are a number of air ambulance services available but two of the largest established ones are based in Switzerland. They are:

Swiss Air Rescue Organization
Mainaustrasse 21
CH-8008 Zurich
Tel: 41-1-385 8585

SOS Air Ambulance
12 Chemin Riantbosson
1217 Meyrin 1
Geneva
Tel: 41 22 736 3333 or 41 22 347 6161

Before departure, or the establishment of an overseas operation, arrangements should be made with one of these, or a similar organization, for the emergency evacuation of sick and injured personnel.

Peoples' behaviour changes as soon as they are overseas. The different culture, climate, food and social activities produce psychological and physiological changes which often affect health. Even the most demure people seem to relax their usual standards of conventional sexual behaviour when abroad, particularly if they are not accompanied by their usual sexual partners.

Some people will seek overseas employment to escape from domestic or financial crises or because they have drinking problems or established psychiatric conditions. Such persons are likely to be disastrous choices for overseas assignments and should be rigorously excluded. The enquiries of the pre-departure medical examiner should be particularly oriented towards revealing these factors.

While staying well in Western countries is taken for granted, because of their excellent public health and medical care systems, staying well in many Third World and tropical countries requires strict self-discipline and personal vigilance. Standards of personal and domestic hygiene must be greater and risks which may be quite acceptable in Europe or North America may lead to dire consequences in tropical Africa. People who may have difficulty in adjusting to this very different environment should be counselled before departure. A trivial and easily managed illness in the United Kingdom can be a major problem for the patient, his family and his employers when it occurs overseas. In no other circumstance is the hackneyed cliché 'prevention is better than cure' more true, while the emergency evacuation of a sick employee is often a hazardous experience for the patient and always an expensive, worrying and very time-consuming predicament for those responsible for the organization of the repatriation.

The essential medical examination should be arranged well in advance of departure and should be conducted by a doctor experienced in travel medicine who is instructed to perform the examination on behalf of the company and to which he should make his report. This should preferably be in confidence to the company's own medical adviser but, if not, it should be in the form of a non-confidential report to the personnel manager or other appropriate senior person. As long as the report is made by a person who has not had clinical care of the employee it will not fall within the Access to Medical Reports Act.

The examining doctor must be aware of the local conditions at the overseas place of residence, preferably through first-hand experience. It may be quite acceptable to transfer someone with quite significant health problems to a location where medical care of an equivalent standard to that at the home base is available, while the same health problem would be an absolute bar to transfer to other places. A totally different standard of medical fitness must be expected in, say, a geologist who may be moving to an office job in Chicago to one who is to lead a survey party in Niger.

The medical examination should be designed and performed to reveal actual or potential health problems which may occur during the course of the overseas assignment. In this respect the examination for transfer overseas differs from a pre-employment examination which is designed to determine only a person's fitness for work. Because of the different environmental and physiological demands many employees who are perfectly fit to work in the United Kingdom would not be fit to do the same work overseas. The examination must also be performed sufficiently ahead of departure so that remediable conditions can be treated.

Any person who is suffering from a medical condition which requires regular medical supervision should not be permitted to transfer overseas unless the examining doctor is quite certain that such supervision, and of an acceptable standard, is available.

If companies with international operations keep their employees under regular health surveillance staff can be very rapidly processed for overseas service and may not even need an examination. However, unless the doctor who has to decide on the potential expatriate's fitness for overseas work is very familiar with his current medical state or has access to notes of a recent examination, the employee must have a comprehensive medical review including a physical examination. In the author's experience screening by questionnaire is not adequate.

Even more important is the examination of family members if the employee is to be accompanied, although there is an increasing tendency for employees to transfer overseas on 'bachelor status' with two weeks' home leave every three months. Children normally adapt to living overseas very well but may have medical conditions which could be a liability, and in many Third World countries the facilities for the medical care of children are even less adequate than those for adults, so that children who are ill must either be nursed at home or repatriated. Expatriate mothers must, therefore, be not only capable, confident, resourceful, and very adaptable, but they must also be very fit. Thorough and detailed review and examination of spouses is just as important as for employees.

When the family have been deemed 'fit to travel' appropriate prophylactic immunizations must be administered and essential emergency medical equipment in the way of drugs, dressings and other items must be provided. Medicines and other medical items readily available and taken for granted in the United Kingdom, are often unavailable or of very inferior quality in developing countries and every expatriate and family should carry essential supplies from their home base. The exact list should be provided by the company medical officer and will depend upon the location and the anticipated requirements of the family. The course of immunizations should also be completed in good time so that any untoward reactions have ceased before departure.

Detailed advice about recommended immunizations can be obtained from any of the centres listed at the end of this appendix. Comments on some of the latest vaccines are:

*Hepatitis A.* Hepatitis A vaccine should be given to all long term assignees (i.e., more than six months' stay) and all regular travellers. Immune globulin ($\gamma$ globulin) should now only be given to unprotected travellers departing at short notice.

*Hepatitis B.* Hepatitis *B* vaccine should be given to all regular travellers and long term assignees (i.e., more than six months' stay) to all areas of the world except North America, Australia, New Zealand and Northern Europe.

*Rabies.* The modern rabies vaccine is safe and effective and it should be given to all travellers to developing areas of the world. By administering this vaccine prophylactically it obviates the need for giving a blood product (rabies immunoglobulin) in the event of a bite, which is particularly reassuring in the current AIDS climate.

*Meningitis.* While Group B meningitis, for which there is no available vaccine, is the commonest strain in the United Kingdom, the other strains, A and C, for which there is an effective vaccine, are commoner in some areas of the world. Meningitis vaccine should be given to overseas assignees or regular travellers to East, West and Central Africa, the Delhi area of India, Nepal, and the whole of the Middle East.

*Japanese encephalitis.* Vaccination against this disease should be considered for persons embarking on rural travel in Asia from India to Japan but individual advice should be sought from one of the centres listed in Appendix 9.

*Yellow fever.* This is not a new vaccine but it is essential for anyone travelling to tropical Africa or South America. A single injection lasts for 10 years, but it is so often neglected until immediately before urgent travel that it is mentioned here to emphasize the importance of taking the vaccine if there is any possibility, at any time, of travelling to a yellow fever area.

*AIDS.* AIDS is covered elsewhere in this book Chapter 22, p. 413 but it is spreading rapidly in both sexes in some areas of Africa, Asia, and the Caribbean and the importance of not taking risks cannot be overemphasized for the regular traveller or overseas assignee.

As a side issue, some international operators, in areas of the world where the prevalence of HIV positivity is reported to be as high as 40 per cent of the population, may have to consider whether it would be of any advantage to screen local employees for HIV prior to employment. For more detail on pre-employment screening see Chapter 22.

**The medical processing of potential expatriates is an essential prerequisite which should be completed well in advance of departure and must include every member of the family who is travelling. The cost of such a procedure is small compared with the cost of medical repatriation which such screening could have prevented.**

### Summary

1. Local medical facilities must be reviewed.
2. Appoint a local doctor.
3. Establish liaison between the local overseas doctor and the company's occupational physician.
4. Arrange adequate medical insurance cover.
5. Prepare contingency plans for medical evacuation/repatriation.
6. Arrange thorough medical examinations, well in advance of departure, for all members of the family who are going.

## Acknowledgement

I am greatly indebted to Dr Gill Lea of Trailfinders and The Centre for Communicable Disease, Colindale, for help in the preparation of this appendix.

## Suggested reading

Walker, E. Williams, G. and Raeside, F. (1993). *The ABC of healthy travel*. BMJ, Publishing, London.

Dawood, R. (ed.) (1992). *Travellers health*. Oxford University Press.

Werner, D. (1979). *Where there is no doctor*. Macmillan, London.

DOH (Department of Health) (1992). *Immunisation against infectious disease*. HMSO, London.

The US Department of Health and Human Services, Public Health Service (1992). *The yellow book. Health information for international travel*. [But beware of significant differences in recommended practice between the United States and Europe].

DOH (Department of Health). *Health advice for travellers*. Published annually. HMSO, London.

Turner, A.C. (1985). *The travellers health guide*. Roger Lascelles, 47 York Road, Brentford, Middlesex TW8 0QP.

## Reference

1. Howell, N. (1990) *Surviving fieldwork*. A report on health and safety in fieldwork. American Anthropological Association, Washington D.C.

# Appendix 6

# Ethics for occupational physicians

## Introduction

When the Guidelines were first published by the Faculty of Occupational Medicine (the Faculty) in 1980, the Introduction stated that they "… may have to be revised from time to time as attitudes in society continue to change".

Each section of this new fourth edition has been revised in the light of these changing attitudes and also changes of values in society, changes in the law, and the enquiries and comments received by the Faculty's Ethics Committee. The fundamental principles governing the ethics of occupational medicine remain largely unchanged although detailed emphasis has altered with new developments, improved knowledge and new technologies for handling data.

The second edition, which was published in 1982, took account of other publications of direct relevance[1,2,3,4] and also a number of comments made about the first edition, notably by Paul Sieghart.[5] Since that time the BMA revised and published a new edition of its handbook which was renamed 'Philosophy and Practice of Medical Ethics'[6] and has recently produced a further publication entitled 'Medical Ethics Today: its practice and philosophy'[(7)], the GMC has published a new edition of its booklet "Professional Conduct and Discipline: Fitness to Practise'[8], and the International Commission on Occupational Health has published an 'International Code of Ethics for Occupational Health Professionals.[9]

Annexes have been added to this appendix which give information about services for sick doctors, and a suggested confidentiality agreement for non-medical personnel employed in occupational health departments.

## Section 1   General Principles

1.1. Attitudes and behaviour in society are changing rapidly and for physicians working in industry and commerce the changes tend to be quicker and more radical than elsewhere. Ethics, as a code of conduct, must take account of these changing attitudes and also of legal standards. The need for special consideration of ethical standards in occupational medicine arises largely because doctors may find themselves in a position where there are conflicts of interest and loyalty derived from the different roles they are required to play. It is in the nature of these conflicts that, because ethical axioms are not always universally agreed, answers to ethical problems cannot always be logically deduced; often there is more than one 'correct' course of action. Nevertheless, some aspects of ethics in medicine receive such widespread support inside and outside the profession that their observance is sanctioned by the General Medical Council. There remain, however, many circumstances in which the answers to ethical questions cannot be codified and it is in such circumstances that these guidelines should be consulted.

1.2. Ethical behaviour is largely self-imposed by each doctor who will take many decisions and act according to individual conscience. However, these guidelines drawn up by the Faculty should help occupational physicians to deal with most ethical difficulties and dilemmas. When in doubt, discussion and consultation with appropriate senior medical colleagues can be invaluable and advice may be obtained from the Faculty's Ethics Committee or from other professional associations.

1.3. Doctors may have three forms of contact with patients: as the traditional therapeutic doctor–patient relationship; as an impartial medical examiner reporting to a third party; and as a research worker. In the course of their day-to-day duties, occupational physicians also adopt these roles, but additionally may be required to give expert advice to managers and to employees or their representatives, including trades unions. In all their relationships with people in the workplace, occupational physicians must demonstrate by their behaviour and their conduct that they clearly appreciate in which capacity they are acting at that time and should ensure that others involved fully understand the position.

1.4. Doctors giving occupational medical advice to companies which employ individuals for whom those same doctors also provide primary care should be careful to separate these roles and ensure that this is understood by the company and also by their patients who are employees.

1.5. Occupational physicians should appreciate that when advising on the nature or extent of a work-related health risk and the means by which it may be controlled, they should not presume to decide for others whether or not that risk is acceptable. Furthermore, the consent of workers' representatives to a medical procedure must not be taken to imply the consent of all the individuals concerned.

1.6. The status of an occupational physician in an organization must be that of impartial professional adviser, concerned primarily with safeguarding and improving the health of employed persons. Demonstrable professional competence, independence, and integrity, as well as openness in matters of concern, are necessary to command the confidence of management, employees, and their representatives.

### Section 2   Confidentiality concerning access to and the release of clinical information about individuals

2.1. The occupational physician and occupational health nurse are, jointly or separately responsible for all clinical information whether kept manually or electronically.

*Guardianship of records*

2.2. Unrestricted access to clinical data should be confined to the occupational physician and the occupational health nurse. However, it is recognized that clinical data may also need to be seen, at the discretion of the physician or nurse, by such people as clerical support staff and other members of the occupational health department, including temporary staff. It is the duty of the physician or nurse to ensure that these persons are made fully aware of their personal responsibility to keep all clinical information confidential. This should be explained orally by the physician or nurse and confirmed in writing and a signed undertaking given by each individual concerned (see Annex B).

*Disclosure of records*

2.3. Normally, the informed written consent of the individual is required before access to clinical data may be granted to others, whoever they may be and whether professionally qualified or not, e.g., solicitors, insurers, managers, trades union representatives, employment medical advisers, etc. To give informed consent the individual should understand clearly what information will be imparted, to whom, for what purpose, and the possible outcomes which may result.

2.4. Clinical data or other information obtained by occupational physicians in the course of their professional activities must not be disclosed except in the following circumstances:
    (a) with the consent of the individual;
    (b) if the disclosure is clearly in the patient's interest but it is not possible or is undesirable to seek consent;
    (c) if it is required by law;
    (d) if it is unequivocally in the public interest;
    (e) if it is necessary to safeguard national security or to prevent a serious crime;
    (f) if it will prevent a serious risk to public health; or
    (g) in certain circumstances for the purposes of medical research.

2.5. In circumstances other than when the individual has given consent to the disclosure of information or when it is required by law, disclosure should only be made after very careful consideration of all the facts.If the doctor is in any doubt, the matter should be discussed and advice obtained from an experienced colleague, a medical defence organization or a professional body. The doctor should also recognize that the final decision may need to be justified at some time in the future.

2.6. The answers given to detailed health questionnaires, the results of health assessments or medical examinations, and health information on individuals obtained from third parties, should be passed directly to and retained by a relevant health professional to ensure confidentiality. Medical records of this nature should not be passed through or held by personnel or other non-medical departments. This need not apply to general questions on health included in some initial job application forms.

*Access to records*

2.7. Since November 1991, under the Access to Health Records Act 1990, an individual has had a statutory right of access to health records made 'in connection with the care of that individual'. Occupational health records which relate to the physical or mental health of employees may be subject to the Act.[10] Data protection legislation gives an individual access to electronically maintained data (see 2.14–19).

2.8. Occupational physicians should consider the development of a clear policy to cover requests by individuals for access to their health records which are outside the statutory requirements, recognizing the possible legal implications.

2.9. Personal health information for the purposes of audit or quality control does not require the informed consent of each individual provided that records are anonymized prior to their use in the audit process and confidentiality is assured. Alternatively, employees or patients should be informed of the possible use of information about them and of their right to withhold consent to disclosure. The requirement for anonymity must also extend to occupational physicians and all other health professionals. Reports to management should not contain information which might allow identification of any individual whether patient, employee, or health professional and should be limited to general conclusions and group results. The Conference of Medical Royal Colleges issued interim guidelines on confidentiality and medical audit in 1991.[11] Further information may be found in two reports on medical audit published by the Royal College of Physicians in 1989[12] and 1993[13] and the General Medical Council's pamphlet.[8]

2.10. Occupational physicians should remember that, with regard to their own colleagues or staff, when they are acting as line managers they must claim no special privilege of access to medical information over and above that which is available to other managers.

*Security of records*

2.11. The responsibility for the confidentiality of clinical data is that of the occupational physician and the occupational health nurse. Arrangements must be made for the proper transfer of data to another physician or nurse when the record holder leaves, retires, or dies. Similar constraints should be applied to medical data of employees moving to another organization, and their consent must be obtained before their clinical data may be transferred. If the organization is to be closed and will cease to exist, it will be necessary to ensure that records are transferred with the individual's consent either to each employee's own doctor or to another medical adviser for safe keeping. In certain circumstances it may be desirable to pass the records to the employee to retain, particularly when the employee is known to have been exposed to hazards having long-term implications for health or when periodic examinations have been undertaken.

2.12. As a last resort the physician should ensure that the records are completely destroyed by shredding or incineration, but care must be taken to ensure that records are retained where retention is required by statute.

2.13. Occupational physicians should consider the development of guidelines for the retention of medical records for their particular circumstances taking into account statutory requirements and potential litigation claims.

*Computerized medical records*

2.14. Computerized health information systems are now common in occupational health practice. Systems range from simple personal computer databases to large networked corporate systems using telecommunication links over long distances. The ethical principles for managing the security and confidentiality of computerized medical records are identical to those for manually maintained paper record systems.

2.15. Computer equipment and stored data should be kept secure in accommodation which should be locked when unattended. The maintenance of computer software and hardware should be supervised to ensure that there is no inappropriate access to employee medical information. Similarly, telecommunication links should be protected to prevent unauthorized access. Suitable identity and password systems should be instituted to control access to employee medical information.

2.16. A policy statement detailing procedures for security and confidentiality should be prepared. All staff with access to the occupational health unit should receive adequate training and sign the policy statement to acknowledge their responsibilities (See 2.2 and Annex B).

2.17. A regular updated copy of the computer records should be taken and kept in a separate and secure location. This back-up will allow the record system to be restored in the event that the computer or records database is damaged. No unauthorized software should be used on the system to prevent the risk of computer viruses being introduced which can corrupt information.

2.18. The Data Protection Act 1984 applies to all computerized occupational health information other than that used only for research or statistical purposes where the individual cannot be identified. The Act requires that the information stored about identifiable personnel must be accurate and managed in a confidential manner. Employees have a right of access to all their computer records with limited exceptions. Although there is no legal requirement, occupational physicians should be prepared to interpret and explain this information.

2.19. The Access to Medical Reports Act 1988 applies both to manual reports and information prepared from computerized records.

*Disclosure of records in litigation cases*

2.20. In any case of litigation brought by or against the employer or by or against the occupational physician, the occupational physician should not release any medical information or records relating to any employee without that employee's informed consent in writing. In any such case, the release of such information should be made only to the named individual authorized by the employee, i.e., the lawyer, doctor, or trades union officer identified on the consent form.

*Disclosure to employers' legal advisers*

2.21. Lawyers employed by a company or an employer's external lawyers have no automatic right of access to any medical records or reports and must first obtain the written informed consent of the individual (see 2.3). Other doctors or nurses should be consulted before such disclosure is to be made if those records include notes or reports made by them. However, occupational physicians who are in doubt about the terms of disclosure in a specific case may find it useful to consult their medical defence society. Useful advice on such medicolegal problems can be found in the report prepared by the Joint Committee representing the Legal and Medical professions.[1] There is a legal obligation to release information when ordered to do so by virtue of an Order for Discovery of Documents issued either by the County Court, High Court, or Industrial Tribunal. However, the duty is restricted to releasing only that information so specified within the terms of the Order.

2.22. An occupational physician may be asked by a solicitor for the disclosure of all medical records held about a patient in the course of litigation about a specific incident, such as an injury. Even if the patient has consented to this disclosure, it may not have been appreciated that the full records may include information about a consultation on other matters unrelated to the injury in question. Under these circumstances the occupational physician should clarify the consent with the patient and whether all records are to be disclosed, or only those relevant to the injury. The patient's wishes may be overruled by a formal court order, but physicians should not be misled by solicitors who state that an application for a court order has been made. The patient's written consent is essential except for disclosure to the patient's own solicitor at the verbal request of the patient, and even then it is advisable.

2.23. Medical notes, reports, and records may also be required to be produced to an industrial tribunal in cases of dismissal on the grounds of ill health, poor performance, excessive absenteeism, or redundancy. Such data may also be used as evidence in discrimination claims and commonly in claims of sexual or racial harassment. Here the occupational physician must follow the normal ethical practice of obtaining the informed consent of the individual concerned and must check exactly which records the individual wishes to be disclosed.

2.24. A different type of problem can arise if an employee or his solicitor asks for the release of only one part of a clinical record but refuses release of other equally relevant parts, for example, a recent audiogram showing deafness but not earlier ones showing perhaps a similar degree of hearing loss. Under these circumstances the physician should consider advising the solicitors of both parties that all the records relevant to the case should be made available to both sides. It would then be up to either or both the solicitors concerned to obtain the plaintiff's agreement to the release of all relevant records, or failing that, to apply to a court for an order. On the other hand, a report specifically commissioned by a solicitor in connection with a legal case must be kept in confidence to that solicitor only as it is protected by absolute legal privilege.

2.25. The rules and other considerations about disclosure of records to a court apply equally to industrial tribunals.

2.26. In many cases occupational physicians may be put under considerable pressure by their employer's own lawyers or insurers to disclose the clinical records of an employee, especially in a case where a claim for personal injuries is being pursued against the employer. The basis for such requests often lies in the belief that the employer owns the medical records. However, while the employer may own the paper, the folder and the filing cabinet, etc., the information which is recorded is considered to be the property of the author. The employer enjoys no automatic rights to such information.

2.27. The occupational physician would be in clear breach of the duty of confidentiality if any such unauthorized disclosure were to be made. All such attempts to require unauthorized disclosure of this nature should be vigorously resisted.

2.28. The correct procedure must be to insist that employees provide informed consent to the disclosure of such information to named individuals.

2.29. The occupational physician should ensure so far as possible that no pressure has been exerted upon the individual in order to obtain such consent.

2.30. Any medical notes which contain codes or abbreviations may be judged to be inadequate and the occupational physician may be required to supplement the information in order that the notes can be understood.

*Disclosure required by law*

2.31. Orders for disclosure are made under the authority of the Administration of Justice Act 1970, Sections 31 and 32, and the Administration of Justice (Scotland) Act 1972, Section 1. Under the Supreme Court Act 1982, the courts will order disclosure to the applicant, the applicant's legal advisers, or to his medical advisers.

2.32. Disclosure of documents and information is, however, subject to 'qualified privilege' and any medical reports prepared for the dominant purpose of bringing or defending legal proceedings may be protected from disclosure—but only in very rare cases. Occupational physicians should be aware that in most cases reports prepared by them in any case of industrial injury or occupational disease will have to be disclosed in any legal proceedings.

2.33. If the occupational physician is likely to be a party to the action because of alleged negligence the order will be made under Section 33 of the Supreme Court Act 1981, but where the physician is involved only as a witness the order will be made under Section 34.

**Occupational physicians are advised to take and maintain full factual, contemporaneous, dated notes. Not only is this good practice, but these notes may be required in the light of possible disclosure or litigation.**

### Section 3    Fitness for work

3.1.  There are many instances in occupational medicine where limited information on the health or fitness of an individual has to be given to people outside the confines of the normal doctor–patient relationship. Occupational physicians' duties involve a wide range of assessments concerning the effects of health on the capacity to work and the effects of work on health. Within these broad categories there are many differing circumstances with correspondingly differing ethical obligations.

*Pre-employment health assessment*

3.2.  In this circumstance the primary responsibility of the occupational physician is to the employer rather than the applicant but the physician has a number of ethical constraints. Any health assessment should be appropriate to the task requirement. Medical examinations are normally justified only when the job involves working in hazardous environments, requires high standards of fitness, is required by law, or when the safety of other workers or of the public is concerned.[14] Generally a health assessment by questionnaire should suffice and physicians should advise against the application of physical or mental standards which are not relevant to the requirements of the job. While employers will naturally wish to recruit able-bodied staff, physicians should encourage the employment of disabled or handicapped applicants into suitable positions,[15] and should not allow unreasonably stringent standards to be used as a way of discriminating against such people.

3.3.  A practice which has been observed in some organizations is to request routinely the consent to full disclosure of general practitioner or other medical records at the pre-employment stage. Few job applicants will refuse such a request in case it jeopardises their prospects. Occupational physicians working within an organization should not condone such a practice and should only be party to requesting disclosure if it can be justified in the light of specific job requirements.

3.4.  General practitioners and other doctors may occasionally receive requests for medical reports from management or from personnel departments. The doctor should not release full medical details to a lay source, but rather should agree to provide a report providing broad conclusions and employment implications and express willingness to communicate in more detail to a nominated physician, provided that the informed written consent of the individual is obtained.

*Assessment for joining a pension scheme*

3.5.  Normally fitness for work is regarded as fitness for membership of the pension scheme but sometimes a fund manager will question the employment of a handicapped applicant or one with an established medical problem. In these circumstances the physician should avoid making firm predictions of prognosis, unless there is a reasonable degree of certainty. As with any other medical assessment, the physician should be aware of any established criteria and the rules of the pension fund and should consider it paramount that both the physician and the company act in good faith.

*Assessment of employees with recurrent absence attributable to sickness or on return to work after illness*

3.6. In these circumstances the primary responsibility of the occupational physician is to each individual being assessed, while taking into account the needs of the organization. Occupational physicians must maintain objectivity and approach employees with a constructive and caring attitude, advising them in their best interests. Some employers erroneously view the occupational physician as a means of controlling sickness absence. The control of sickness absence is the responsibility of line management and the role of the physician is to provide advice to both the employee and the employer. Care should be taken to ensure that the employee understands the physician's duty to the employer and physicians are advised to consider obtaining the employee's written consent to be examined in such circumstances.[8] Occupational physicians should take care not to allow any preconceived views of others to colour their clinical judgement.

3.7. There are occasions when the employee is seen subject to a formal process, such as part of a sickness absence or substance abuse policy, and this may be on the instruction of line management or a personnel department. In these circumstances the occupational physician should take particular care to explain precisely the purpose of the assessment, make it clear to the individual that the physician is acting as an impartial medical adviser, and ensure that the employee agrees to the assessment. A misunderstanding is less likely when the purpose of such a referral has been defined in a company policy agreed between management and the workforce.

**As far as possible a climate should be created in which many referrals to the occupational health service are informal and at the request of the individual.**

*Ill-health retirement*

3.8. Retirement from work on the grounds of ill health is, for some, an inevitable outcome. Retirement on such grounds may be advantageous to the mature employee who has coped with disability and increasing job demands and has many years in a good pension scheme. However, this is not always the case.

3.9. Occupational physicians should not be party to the misuse of their services to assist with the shedding of labour. They should be familiar with the various provisions of the company's pension scheme and should provide impartial professional advice. In cases where premature medical retirement due to incapacity may be necessary the physician should be fully satisfied that there are justifiable medical grounds either by seeing and examining candidates personally or by the examination of full medical reports supplied by others. They should also consider whether suitable alternative work is available.[15] General practitioners should, with the consent of the individual, be kept aware of the position and in those cases where they have not initiated the process should preferably support the decision that retirement is justified.

*Health screening and executive medical examinations*

3.10. Occupational physicians are involved in various aspects of health promotion in the workplace which may involve collaboration with other non-medical agencies, both within and outside the organization. They should ensure that any screening or other procedures are ethically and clinically justifiable, that they fulfill the usual criteria for a valid screening procedure,[16] that there is adequate quality control of procedures performed, that participation is voluntary, and that the process for dealing with employees in whom abnormalities are discovered is established and clearly understood.

3.11. Detailed clinical information resulting from such screening procedures or from so-called executive medical examinations should not be passed to the employer where it would be open to misinterpretation, but only to a medically qualified adviser, and even then only with the informed consent of the individual. It is for the employee to decide what information, if any, is to be disclosed, and to whom. Management may only be supplied with the results of examinations with the informed consent of the individual given without coercion. However, employers may be given group anonymized data but only for large groups where anonymity is more readily guaranteed. Public communication of such company data should only be made with consent from the employer and employees or their representatives.

*Testing for alcohol and drugs*

3.12. Occupational physicians may be involved in screening and testing programmes for alcohol and other drugs in situations including pre-employment screening, following an accident or incident ('for-cause' testing), or at random. Additionally, occupational physicians may include similar procedures for clinical reasons, and it is important that a clear distinction is made between tests which are part of a company programme and those which are carried out for purely clinical purposes.

3.13. Clinical tests demand the same degree of confidentiality as any other medical examination. However, where the results indicate that the patient is currently affected by drugs or alcohol, the occupational physician will have a responsibility to ensure that the safety of other workers or the public is properly considered, and such considerations may override the duty of confidentiality to the individual (see 2.4).

3.14. Where tests are instituted as part of a company programme it is important that the role of medical and nursing staff is clearly defined in advance and that the handling of the results of such tests is clearly understood by medical and nursing staff, by the subjects being tested, and by managers. Such tests still require informed consent and it is important that this is assured by proper contractual arrangements in advance of the test programme. It remains important that the occupational physician receives assurance from the subject at the time of the test that these arrangements are understood.

3.15. It should not be necessary or appropriate to involve medical or nursing staff in procedures such as breath analysis for alcohol where these are undertaken as part of a company programme. The involvement of health staff in 'policing' procedures may undermine their role as confidential medical advisers and any possible confusion should be avoided.

3.16. Where medical staff are unavoidably involved in taking and processing biological samples for test purposes as part of a company programme they are acting as the agent of the employer. Medical staff should not use such an occasion for giving individuals medical advice. This should avoid the risk of confusion between their role as an agent of the employer and their role as confidential medical adviser. It is important to ensure that strict procedures are in place for the handling of samples, for their transmission to laboratories, and for handling the results.

*Biological monitoring*

3.17. Many people in hazardous work may be subject to various forms of biological monitoring. The nature and any possible risk involved in such investigations, such as X-rays, must be explained to each person. The results of such tests and their significance should also be explained by the doctor either orally or in writing.

3.18. Where relatively minor but clinically significant abnormalities are revealed, such as pleural thickening in an asbestos worker, the doctor should err on the side of communicating more, rather than less, fully. Individual results should not be released to others without the agreement of the employee (see 2.3). Group results without individual identification may be given to the employer and to other interested parties when relevant to legislative requirements, for example the Control of Substances Hazardous to Health Regulations 1988, or to the provision and/or the effectiveness of preventive measures (see 3.11).

*Genetic screening*

3.19. The area of genetic screening is as yet poorly developed. If in future a highly reliable genetic screening test is developed with the predictive power to identify individuals at risk of developing an occupational disease, its use is likely to be encouraged as a part of a preventive strategy. The implementation of a genetic screening programme should be subject to the same ethical constraints as any other form of screening (see 3.10–11).

*Testing for hepatitis B*

3.20. Some occupational physicians will be involved in screening medical, dental, nursing, and midwifery students and staff due to the risk of the transmission of hepatitis B to patients during invasive procedures. Those health care workers without natural immunity will need to be immunized and their response to immunization checked.

3.21. Ethical problems may arise over screening and immunization, particularly when the results indicate the need for a change of duties. Clear procedures should be in place in advance to deal with such eventualities, including the provision of counselling, the release of information, and the procedure to be adopted when the employee or student declines to be tested or immunized. Staff whose HBV status may place patients at risk of infection should be given every encouragement to reveal that status to their employer, as the occupational physician will not normally do so without the health care worker's informed consent. However, where patients are, or have been, at risk it may be necessary for the employer to be given access to relevant confidential information to safeguard public interest.

3.22. The situation when an individual refuses to be tested or immunized should ideally be covered by prior written agreement between the employer and all those concerned or their representatives. This agreement should include a recognition of the possible consequences for the individual.

3.23. The Department of Health issued guidance on this topic in 1981,[17] and an extensively revised edition will appear shortly. Occupational physicians with responsibilities for health care staff should study current guidance and follow it with care.

*Testing for HIV*

3.24. In the absence of effective immunization and treatment, screening for HIV in the occupational setting can seldom be justified. However, some countries require proof of freedom from infection before allowing visitors to work in that country.

3.25. Where testing is essential, appropriate and skilled counselling should be given to ensure the individual's fully informed consent. Counselling must also be available in the event of a positive test.

3.26. Occupational physicians who are asked to undertake screening or testing for HIV are strongly advised to seek expert advice before embarking on such procedures, to ensure that the justification would stand up to peer review.

*HIV and health care workers*

3.27. Included in the interim guidance on the management of HIV-infected health care workers published by the Department of Health in 1993[18] is a section on the role and responsibilities of the occupational physician. Annex A of this document gives an extract from the General Medical Council's Statement on 'HIV infection and AIDS: the ethical considerations' which were first circulated in 1988 and revised and reissued in 1993. Two paragraphs taken from the 1993 version of this statement concerning the duties and rights of doctors infected with the virus are as follows:

10. It is unethical for doctors who know or believe themselves to be infected with HIV to put patients at risk by failing to seek appropriate counselling or by failing to act upon it when given. Such behaviour may result in proceedings by the Council which could lead to the restriction or removal of a doctor's registration if this were necessary to protect patients or the doctor's own health. The Council has already given guidance, in paragraph 63 of the booklet 'Professional conduct and discipline: fitness to practise', on doctors' duty to inform an appropriate person or authority about a colleague whose professional conduct or fitness to practise may be called in question. A doctor who knows that a health care worker is infected with HIV and is aware that the person has not sought or followed advice to modify his or her professional practice, has a duty to inform the appropriate regulatory body and an appropriate person in the health care worker's employing authority, who will usually be the most senior doctor.

11. Doctors who become infected with the virus are entitled to expect the confidentiality and support afforded to other patients. Only in the most exceptional circumstances, where the release of a doctor's name is essential for the protection of patients, may a doctor's HIV status be disclosed without his or her consent.

3.28. Further information and guidance regarding HIV and AIDS and employment is given in an earlier Department of Health guidance note[19] and a booklet published by the Society of Occupational Medicine.[20]

## Section 4 Communications of information

4.1 While clinical findings should not be disclosed to a third party (including the general practitioner) without the individual's written informed consent (see 2.3), the individual has the right to be informed of the findings of medical assessment and screening procedures. This is formalized in the Access to Medical Reports Act 1988 and Access to

Health Records Act 1991. The ethical principles that are embodied in the Access to Medical Reports Act are recognized as good practice and should be considered even when the Act is not formally applicable.

*Advice to management*

4.2. Advice given to management about the results of a medical assessment should generally be confined to advice on ability and limitations of function. Clinical details should be excluded and even when the individual has himself given clinical information to management, the occupational physician should exercise caution before confirming any of it. If a report on the health or fitness for work of an employee is to be communicated to management it is important to ensure that the employee understands the physician's duty to the employer. The contents of the proposed report should be discussed with the employee and consideration should be given to obtaining the signed consent of the employee to be examined in such circumstances.[8]

4.3. Discussions with management on further courses of action consequent upon the medical assessment should take account of possible alternatives, with emphasis on those likely to be of most benefit to the individual. Statements such as 'fit for light duties' should be avoided as their interpretation can cause misunderstandings and even resentment. A statement of work that is suitable and activities which should be avoided is preferable. Advice to management on fitness for work should be submitted in a formal manner not only as a matter of principle, but also because documents may at some future time have to be disclosed to a court or industrial tribunal (see 2.21–25). The physician should bear in mind that it is the employer who is responsible for allocating duties even though the decision should take account of constructive professional advice wherever practicable.

4.4. Occasionally an occupational physician, when acting in a role other than that of independent examiner (e.g. in a screening, therapeutic, or research role), may find that an individual is unfit for a job where the safety of other workers or of the public is concerned. Great care should then be taken to explain fully why disclosure of unfitness is necessary. If sufficient time is taken in explanation, there is rarely difficulty in obtaining agreement. When this is not obtained the occupational physician is faced with an ethical dilemma. No firm guidance is possible and each case must be considered on its merits. On such occasions it may be useful for the occupational physician to discuss the issue with an experienced colleague. Ultimately the safety of other workers and the general public must prevail as one of the exceptions to the duty of confidentiality (see 2.3).

*Communication with professional colleagues*

4.5. Communication with general practitioners and other colleagues is often needed. When reports are sought from a general practitioner or consultant the requirements of the Access to Medical Reports Act 1988 must be followed. These include informing employees about their entitlements under the Act, obtaining their informed consent, and ensuring that they understand their entitlement to see and object to or obstruct any report being sent to the occupational physician. If occupational physicians wish to discuss an employee's health in a telephone conversation with the general practitioner or other doctor, they should normally have obtained the employee's consent in writing, unless in exceptional circumstances such as in medical emergencies or accidents. In some circumstances, as in the case of long-term absence, the occupational physician and the other doctor may not agree about an employee's fitness. Then the occupational physician may find it helpful to obtain a further assessment from an independent consultant and keep the general practitioner fully informed. When agreement cannot be reached, the advice of the occupational physician to the employer and employee will generally prevail.

## Section 5  Commercial secrecy

5.1. Employers and manufacturers are required to disclose information concerning products, processes, or practices which may be a risk to health at the place of work under Section 2(2)(c) and Section 6 of the Health and Safety at Work, etc. Act 1974 and the Safety Representatives Regulations.[21] Normally the employer will disclose this information. However, should such information concerning the injurious nature of a new material, process, or procedure come into the possession of the occupational physician, the employer should be informed and reminded of the statutory responsibilities. Only if the management of the organization refuses permission for such specific disclosure will the occupational physician have to consider whether to inform the workforce and other doctors who may need to know of the potentially harmful effects. The responsibility for the health of workers exposed to hazards should take precedence over management's refusal to disclose. However, the physician would be wise to seek the views of other senior occupational physicians or the Faculty before taking further action. Management should always be informed of what steps are proposed.

5.2. Such a situation is now unlikely to arise as a result of the Management of Health and Safety at Work Regulations 1992 and other legislation under which the employer is required to assess risks in the workplace, establish effective controls, monitor exposure, and provide health surveillance. In all of these the occupational physician is likely to have a role.

5.3. Should unforeseen ill-effects become apparent following the introduction of a new process, the situation should be carefully explained to the workers involved while the nature of the hazard is being investigated with all reasonable speed.

5.4. It is appreciated that difficulties might occur when these guidelines are applied to processes subject to the Official Secrets Act, and sometimes to commercial secrets. In these circumstances, occupational physicians should make their concerns clear in writing to senior management, and request that sufficient information be released to the employees to enable them to protect themselves. This information need not include, for example, detailed chemical composition. If employees remain concerned they could be referred to Section 28 of the Health and Safety at Work, etc. Act 1974.

5.5. The occupational physician may be in an advantageous position to assist in identifying potential health risks in relation to product safety or damage to the environment. Where appropriate, management's attention should be drawn to potential or actual hazards.

## Section 6  Clinical investigation for the purpose of research

6.1. The ethical considerations associated with research and resulting publication in occupational medicine are in general terms the same as those encountered in all medical research. At the outset occupational physicians should make clear their role as research investigators (see 1.3). Points to be borne in mind are:

1. Guidelines on this subject produced by various professional bodies should be consulted.[6,22-5] Badly designed research can be considered unethical.

2. The content of the research procedures should avoid any questions or procedures which might be distressing or carry a risk to health.

3. Occupational physicians may be perceived by workers to be part of management and therefore it is particularly important to ensure that informed agreement is given freely and that individuals recognize that they are free to withdraw at any time without detriment. Consent of trades unions to participate in research projects must not be taken to imply the consent of all individuals involved.

4. Whenever research is proposed, whether of a clinical or an epidemiological nature, the occupational physician should consult an appropriate Local Research Ethics Committee to discuss the protocol before starting the project. If no such committee is available, the Faculty may be approached.

5. When all the above factors have been considered it remains true that experimental procedures may be too technical for patients and non-experts to understand fully; the doctor still carries a moral responsibility for the investigations that are proposed.

6. Mortality studies have made invaluable contributions to occupational medicine. Nevertheless, consent by both employers and employees (or their representatives) to such studies, particularly when outside investigators are involved, should normally be obtained before commencing the research. One problem concerns the tracing of those who have left their workplace for any reason, to find out whether they are alive or dead. Although death certificates are public documents, the name, age, and last known address must be passed to the researchers in order to trace such people. It is considered that provided this information is passed in strict confidence, to be used only for purposes of establishing the fact of life or death, and provided that any final report contains no identifiable personal data, this procedure is acceptable.

7. The principles included in the above paragraphs should also apply to epidemiological research projects conducted using current medical records.

6.2. Different ethical problems may arise when information about patients with cancer is obtained from the National Cancer Registry. Most of these individuals are of course alive and any investigation of this nature must be approved by a Local Research Ethics Committee before any investigation can commence.

### Section 7    Relationships with others

7.1. Occupational physicians, like other doctors, have an ethical responsibility to put the interests of individual patients first. However, their obligations to their employers, to the workforce in general (and their representatives), and to the general public must also be recognized.

*Doctors*

7.2. In normal circumstances, the occupational physician should inform the general practitioner of work-related facts which may have a bearing on the health of an individual. It would be unusual for this to occur without the prior agreement of the individual.

7.3. When occupational physicians wish to obtain medical information on an individual from the general practitioner, from hospital medical staff, or from a private consultant, this should normally be done with the individual's written consent (see 2.3). A copy of the consent should be sent to the physician of whom the enquiry is being made. The consent applies only to the time, condition, and circumstances when it was obtained.[10,26] Where applicable, the requirements of the Access to Medical Reports Act 1988 should be met.

7.4. Except in an emergency, referral to a hospital consultant will normally be the responsibility of the general practitioner, rather than of the occupational physician. The latter may sometimes make such a referral with the agreement of the general practitioner. In the case of the occupational physician working in the NHS, it is particularly important that the general practitioner is not by-passed. In such circumstances, it is also important that ethical considerations should not be blurred by the potentially close working relationships between consultant, patient, and occupational physician.

7.5. Visits by other doctors (including consultants in occupational medicine, employment medical advisers, general practitioners, and others) to industrial, commercial, and other workplaces should be subject to proper professional courtesy. The visiting doctor should normally ascertain whether there is a whole or part-time occupational physician to the organization concerned who should be informed of the intention to visit. Sensitive industrial relations may be involved and visiting doctors should make every effort to collaborate closely with the occupational physician to the company. It is accepted that doctors who have a statutory right to enter a place of work may, on occasions, need to visit the establishment unannounced. On arrival, the visitor should suggest that the company's occupational physician is informed.

*Nurses*

7.6. Ethical guidance to occupational health nurses is given by the Royal College of Nursing.[27] Occupational physicians should familiarize themselves with current guidance and should discuss ethical issues openly with nursing staff. It is particularly important that ethical issues are properly addressed when the occupational physician is employed on a part-time or sessional basis and nursing staff are full-time, and may have managerial responsibility for an occupational health department.

*Occupational hygienists, safety engineers, and others working in the health and safety field*

7.7. Maintenance of a healthy working environment depends largely on team effort. The occupational physician needs to work closely with occupational hygienists, safety engineers, other health and safety practitioners, and with management. Exchange of information is essential if members of the team are to be effective. However, the doctor must safeguard confidential medical information about individual employees. Individuals are entitled to expect that such information, and medical records, remain confidential to doctor and patient, although occupational health nurses and other staff in the occupational health department will have access to medical records. Other staff may not have such access without the informed consent of the individual (see 2.3). Occupational physicians should discuss with employees the need to share confidential clinical information, such as biological monitoring results, with other members of the occupational health team. It will generally only be necessary to share information regarding groups rather than individuals (see 3.11).

*Management*

7.8. The relationship between occupational physicians and management can raise problems. Not all managers may readily appreciate the physician's duty to the individual patient and independent position on clinical matters. Nevertheless, the occupational physician has a duty of service to the employer and in this respect is in the same position as a doctor working within the NHS. Although employed in an organization, it is important to emphasize that, as an impartial professional adviser, the physician has a responsibility to employees as well as to management and there is an ethical duty to put the interests of patients first.

7.9. The distinction between the responsibilities and duties to the employer and the professional ethical obligations and principles concerning such matters as confidentiality and disclosure should be clarified. Consideration should be given to the inclusion of a clause in the contract of employment of the occupational physician which recognizes those matters to mutual advantage. Such a clause could be phrased as follows:

> The company recognizes the clinical independence of the physician, his duties to his patients and his right to maintain the confidentiality of the personal medical records for which he is responsible. In turn, the physician, as employee, recognizes that he is subject to the normal duties to protect the company's confidential information, to the extent that these duties do not conflict with his professional ethics.

7.10. In cases of conflict which cannot easily be resolved it will be found helpful to establish clearly the real needs of those who require to be served. Possible objections to a proposed course of action should be considered carefully and reasonable expectations should be met as far as possible. After discussions with all those concerned decisions should be made openly so that everyone knows what to expect.

7.11. There is a legal requirement for management to maintain certain health records. It is important that a clear distinction is made between such records and clinical medical records, the former being maintained by management, preferably outside the occupational health department. The information provided for these records by occupational health departments should be that which is statutorily required, and exclude clinical information relating to individuals.

*Safety representatives and trades unions*

7.12. Occupational physicians should be prepared to discuss matters relating to health and work with trades unions and safety representatives. They must also be ready to explain their rationale for advice on matters of occupational health. Legislation entitles safety representatives to inspect and take copies of relevant documents required to enable them to perform their functions under the Health and Safety at Work Act 1974. This applies only to documents which the employer is required to keep according to the provisions of the Act and of regulations made under the Act.

*Government and official agencies*

7.13. The work of occupational physicians will often bring them into direct contact with government and official agencies. Ethical relationships with such bodies should be governed by the principles set out in this document. Occupational physicians should be prepared to assist representatives of these bodies, particularly on matters affecting the health and safety at work of individuals or groups.

*The public and the environment*

7.14. In common with other members of the medical profession the occupational physician has a duty to society, and situations may occur in which the public interest may have to be put before that of the individual patient. When safety or public health may be endangered the physician may sometimes find that there are obligations under the law. Various statutory obligations require doctors to notify certain diseases, abortion, and drug addiction.[28] In other cases it can only be the physician's conscience which dictates action and advice should be taken from professional colleagues and associations, including, when appropriate, the local public health physician. Whenever possible, those likely to be directly affected either by what is proposed, or by what has been done, should be informed.

7.15. Increasingly, occupational physicians are involved not only with the health of the workforce, but with the effect of a company's products, processes, and practices on the health of customers and the general public, and on the environment. Conflicts of interest may arise if the information provided by the company is not soundly based, accurate, and openly available when required. The physician's responsibilities as an employee may clash with concern for public health, and it may be valuable to seek the counsel of professional colleagues in such circumstances, particularly before entering public debate. Physicians may find themselves drawn into debate on television or radio on such issues and will need to be properly prepared. Any information given should be limited to scientifically based facts and the health of named individuals should not be discussed in such circumstances.

## Annex A    Services for sick doctors

Doctors who are aware of their own incapacity through sickness may have difficulty in seeking medical help. Others who are sick may not be aware of or be willing to admit to incapacity. There are, thus, ethical problems for colleagues who may also have difficulty in knowing what, if any, action to take and yet have a joint responsibility to ensure that patients and others are not put at risk. The majority of these problems are related to mental illness or alcohol or drug abuse.

The General Medical Council places a duty upon doctors to 'inform an appropriate person or authority about a colleague whose professional conduct or fitness to practise may be called into question', where the circumstances warrant this. There are a number of mechanisms for dealing with sickness in the medical profession.

Informal help may be obtained from the National Counselling Service for Sick Doctors which was set up in 1985. Unlike the NHS and GMC procedures described below, the service has no powers to restrict employment or registration; it is fully confidential and non-coercive and operates through a system of national advisers. These advisers are senior members of the same specialty and there are two in the field of occupational medicine. No permanent records are kept of names and under no circumstances are names disclosed to statutory medical bodies. The service can be contacted via a special telephone number 0171-935 5982, which is dedicated to the service.

For doctors in NHS employment, advice about appropriate action may be sought from a senior officer of the health authority. For general practitioners, advice may be sought from the Local Medical Committee or the Family Health Services Authority. These bodies have procedures for handling cases of sickness in the profession.

For all registered doctors, the General Medical Council's health procedures offer a confidential system for tackling problems of illness. The primary purpose of those procedures is to protect patients, but they also offer medical supervision with the aim of rehabilitating the doctor and returning him or her to full practice. Wherever possible, doctors are permitted to remain in practice while subject to the procedures. Further advice, on a confidential and, if necessary, anonymous basis, may be obtained from the GMC's health section.

### Annex B     Suggested wording of medical confidentiality agreement for non-medical personnel

'During the course of your employment you may have access to, gain knowledge of, or be entrusted with medical and/or personnel information concerning individual members of staff. This information may contain matters of a highly sensitive and/or personal nature.

You understand that access to these data, whether computerized or manual records is made available only to those members of staff who have an absolute right and need to know — that is professionally qualified medical and nursing personnel. As a direct consequence of carrying out your duties (clerical, administrative, security, or maintenance), you may at some time have or gain access to an individual's medical records.

You agree, not at any time, whether during or after the end of your employment with the company, to disclose to any person or make any use of such confidential information as described above.

This duty includes keeping the names and other details strictly confidential relating to those individuals making and keeping appointments within the department.

If such disclosure or misuse of information occurs during your employment the penalty for so doing will be summary dismissal and this is described in the disciplinary procedure which forms part of your contract of employment.'

### References

1.  BMA (British Medical Association) (1981). *Medical evidence*. The report of a Joint Committee of the British Medical Association, the Senate at the Inns of the Court and the Bar, and the Law Society. BMA, London.
2.  Kennedy, I. (1981) *The unmasking of medicine*. George Allen & Unwin, London.
3.  Lord Scarman (1981). Legal liability and medicine. *J. Roy. Soc. Med., 74*, 11–15.
4.  GMC (General Medical Council) (1980). *Annual Report of General Medical Council*, GMC, London.
5.  Sieghart, P. (1982). Lucas Lecture, Faculty of Occupational Medicine, Royal College of Physicians of London. Professional ethics—for whose benefit? *J. Soc. Occup. Med., 32*, 4–14.
6.  BMA (British Medical Association) (1988). *The philosophy and practice of medical ethics*. BMA, London.

7. BMA (British Medical Association) (1993). *Medical ethics today: its practice and philosophy.* BMA, London.
8. GMC (General Medical Council) (1993). *Professional conduct and discipline: Fitness to practise.* GMC, London.
9. (ICOH) International Commission on Occupational Health (1992). *International code of ethics for occupational health professionals.* ICOH, Singapore.
10. BMA (British Medical Association) (1992). *Rights and responsibilities of doctors.* BMA, London.
11. Conference of Medical Royal Colleges and their Faculties in the United Kingdom. (1991). Interim guidelines on confidentiality and medical audit. *Brit. Med. J.* **303**, 1525.
12. Royal College of Physicians (1989). *Medical audit. A first report: What, why and how?* Royal College of Physicians, London.
13. Royal College of Physicians (1993). *Medical audit: A second report.* Royal College of Physicians, London.
14. HSE (Health and Safety Executive) (1982). *Pre-employment health screening. Guidance note MS20*, HMSO, London.
15. Edwards, F.C. McCallum, R.I. and Taylor, P.J. (1988). *Fitness for work: The medical aspects*, Royal College of Physicians of London and Faculty of Occupational Medicine. Oxford University Press.
16. Farmer, R. and Miller, D. (1991). *Lecture notes on epidemiology and public health medicine.* Blackwell, Oxford.
17. DOH (Department of Health) (1981). *Hepatitis B and NHS staff.* CMO Letter–CMO (81)11. DOH, London. (in revision).
18. DOH (Department of Health) (1993). *AIDS–HIV infected health care workers: Guidance on the management of infected health care workers.* DOH, London.
19. DOH (Department of Health)(1991). *AIDS/HIV infected health care workers— Occupational guidance for health care workers, their physicians and employers.* Expert Advisory Group UK Health Departments. DOH, London.
20. Society of Occupational Medicine (1992). *What employers should know about HIV and AIDS.* London: Society of Occupational Medicine, London.
21. The Safety Representatives and Safety Committees Regulations 1978 SI 1977, No. 500. HMSO, London.
22. Royal College of Physicians (1990). *Guidelines on the practice of ethics committees in medical research involving human subjects.* A report. Royal College of Physicians, London.
23. Royal College of Physicians (1990). *Research involving patients.* A report. Royal College of Physicians, London.
24. DOH (Department of Health) (1990). *Local research ethics committees.* HSG991 S. DOH, London.
25. Royal College of Physicians (1986). *Research on healthy volunteers.* Royal College of Physicians, London.
26. Toon, P. D. and Jones, E.J. (1986). Serving two masters: A dilemma in general practice. *Lancet,* 1986; May 24: 1196–8.
27. Royal College of Nursing (1987). Information leaflet No. 13. Royal College of Nursing, London.
28. Medical Confidence and the Law (1981). *Brit. Med. J.,* **283,** 1062.

# Appendix 7

# European Community directives affecting health and safety and employment

*W.J. Hunter*

## Introduction

Legislation emanating from the European Commission is a constantly evolving scene but the following is a list of the directives relevant to health, safety, and employment current at the time of going to press. Full copies of the directives are obtainable from HMSO Publication Centre (see Appendix 9 for the address).

*Council Directive 77/756/EEC of 25 July 1977 on the approximation of the laws, regulations and administrative provisions of the member states relating to the provision of safety signs at places of work* (O.J. No. L229 of 7.09.1977, p. 12) abrogated by the ninth individual directive: Directive 92/58/EEC of 24 June 1992.

*Council Directive 78/610/EEC of 29 June 1978 on the approximation of the laws, regulations, and administrative provisions of the member states on the protection of the health of workers exposed to vinyl chloride monomer* (O.J. No. L197 of 22.07.78, p. 12). This directive applies to workers exposed to VCM, particularly in works where it is produced, reclaimed, stored, or converted into polymers. The directive sets down a set of specific measures for health protection.

*Council Directive 79/640/EEC of 21 June 1979 amending the Annexes to the Council Directive 77/576/EEC on the approximation of the laws, regulations, and administrative provisions of the member states relating to the provision of safety signs at places of work* (O.J. No. L183 of 19.07.1979, p. 11) abrogate by the ninth individual directive: Directive 92/58/EEC of 24 June 1992.

*Council Directive 80/1107/EEC of 27 November 1980 on the protection of workers from the risks related to exposure to the chemical, physical, and biological agents at work* (O.J. No. L327 of 2.12.1980, p. 8). This directive provides a general framework for the control of risks to health at work from chemical, physical, and biological agents, including the preventive measures required.

*Council Directive 82/605/EEC of 28 July 1982 on the protection of workers from the risks related to exposure to metallic lead and its ionic compounds at work* (O.J. No. L247 of 23.08.1982, p. 12). This directive makes provision for preventive measures, including health surveillance. It sets limit values for lead in air and in biological fluids.

*Council Directive 83/447/EEC of 19 September 1983 on the protection of workers from the risks related to exposure to asbestos at work* (O.J. No. L263 of 24.09.1983, p. 25). This directive provides for the protection of workers from exposure to all forms of asbestos, including demolition work. It prohibits asbestos spraying. Preventive measures, including health surveillance, are prescribed. Limit values are established.

*Council Directive 86/188/EEC of 12 May 1986 on the protection of workers from the risks related to exposure to noise at work* (O.J. No. L137 of 24.05.1986, p. 28). This directive aims to reduce the exposure to noise, to reduce the risks of loss of hearing, to give priority to reducing the level of noise at source, and complementarily the use of individual hearing protectors.

*Council Directive 88/364/EEC of 9 June 1988 on the protection of workers by the banning of certain specified agents and/or certain work activities* (O.J. No. L179 of 9.07.1988, p. 44). This directive prohibits the production and use of four dangerous substances which present serious risks for workers and for which the precautions to avoid exposure do not guarantee satisfactory protection of safety and health. The four substances are:

(1)    2-naphthylamine and its salts
(2)    4-aminobiphenyl and its salts
(3)    benzidine and its salts
(4)    4-nitrodiphenyl

*Council Directive 88/642/EEC of 16 December 1988 amending Directive 80/1107/EEC on the protection of workers from the risks related to exposure to chemical, physical, and biological agents at work* (O.J. No. L356 of 24.12.1988, p. 74). This directive strengthens the provisions of Directive 80/1107/EEC by providing for the establishment, at Community level, of indicative limit values to be taken into account by member states when setting national limit values.

*Council Directive 89/391/EEC of 12 June 1989 on the introduction of measures to encourage improvements in the safety and health of workers at work* (O.J. No. L183 of 29.06.1989, p. 1). This general framework lays down the principles regarding the obligations and responsibility of employers in respect of the safety and health of workers. Employers' obligations are clearly defined, as are the procedures for information, training, consultation, and participation in this field.

*Council Directive 89/654/EEC of 30 November 1989 concerning the minimum safety and health requirements for the workplace* (O.J. No. L393 of 30.12.1989, p. 1). This directive lays down the minimum safety and health requirements for the design and equipment of workplaces, whether they are new, being modified, or already in use.

*Council Directive 89/655/EEC of 30 November 1989 concerning the minimum safety and health requirements for the use of work equipment by workers at work* (O.J. No. L393 of 30.12.1989, p. 13). This sets out the minimum health and safety requirements regarding the choice, introduction, use, and maintenance of equipment whether new, second-hand, or modified since manufacture (reference: date of entry into force of the directive).

*Council Directive 89/656/EEC of 30 November 1989 concerning the minimum health and safety requirements for the use by workers of personal protective equipment at the workplace* (O.J. No. L393 of 30.12.1989, p. 18). This directive indicates the minimum health and safety requirements for the judicious choice and use of personal protective equipment. Certain provisions also set out the conditions under which personal protective equipment must be provided and the employers' and workers' obligations in this area.

*Council Directive 90/296/EEC of 29 May 1990 on the minimum health and safety requirements for the manual handling of loads where there is a risk particularly of back injury to workers* (O.J. No. L156 of 21.06.1990, p. 9). This directive contains provisions recommending the replacement wherever possible of manual handling by mechanical handling. Where the latter is not possible the directive provides for a detailed analysis of the risks associated with the job in question and of various intervening factors, and sets out the minimum safety and health requirements applicable in such cases.

*Council Directive 90/270/EEC of 29 May 1990 on the minimum safety and health requirements for work with display screen equipment* (O.J. No. L156 of 21.06.1990, p. 14). This lays down the minimum requirements in respect of the ergonomics, design, and organization of workstations with display screen equipment. It includes provisions on the organization of working time and medical supervision of the eyesight of workers.

*Council Directive 90/394/EEC of 28 June 1990 on the protection of workers from the risks related to exposure to carcinogens at work* (O.J. No. L196 of 26.07.1990, p. 1). This directive establishes a system of worker protection to reduce the health risks of exposure to carcinogens.

*Council Directive 90/679/EEC of 26 November 1990 on the protection of workers from risks related to exposure to biological agents at work* (O.J. No. L374 of 31.12.1990, p. 1). This directive sets out the criteria for drawing up lists of biological agents and lays down a series of provisions to avoid health risks arising from exposure to these agents.

*Council Directive 91/322/EEC of 29 May 1991 on establishing indicative limit values for implementing Council Directive 80/1107/EEC on the protection of workers from the risks related to exposure to chemical, physical and biological agents at work* (O.J. No. L177 of 5.07.1991, p. 22). This directive establishes a first list of indicative limit values under the provisions contained in Directives 80/1107/EEC as amended by Directive 88/642 EEC.

*Council Directive 91/382/EEC of 25 June 1991 amending Directive 83/477/EEC on the protection of workers from the risks related to exposure to asbestos at work* (O.J. No. L206 of 29.07.1991, p. 16). The Commission proposed to Council on 6 June.1990 a directive amending Directive 83/477/EEC to comply with the provisions of Article 9 of that Directive. The revision relates to the levels of action and limit values for occupational exposure to asbestos and takes account of progress in scientific knowledge and technology, and of the experience gained in applying the earlier directive.

*Council Directive 92/29/EEC of 31 March 1992 on the minimum health and safety requirements for improved medical treatment on board vessels* (O.J. No. L113 of 30.04.1992, p. 19). Work on board ship entails very specific hazards. The results of accidents are often made worse by the fact that the medical equipment on board is inadequate and the time taken to get outside help is long. The purpose of this directive is to improve the safety and health of workers on board ship by improving the medical facilities on board.

*Council Directive 92/57/EEC of 24 June 1992 on the implementation of minimum health and safety requirements at temporary and mobile work sites* (O.J. No. L245 of

26.08.1992, p. 6). Work on temporary and mobile work sites involves major risks. The directive provides for the inclusion of safety and health requirements at the initial stage of planning of work sites; it defines the health and safety responsibilities of all the persons involved in work on such sites and sets out safety requirements for certain jobs.

*Council Directive 92/58/EEC of 24 June 1992 concerning the minimum requirements for the provision of safety and/or health signs at work* (O.J. No. L245 of 26.08.1992, p. 23). The workplaces directive sets out the minimum requirements for workplaces but does not refer specifically to safety signs. Some were provisions included in Council Directive 77/575/EEC and Commission Directive 79/640/EEC. This directive is a revision and an extension of those two directives. It incorporates updated extracts for the older legislation and adds a number of measures arising from technical progress.

*Council Directive 92/85/EEC of 19 October 1992 concerning measures to encourage improvements in the safety and health of pregnant workers, women workers who have recently given birth, and women who are breastfeeding* (O.J. No. L348 of 28.11.1992, p. 1). Since none of the existing Community legislation on the protection of workers has taken sufficient account of the specific problems of pregnancy, the Commission has filled this gap by proposing the above directive to Council. The directive takes account of both the wide variety of types of work, and the need to avoid creating obstacles to the employment of women.

*Council Directive 92/91/EEC of 3 November 1992 concerning the minimum requirements for improving the safety and health protection of workers in the mineral-extracting industries through drilling* (O.J. No. L348 of 28.11.1992, p. 9).

*Council Directive 92/104/EEC of 3 December 1992 on the minimum requirements for improving the safety and health protection of workers in surface and underground mineral-extracting industries* (O.J. No. L404/92 of 31.12.1992, p. 10).

The aim of these directives is to prevent accidents such as those which occurred:
–   on the Piper Alpha rig in the North Sea, in which 167 workers were killed on 6 July 1988 as a result of explosions and fires; and
–   at the Stolzenbach mine in Germany, where 51 miners were killed on 1 June 1988 by explosions of lignite dust.
These directives cover all the extractive industries. The first refers specifically to exploration and exploitations by means of boreholes, the second on mines and quarries (the second will be adopted by the Conseil by 3.12.1992).

Useful information on impending legislation in the European Community can be found in two publications, *Social Politics in the Community* and *Social Europe*, obtainable from HMSO.

# Appendix 8

# Ill-health retirement guidance
## *K.J. Pilling*

From time to time all doctors are called upon to offer an opinion on fitness to work and on retirement on medical grounds, but advising managers and employees on these issues is a regular responsibility of occupational physicians. For an employee, ill-health retirement is a major life event which hinges on the doctor's opinion and clinical judgement and on a manager's interpretation of this advice after taking account of company policy. Some cases will be straightforward but others will require careful consideration of all the circumstances. Most companies do not have a clear and detailed set of rules available to help those involved in the ill health retirement process to reach a fair, consistent, and auditable decision.

This subjective approach introduces bias which can significantly influence company ill health retirement rates. The following guidance is intended to help all parties involved in decision-making and to promote equity and confidence in the process.

**Nine key questions**

1. What written criteria, if any, does the pension scheme provide for guidance and, in particular, what do the pension scheme rules state about ill-health retirement?

2. Is the employee currently able to perform the duties for which he was most recently employed?

3. Is this situation likely to be permanent or continue for the foreseeable future?

4. Is the employee's medical condition likely to be aggravated by remaining in the present post?

5. Does the medical condition make it unsafe, either for himself or others, for the employee to continue as before?

6. Can the content, working hours, or location of the employee's job be changed, within the terms of his contract, or is the employee fit for any other post that the company may reasonably offer having regard to the individual's skills and experience?

7. Has the employee been accurately informed about the financial consequences of ill-health retirement and by whom?

8. Is the employee in favour of ill-health retirement?

9. Is the employee's general practitioner in favour of ill-health retirement and has he or his specialist sent written comments on the employee's current medical condition and prognosis?

## Guidance notes

*Question 1: What criteria, if any, does the pension scheme provide in relation to criteria for eligibility and for guidance?*

Pension scheme medical advisers should always know what the criteria and rules are for eligibility for a pension, and should use them in order to guide them in making their ill health retirement decisions. Where pension scheme guidance is unclear or requires only a yes or no answer the following eight additional questions will help the examining physician to provide fair and considered advice to management, who ultimately have to decide whether or not to retire an employee on ill-health grounds.

*Question 2: Is the employee currently able to perform the duties for which he was most recently employed?*

It is important to have an accurate knowledge of the current work content of the post, especially the physical and psychological demands and skills required to enable the employee to work effectively. It is important to discuss these matters with the employee and management. Managers will often be in the best position to assess performance. It is important for physicians to be familiar with an employee's work **but** it is impossible to know how an individual is coping when he is not being observed.

*Question 3: Is this situation likely to be permanent or continue for the foreseeable future?*

Some physicians are expected to work to extremely strict criteria and have to state that in their opinion an employee will never work again. If this is taken literally then an ill-health retirement pension can only be awarded to those with extreme ill health or disability. Even in these cases it is sometimes impossible, as a result of improved treatments, to state that a return to work is impossible. For example, advanced heart disease, liver disease, and kidney disease treated by transplantation can result in individuals making a successful return to their original jobs. A more pragmatic approach is to consider whether a return to any type of available work is likely in the foreseeable future. Clearly, employers are unable to keep posts open indefinitely and sick, pensionable employees should not remain on sick leave for prolonged periods if improvement is not observed or likely.

*Question 4: Is the employee's medical condition likely to be aggravated by remaining in the present post?*

When workplace occupational factors may have contributed to the poor health of an employee considered for ill-health retirement it is obviously unsound practice to allow the employee to remain in the same post. Similarly, those workers who have developed non-occupational conditions which could be aggravated by the workplace should also be transferred to alternative work whenever practicable. If no suitable alternative work is available termination of contract on ill-health grounds may be a fair reason for dismissal under employment protection legislation.

*Question 5: Does the medical condition make it unsafe, either for himself or others, for the employee to continue as before?*

When the health of an employee impairs performance in such a way that the individual is unable to work safely and risks injuring himself or colleagues it is inappropriate and possibly unlawful for that person to continue as before. A credible attempt at finding alternative work should be made. Employers should be mindful of their common law duty not to be negligent by placing the employee or others at risk.

*Question 6: Can the content, working hours or location of the employee's job be changed or is the employee fit for any other post that the company may reasonably offer having regard to the individual's skills, experience and terms of his contract?*

The majority of companies have some provision for alternative employment or in-house rehabilitation for employees returning to work after illness.

In general:

1. Occupational physicians, managers and the employee should communicate as openly as possible and share the responsibilities, difficulties, and successes of the rehabilitation process.

2. Short-term redeployment is much easier for most companies to support than long-term, and employers should be given the best possible medical advice on the likely duration of an employee's reduced capacity.

3. Arrangements for employees to return to work on shorter hours and lighter duties can frequently be offered. Careful observation, support, and modification of duties are essential so that targets can be set, attained, and reset. Where progress is unsatisfactory ill-health retirement can be considered.

4. In practice, an employee's personal qualities, qualifications, past attendance record and performance will have an impact upon how much effort and support is provided for rehabilitation. In times of economic hardship, recession, contracting labour force and use of contractors in non-critical jobs, rehabilitation is becoming more difficult. These days it is rare for companies to operate redeployment panels or have in-house convalescent facilities.

5. A reasonable alternative post should, as a rough guide, have a job value of not less than 66 per cent of the original post. This arbitrary rule of thumb prevents any pressure on workers to accept a job which might damage self-esteem.

*Question 7: Has the employee been accurately informed about the financial consequences of ill-health retirement?*

It is important for sick employees to be aware not only of the financial benefits that will accrue on accepting ill-health retirement but also the implications of remaining at work if this is a credible alternative.

For employees attempting to remain at work or on rehabilitation programmes temporary reduction of hours or modification of duties when recommended by a medical adviser and supported by management should not normally incur financial penalty. If an employee is ultimately down-graded employers should not reduce salary but freeze income until the job value increases to equal the frozen salary. A decision should be made on whether company benefits, such as a company car, would be retained. Shift workers who move on to day work would expect to lose the shift allowance. Although understandable, this may have serious consequences from loss of earnings.

The financial consequences *must* be explained if there are valid medical and performance reasons for retiring an employee.

*Question 8: Is the employee in favour of ill-health retirement?*

Wherever possible it is best that all parties involved in the ill-health retirement decision are in agreement. The majority of sick employees initiate the ill-health retirement option. Some employees are ill-health retired without their consent but employers must behave responsibly and reasonably if this course of action is pursued as it is likely that in these circumstances the employee will seek legal advice on the matter.

In practice, this question is of interest only if the medical grounds for ill-health retirement are in doubt. If an individual cannot perform such duties as are available there may be no other option but to terminate service. However, Permanent Health Insurance (PHI) schemes may offer one alternative.

*Question 9: Have the employee's general practitioner and/or specialist been properly informed and sent written comments on the employee's current medical condition and prognosis?*

In cases of ill-health retirement occupational physicians should be aware of all relevant medical details before advising management. Once the employee's written consent has been given this may involve the occupational physician discussing the case with the employee's general practitioner and/or consultant. A consensus view on the appropriateness or otherwise of ill health retirement from all medical practitioners involved is to be recommended, and this is even more important if the employee is to be ill-health retired against his wishes. Where there are two conflicting medical opinions pension schemes tend to take the advice of their medical adviser. However, in disputed cases there are three situations where a reasonable employer ought to take a third medical opinion from another specialist:

1. Where the occupational physician's report is vague or unhelpful.

2. Where the occupational physician or the general practitioner has looked only at the medical files and has not interviewed or carried out a medical examination on the employee.

3. Where the employee is undergoing specialist treatment and that specialist has not been asked to give an opinion. Even in cases where the employee's general practitioner and the company medical adviser agree, an employee may wish to present his specialist's report when this may make a significant difference to the prognosis.

# Appendix 9

# Address list

*Anna McNeil*

---

**Chapter 1   Introduction**

Benefits Agency Medical Services (BAMS)
Department of Social Security
Room 6/25, The Adelphi
1/11 John Adam Street
London WC2N 6HT
(Tel: 0171 962 8757)

Employment Medical Advisory Service (EMAS)
Field Operations Division
Health and Safety Executive
Daniel House
Trinity Road
Bootle
Merseyside L20 7HE
(Tel: 0151 951 4000)

The National Council for Voluntary Organisations (NCVO)
Regent's Wharf
8 All Saints Street
London N1
(Tel: 0171 713 6161)

**Chapter 2   Legal aspects and services for the disabled**

The Royal Association for Disability and Rehabilitation (RADAR)
12 City Forum
250 City Road
London EC1V 8AF
(Tel: 0171 250 3222)
(Minicom: 0171 250 4119)

The Disabled Living Foundation
380–384 Harrow Road
London W9 2HU
(Tel: 0171 289 6111)

Skill: National Bureau for Students with Disabilities
336 Brixton Road
London SW9 7AA
(Tel: 0171 274 0565 voice/minicom)

Opportunities for People with Disabilities
1 Bank Buildings
Princes Street
London EC2R 8EU
(Tel: 0171 726 4961)
(Minicom: 0171 726 4963)

Health and Safety Executive
Information Centre
Broad Lane
Sheffield S3 7HQ
(Tel: 0114 289 2345)

Disability Information Trust
Mary Marlborough Lodge
Nuffield Orthopaedic Centre
Headington
Oxford OX3 7LD
(Tel: 01865 227592)

Disability Information Advice Service (0171 275 8485)

The Employers' Forum on Disability
5 Cleveland Place
London SW1Y 6JJ
(Tel: 0171 321 6591)

**The four residential training colleges for people with disabilities are:**

Finchale Training College
Durham DH1 5RX
(Tel: Durham (019138) 62634)

Portland Training College for People with Disabilities
Nottingham Road
Mansfield
Nottingham NG18 4TJ
(Tel: Mansfield (01623) 792141)

Queen Elizabeth's Training College
Leatherhead Court
Woodlands Road
Leatherhead
Surrey KT22 0BN
(Tel: 0137 284 2204)

St. Loye's College Foundation
Topsham Road
Exeter
Devon EX2 6EP
(Tel: Exeter (01392) 55428)


**Chapter 3    Medication**

The Liverpool School of Tropical Medicine
38 Pembroke Place
Liverpool L3 5QA
(Tel: 0151 708 9393)

The Malarial Reference Laboratory
The Ross Institute
London School of Hygiene and Tropical Medicine
Keppel Street
London WC1E 7HT
(Tel: 0171 636 8636)

Birmingham Heartlands Hosptial
Bordesley Green East
Bordesley Green
Birmingham B9 5SS
(Tel: 0121 766 6611)

British Airways Travel Clinics
156 Regent Street
London W1R 5TA
(Tel: 0171 434 4718)

MASTA–Medical Advisory Service for Travellers Abroad
(Tel: 0171 631 4408)


**Chapter 4    Hearing and vestibular disorders**

Department of Health
Medical Devices Directorate
14 Russell Square
London WC1B 5EP

Royal National Institute for Deaf People (RNID) (Headquarters)
105 Gower Street
London WC1E 6AH
(Tel: 0171 387 8033)
(Text: 0171 388 6038)
(Minicom: 0171 383 3154)

Royal National Institute for the Deaf (Residential Training)
Court Grange
Abbotskerswell
Newton Abbot
Devon TQ12 5NH
(Tel: 01626 53401)

Doncaster College for the Deaf
Leger Way
Doncaster
South Yorkshire DN2 6AY
(Tel: 01302 342166)

British Deaf Association
38 Victoria Place
Carlisle CA1 1HU
(Tel: 01228 48844 voice to minicom)

Job Club for Deaf People
The Co-op Centre
Unit 2A
11 Mowll Street
London SW9 6BG
(Tel: 0171 582 0951)
(Minicom: 0171 735 0969)

## Chapter 5    Vision and ocular disorders

Royal National Institute for the Blind (RNIB)
224 Great Portland Street
London W1N 6AA
(Tel: 0171 388 1266)

Royal National Institute for the Blind (RNIB)
Vocational College
Radmoor Road
Loughborough
Leicestershire LE11 3BS
(Tel: 01509 611077)

Royal National College for the Blind (Residential Training)
College Road
Hereford HR1 1EB
(Tel: 01432 265725)

Queen Alexandra College (Residential Training)
Court Oak Road
Harborne
Birminham B17 9TG
(Tel: 0121 427 4577)

International Glaucoma Association
c/o King's College Hospital
Denmark Hill
London SE5 9RS
(Tel: 0171 737 3265)

## Chapter 6    Dermatology

National Eczema Society
4 Tavistock Place
London WC1H 9BA
(Tel: 0171 388 4097)

The Psoriasis Association
Milton House
7 Milton Street
Northampton NN2 7JG
(Tel: 01604 711129)

Acne Support Group
16 Dufours Place
Broadwick Street
London W1V 1FE
(Tel: 0181 743 2030)

Vitiligo Society
97 Avenue Road
Beckenham
Kent BR3 4RY
(Tel: 0181 776 7022)

## Chapter 7   Neurological disorders

The Multiple Sclerosis Society of Great Britain and Northern Ireland
25 Effie Road
Fulham
London SW6 1EE
(Tel: 0171 736 6267)

Parkinson's Disease Society of the United Kingdom
22 Upper Woburn Place
London WC1H ORA
(Tel: 0171 383 3513)

Motor Neurone Disease Association
P.O. Box 246
Northampton NN1 2PR
(Tel: 0345 626262)

ME Association
Stanhope House
High Street
Stanford-le-Hope
Essex SS17 OHA
(Tel: 01375 642466)

British Guillain-Barré Syndrome Support Group
Churchgate House
Old Harlow
Essex CM17 0JT
(Tel: 01279 427148)

The Stroke Association
CHSA House
Whitecross Street
London EC1Y 8JJ
(Tel: 0171 490 7999)


## Chapter 8    Epilepsy

British Epilepsy Association
Anstey House
40 Hanover Square
Leeds LS3 1BE
(Tel: 0113 2439393)

Ridgeside Hostel
Hall Lane
Cookridge Lane
Leeds LS16 7NF
(Tel: 0113 267 2569)

The David Lewis Centre for Epilepsy and David Lewis School
Mill Lane
Warford
Nr. Alderley Edge
Cheshire
(Tel: 01565 872613)

St. Piers Lingfield
St. Piers Lane
Lingfield
Surrey RH7 6PW
(Tel: 01342 832243)

Meath Trust
Meath Home
Westbrook Road
Godalming
Surrey GU7 2QJ
(Tel: 01483 415095)

National Society for Epilepsy
Chalfont St Peter
Gerrards Cross
Bucks SL9 ORJ
(Tel: 01494 873991)

**Chapter 9    Spinal disorders**

National Ankylosing Spondylitis Society
5 Grosvenor Crescent
London SW1X 7ER
(Tel: 0171 235 9585)

National Back Pain Association
31–33 Park Road
Teddington
Middlesex TW11 OAB
(Tel: 0181 977 5477)

Arthritis Care
18 Stephenson Way
London NW1 2HD
(Tel: 0171 916 1500)

The Arthritis & Rheumatism Council for Research
Copeman House
St. Mary's Court
St. Mary's Gate
Chesterfield
Derbyshire S41 7TD
(Tel: 01246 558033)

Banstead Mobility Centre
Damson Way
Orchard Hill
Queen Mary's Avenue
Carshalton
Surrey SM5 4NR
(Tel: 0181 770 1151)

Mobility Advice and Vehicle Information Service (MAVIS)
Department of Transport
TRL
Crowthorne
Berkshire RG11 6AU
(Tel: 01344 770456)

Spinal Injuries Association
Newpoint House
76 St. James's Lane
Muswell Hill
London N10 3DF
(Tel: 0181 444 2121)
(Counselling line: 0181 883 4296)

Medesign Ltd
Clock Tower Works
Railway Street
Southport
Merseyside PR8 5BB
(Tel: 01704 542373)


**Chapter 10   Limb disorders**

Restricted Growth Association
103 St Thomas Avenue
West Town
Hayling Island PO11 OEU
(Tel: 01705 461813)


**Chapter 11   Trauma**

Headway (National Head Injurys Association)
7 King Edward Court
King Edward Street
Nottingham NG1 1EW
(Tel: 0115 924 0800)

The Royal Society for the Prevention of Accidents (RoSPA)
Cannon House
The Priory
Queensway
Birmingham B4 6BS
(Tel: 0121 200 2461)


**Chapter 12   Diabetes mellitus and thyroid disorders**

British Diabetic Association
10 Queen Anne Street
London W1M OBD
(Tel: 0171 323 1531)


**Chapter 13   Gastrointestinal and liver disorders**

National Association for Colitis and Crohn's Disease
98a London Road
St. Albans
Herts AL1 INX
(Tel: 01727 44296)

Ileostomy Association of Great Britain and Ireland
Amblehurst House
Black Scotch Lane
Mansfield
Notts. NG18 4PF
(Tel: 01623 28099)

The British Colostomy Association
15 Station Road
Reading
Berkshire RG1 1LG
(Tel: 01734 391537)

**Chapter 14   Cardiovascular disorders**

The British Pacing and Electrophysiology Group (BPEG)
9 Fitzroy Square
London W1P 5AH
(Tel: 0171 6365994)

British Heart Foundation
14 Fitzhardinge Street
London W1H 4DH
(Tel: 0171 935 0185)

**Chapter 15   Respiratory disorders**

Action on Smoking and Health (ASH)
109 Gloucester Place
London W1H 3PM
(Tel: 0171 935 3519)

National Asthma Campaign
Providence House
Providence Place
London N1 ONT
(Tel: 0171 226 2260)
(Helpline: 0345 010203)

Cystic Fibrosis Trust
Alexandra House
5 Blyth Road
Bromley BR1 3RS
(Tel: 0181 464 7211)

Quit (Smoking)
102 Gloucester Place
London W1H 3DA

Quit – Smokers' quit-line 0171 487 3000

## Chapter 16   Renal and urological disorders

British Renal Association
(c/o Professor J.S. Cameron)
Guy's Hospital
St. Thomas Street
London SE1 9RT
(Tel: 0171 955 4305)

European Dialysis and Transplant Association (EDTA)
European Renal Association
(c/o Professor A.E.R. Raine)
St. Bartholomew's Hospital
West Smithfield
London EC1A 7BE
(Tel: 0171 601 8888)

National Federation of Kidney Patients' Associations
(known as National Kidney Federation)
6 Stanley Street
Worksop
Notts. S81 7HX
(Tel: 01909 487795)

The British Kidney Patient Association
Bordon
Hants. GU35 9JZ
(Tel: 01420 472021/2)

The Association for Continence Advice
(based with the Disabled Living Foundation)
The Basement
2 Doughty Street
London WC1N 2PH
(Tel: 0171 404 6821)

The Coeliac Society of the United Kingdom
P.O. Box 220
High Wycombe
Bucks. HP11 2HY
(Tel: 01494 437278)

## Chapter 17   Haematological disorders

Haemophilia Society
123 Westminster Bridge Road
London SE1 7HR
(Tel: 0171 928 2020)

Lambeth Sickle Cell/Thalassaemia Centre
2 Stockwell Road
Stockwell
London SW9 9EN
(Tel: 0171 737 3588 & 0171 326 1495)

United Kingdom Thalassaemia Society
107 Nightingale Lane
London N8 7QY
(Tel: 0181 348 0437)

Sickle Cell Society
54 Station Road
London NW10 4UA
(Tel: 0181 961 7795)

Leukaemia Research Fund
43 Great Ormond Street
London WC1N 3JJ
(Tel: 0171 405 0101)


**Chapter 18    Women at work**

Wellbeing
27 Sussex Place
Regent's Park
London NW1
(Tel: 0171 723 9296)

Women's Nationwide Cancer Control Campaign
Suna House
128–130 Curtain Road
London EC2A 3AR
(Tel: 0171 729 4688)


**Chapter 19    Surgery**

Department of Health
BACUP (British Association of Cancer United Patients)
3 Bath Place
Rivington Street
London EC2A 3JR
(Tel: 0171 613 2121 or 0800 181199)

Cancer Relief Macmillan Fund
15–19 Britten Street
London SW3 3TZ
(Tel: 0171 351 7811)

The British Colostomy Association
15 Station Road
Reading
Berkshire RG1 1LG
(Tel: 01734 391537)

Ileostomy Association of Great Britain and Ireland
Amblehurst House
Black Scotch Lane
Mansfield
Notts NG18 4PF
(Tel: 01623 28099)

## Chapter 20    Psychiatric disorders

MIND, The National Association for Mental Health
Granta House
15–19 The Broadway
Stratford
London E15 4BQ
(Tel: 0181 519 2122)

Saneline: 0171 724 8000

Association for Stammerers
St. Margaret's House
Old Ford Road
London E2 9PL
(Tel: 0181 983 1003)

## Chapter 21    Stress, alcohol and drug abuse

Accept
724 Fulham Road
London SW6 5SE
(Tel: 0171 371 7477)

Al-Anon Family Groups UK and Eire
61 Great Dover Street
London SE1 4YF
(Tel: 0171 403 0888)

Alcoholics Anonymous
P.O. Box 1
Stonebow House
Stonebow
York YO1 2NJ
(Tel: 01904 644026)

(London helpline: 0171 352 3001)

Institute for the Study of Drug Dependence (ISDD)
1 Hatton Place
London EC1N 8ND
(Tel: 0171 430 1991)

SCODA ltd
Standing Conference on Drug Abuse
1/4 Hatton Place
Hatton Garden
London EC1N 8ND
(Tel: 0171 430 2341)


**Chapter 22    Acquired immune deficiency syndrome (AIDS)**

The Terrence Higgins Trust
52–54 Grays Inn Road
London WC1X 8JU
(Tel: 0171 831 0330 administration
          0171 242 1010 helpline 1200–2200)

Health Literature Line: 0800 555777
for bulk orders, write to:
BAPS–Health Publications Unit
Heywood Stores
Manchester Road
Heywood
Lancs. OL10 2PZ

National AIDS helpline: 0800 567123

Northern Ireland AIDS helpline: 01232 326117
(Monday & Wednesday 19.30–22.00)
The Hope Centre
24 Mount Charles
Belfast BT7 1NZ


**Appendix 1    Driving**

Drivers' Medical Unit (D7)
DVLA, Longview Road, Morriston,
Swansea SA99 1TU
(Tel: 01792 783686)

General Medical Council
55 Hallam Street
London W1N 6AE
(Tel: 0171 580 7642)

Medical Commission on Accident Prevention
35–43 Lincolns Inn Fields,
London WC2A 3PN
(Tel: 0171 242 3176)


**Appendix 2    Civil aviation**

Civil Aviation Authority
CAA House, 45–59 Kingsway,
London WC2B 6TE
(Tel: 0171 379 7311)


**Appendix 3    Seafarers**


**Appendix 4    Offshore workers and divers**

UK Offshore Operators Association
3 Hans Crescent
London
SWIX 0LN
(Tel: 0171 589 5255)


**Appendix 5    Working overseas**

Communicable Diseases (Scotland) Unit and
Department of Tropical Medicine
Ruchill Hospital
Glasgow G20 9NB
(Tel: 0141 946 7120)

PHLS Communicable Diseases Surveillance Unit
61 Colindale Avenue
London NW9 5EQ
(Tel: 0181 200 6868)

Department of Communicable and Tropical Diseases
Birmingham Heartlands Hospital
Bordesley Green Road
Birmingham B9 5ST
(Tel: 0121 766 6611)

Department for Tropical Diseases and Tropical Medicine
Monsall Hospital
Manchester M10 8WR
(Tel: 0161 205 2393)

Hospital for Tropical Diseases
180–2 Tottenham Court Road
London W1P 9LE
(Tel: 0171 637 9899)
('Tropical Hotline' with health advice by country or region
for the general public: 0898 345081)

Liverpool School of Tropical Medicine
38 Pembroke Place
Liverpool L3 5QA
(Tel: 0151 708 9393)

Medical Advisory Service for Travellers Abroad
London School of Hygiene and Tropical Diseases
Keppel Street
London WC1E 7HT
(Tel: 0171 631 4408)

## Appendix 6    Ethics

Faculty of Occupational Medicine
6 St. Andrews Place
Regents Park
London NW1 4LB
(Tel: 0171 487 3414)

## Appendix 7    European Community Directives

HMSO Publications Centre
51 Nine Elms Lane
London SW8 5DR
(Tel: 0171 873 9090)

Office for Official Publications of the European communities
2 Rue Mercier
L2985 Luxembourg
(Tel: Luxembourg 499 281)

## Appendix 8    Ill-health retirement guidance

General Medical Council
55 Hallam Street
London W1N 6AE
(Tel: 0171 580 7642)

*Misc.*
The Patients Association
18 Victoria Park Square
Bethnal Green
London E2 9PF
(Tel: 0181 981 5676)

# Index